# Mesenchymal Tumors of the Breast and Their Mimics

J. Jordi Rowe • Erinn Downs-Kelly
Editors

# Mesenchymal Tumors of the Breast and Their Mimics

## A Diagnostic Approach

Springer

*Editors*
J. Jordi Rowe
Cleveland Clinic, Department of Pathology
Robert J. Tomsich Pathology and
Laboratory Medicine Institute
Cleveland, OH
USA

Erinn Downs-Kelly
Cleveland Clinic, Department of Pathology
Robert J. Tomsich Pathology and
Laboratory Medicine Institute
Cleveland, OH
USA

ISBN 978-3-030-74473-1 ISBN 978-3-030-74474-8 (eBook)
https://doi.org/10.1007/978-3-030-74474-8



This Springer imprint is published by the registered company Springer Nature Switzerland AG
The registered company address is: Gewerbestrasse 11, 6330 Cham, Switzerland

# Preface

Given the overall low incidence of mesenchymal lesions of the breast along with their mimics, surgical pathologists are not consistently exposed to these spindle cell lesions. Compounding this problem is the broad differential that these lesions engender, with entities ranging from reactive/reparative lesions to poorly differentiated spindle cell malignancies. One of the most important rules of thumb to bear in mind is that even seemingly bland spindle cell lesions raise the possibility of a metaplastic carcinoma, and this diagnosis must be excluded when faced with virtually any spindle cell lesion of the breast. Furthering the challenge, the diagnoses may be complicated by fixation issues, sampling method, small sample size, lack of clinical history, and prior treatment effects. When faced with these lesions, the pathologist may struggle with such fundamental questions as: Is this a reactive or neoplastic process? Is this benign or malignant? Is this mesenchymal in origin or a non-mesenchymal mimic? What is the most effective way to approach this case?

This book will use a uniform approach to these lesions in order to provide a framework for the diagnosis of mesenchymal tumors of the breast while highlighting their mimics. An emphasis is placed on a practical approach to the morphologic interpretation and useful ancillary testing while exploring the differential diagnoses in depth. As you familiarize yourself with this text, our objectives are to introduce the reader to the spectrum of these lesions while providing a systematic approach that will help establish accurate diagnoses that in turn drive appropriate clinical follow up and treatment.

Given how morphologically and clinically diverse these lesions are, we hope this text provides a construct for integrating the varied components that go into establishing a diagnosis for this challenging aspect of breast pathology.

Cleveland, OH, USA — J. Jordi Rowe
Cleveland, OH, USA — Erinn Downs-Kelly

# Contents

# Contributors

**Steven D. Billings, MD** Cleveland Clinic, Department of Pathology, Robert J. Tomsich Pathology and Laboratory Medicine Institute, Cleveland, OH, USA

**Darya Buehler, MD** Department of Pathology and Laboratory Medicine, School of Medicine and Public Health, University of Wisconsin-Madison, Madison, WI, USA

**Alison L. Cheah, MBBS** Douglass Hanly Moir Pathology, Department of Histopathology, Macquarie Park, NSW, Australia

**Erinn Downs-Kelly, DO** Cleveland Clinic, Department of Pathology, Robert J. Tomsich Pathology and Laboratory Medicine Institute, Cleveland, OH, USA

**J. Jordi Rowe, MD** Cleveland Clinic, Department of Pathology, Robert J. Tomsich Pathology and Laboratory Medicine Institute, Cleveland, OH, USA

**Paul Weisman, MD** Department of Pathology and Laboratory Medicine, School of Medicine and Public Health, University of Wisconsin-Madison, Madison, WI, USA

# Metaplastic Carcinoma of the Breast

# 1

Erinn Downs-Kelly

## Contents




E. Downs-Kelly (✉)
Cleveland Clinic, Department of Pathology, Robert J. Tomsich Pathology and Laboratory Medicine Institute, Cleveland, OH, USA
e-mail: downske@ccf.org




J. J. Rowe, E. Downs-Kelly (eds.), *Mesenchymal Tumors of the Breast and Their Mimics*, https://doi.org/10.1007/978-3-030-74474-8_1

## Introduction

Metaplastic carcinoma (MC) accounts for roughly 1% of all breast carcinomas and represent a group of breast carcinomas that have marked heterogeneity in tumor morphology as well as in clinical behavior. These unique lesions have differentiation of their glandular epithelial components into metaplastic components that may have squamous or mesenchymal features with spindled, osseous, chondroid, or rhabdoid morphology. The resulting lesion may be entirely composed of the metaplastic elements or there may be an admixture of carcinomatous components as well as metaplastic components. Some of these lesions represent low-grade invasive carcinomas that have a risk for local recurrence but appear to lack metastatic potential, while at the other end of the spectrum are rapidly growing, high-grade invasive carcinomas that will follow an aggressive clinical course. A common feature of these lesions, regardless of grade, is their overall triple-negative status. That said, their prognosis seems to be worse than stage and grade matched triple-negative invasive ductal carcinoma, NOS (IDC-NOS). In the most recent WHO classification of breast tumors (5th edition), these lesions are categorized descriptively based on the metaplastic elements present and will be discussed below. The clinical, imaging, and gross features are described for the overall group of MC, while the microscopic findings, immunohistochemistry, and differential diagnosis are described according to specific metaplastic elements. It bears stating and repeating that in the evaluation of any spindle cell lesion of the breast, irrespective of bland or malignant cytomorphology, MC must be excluded and should be at the top of any differential diagnosis.

## Clinical Features

MC typically presents as a palpable mass, often noted to have grown rapidly. High-grade MC often presents with higher-stage disease than IDC-NOS. The age range is variable with lesions identified in both the premenopausal and postmenopausal settings. The median age at diagnosis for one of the largest studies was 64 years of age.

## Imaging

On imaging, a study by Yang et al. identified that MC more frequently had benign imaging qualities including round- or oval-shaped masses with circumscribed margins, while the more worrisome features of spiculated margins and posterior acoustic shadowing were uncommon.

## Gross Pathologic Features

Low-grade lesions tend to be smaller and have a median size of roughly 25 mm, while high-grade lesions can grow to substantial size and, in extreme cases, involve the majority of the breast. Lesions may appear well circumscribed, mirroring the imaging findings, while areas of irregularity at the tumor border have been described.

## Specific Histomorphologies of Metaplastic Carcinoma

### Low-Grade Adenosquamous Carcinoma

#### Microscopic

As the name implies, low-grade adenosquamous carcinoma (LGASC) has glandular elements as well as areas of squamous differentiation in a background of a bland spindle cell process. The periphery of the lesion has tendrils of tumor that extend outward and infiltrate in and around normal breast epithelial elements (Fig. 1.1). These lesions may arise de novo or in the background of a sclerosing lesion or papilloma (Fig. 1.2). The glands are frequently described as being small with rounded contours or they may have compressed lumens. The glandular cells are cuboidal to columnar and lack significant atypia (Fig. 1.3). The squamous component ranges from solid nests and small clusters of squamous cells to individual squamous cells and even microcysts with keratin debris (Fig. 1.4). Mitotic activity is scarce and necrosis is not typical. Lymphocytic aggregates are frequent at the periphery of the lesion.

#### Immunohistochemistry

LGASC has interesting immunohistochemical findings and a potential pitfall, as p63 and smooth muscle myosin can identify myoepithelial cells surrounding a subset of the glandular structures. This staining is variable, with some glands having complete or incomplete investiture by myoepithelial cells or they may have a total absence of surrounding myoepithelial cells (Fig. 1.5). The spindled stromal cells surrounding the glands have been shown to have a lamellar pattern of staining with

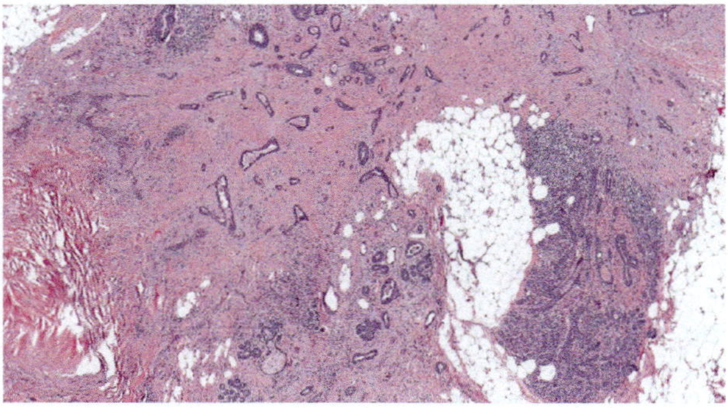

**Fig. 1.1** Low-grade adenosquamous carcinoma (LGASC) at low power showing the infiltrative nature of the lesion. Features include an altered desmoplastic appearing stroma with angulated tubules that infiltrate into the surrounding stroma

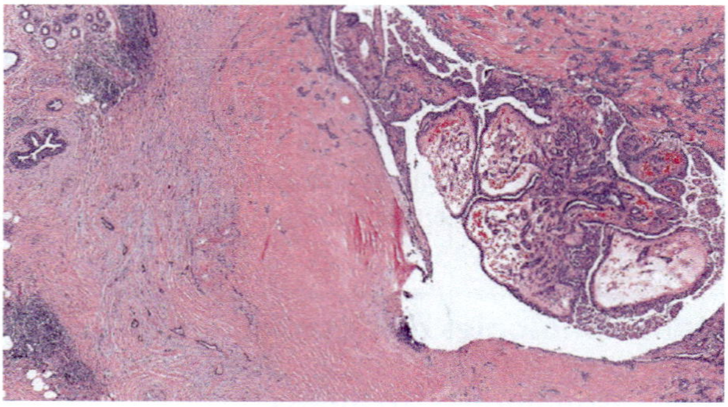

**Fig. 1.2** LGASC arising in the background of a sclerosed papilloma. The papillary architecture is appreciated in the right half of the photomicrograph with surrounding eosinophilic collagenized stroma. Toward the left half of the image, the stroma becomes more basophilic and has rare, angulated tubules

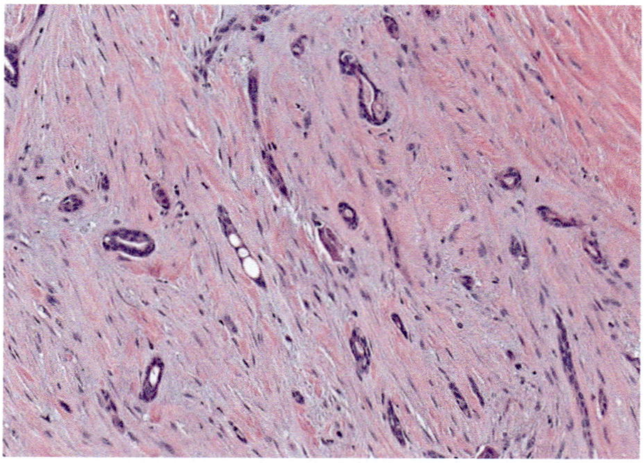

**Fig. 1.3** The typical compressed and angulated glands of LGASC with overall bland nuclei

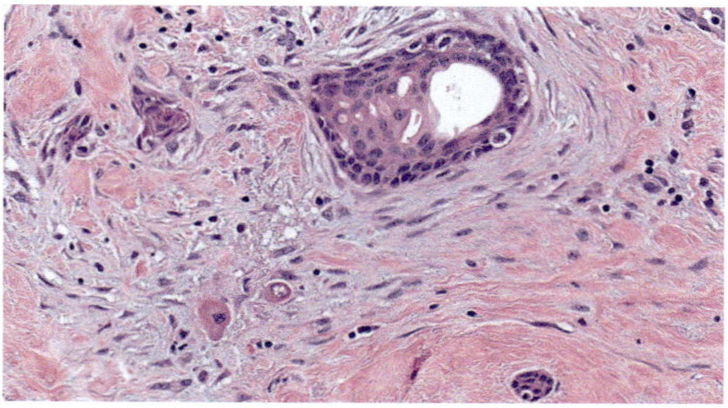

**Fig. 1.4** Squamous differentiation in LGASC may take the form of small nests and clusters of squamous cells to individual squamous cells and even microcysts with keratin debris. In this example, there are rare individual cells and small clusters of cells within the stroma that have the prominent eosinophilic cytoplasm characteristic of squamous differentiation. A gland in the center of the field has developed squamous metaplastic change within its lumen

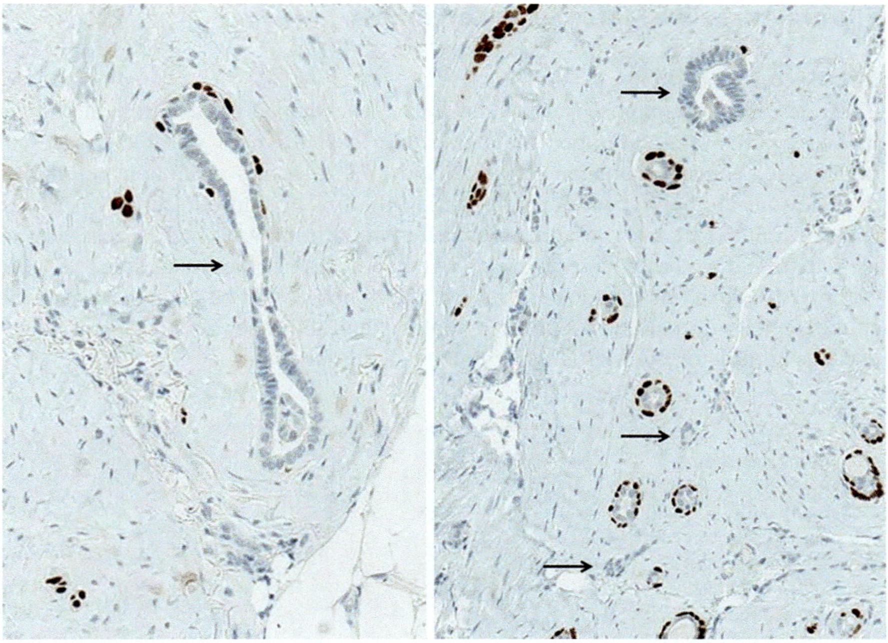

**Fig. 1.5** Variable myoepithelial cell staining is a common finding with respect to the glands of LGASC. Many glands show intact surrounding myoepithelial cells, while incomplete staining (as noted in the left-hand panel and denoted with an arrow) to absent staining (as noted in the right-hand panel and denoted with arrows) is also appreciated

calponin and smooth muscle myosin, but do not express p63. Not surprisingly, the foci of squamous differentiation will be immunoreactive with p63 as well. All lesional components are typically negative for estrogen and progesterone receptor expression as well as HER2.

## Differential Diagnosis

LGASC should be differentiated from tubular carcinoma and syringomatous adenoma. Tubular carcinoma will also be composed of bland glands; however, these glands have an angulated appearance and are lined by a monolayer of cuboidal-shaped cells. Myoepithelial cells will be absent surrounding the infiltrative glands of a tubular carcinoma and a squamous component will not be evident. Tubular carcinomas are also uniformly estrogen receptor positive and HER2 negative, in difference to the usual triple-negative immunophenotype of LGASC. Syringomatous adenoma has significant histologic overlap with LGASC and is typically identified underlying the nipple. Syringomatous adenoma is also composed of small bland glands having tear drop or angulated contours and squamous nests within a fibrotic background. This infiltrative process insinuates between smooth muscle bundles of the nipple and around breast epithelial elements. Many authors have pointed out the similarities between syringomatous adenoma and cutaneous appendageal tumors, and given the location with the nipple dermis, the pervasive thought is that these lesions represent a cutaneous adnexal tumor.

## Fibromatosis-like Metaplastic Carcinoma

### Microscopic

These lesions are composed of spindle- or stellate-shaped cells with bland nuclei having tapered ends, arranged in intersecting fascicles with variable degrees of interspersed admixed collagen (Figs. 1.6 and 1.7). Although variable in cellularity, these lesions are not hypercellular. Atypia is minimal and mitotic activity is scarce (Figs. 1.8 and 1.9). Foci of squamous differentiation may be seen. These lesions may arise de novo or in the background of a papilloma or other sclerosing lesion. In order to establish this diagnosis, >95% of the tumor should be composed of bland spindle cells with pale eosinophilic cytoplasm and thin nuclei with tapered edges and fine chromatin. No high-grade cytology should be seen.

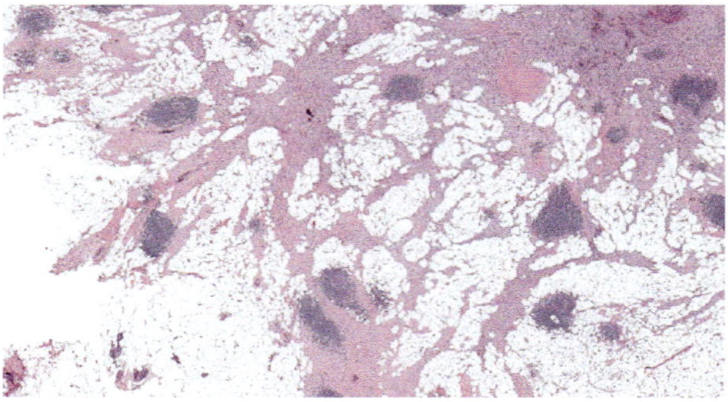

**Fig. 1.6** Fibromatosis-like metaplastic carcinoma from low power is a low to moderately cellular spindle cell population arranged in fascicles that may have associated lymphoid aggregates at the periphery of the lesion, histologically akin to its namesake

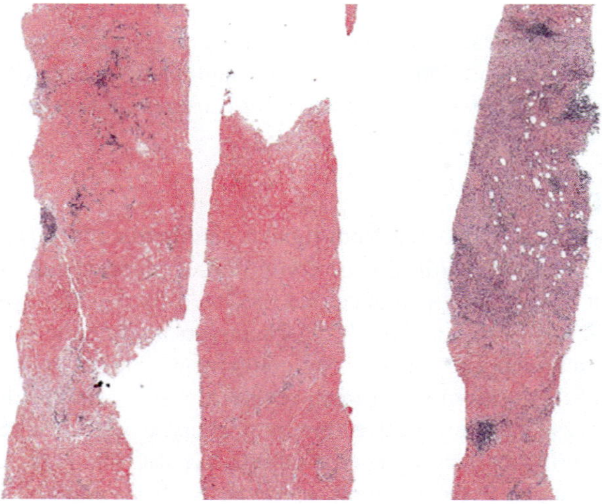

**Fig. 1.7** Fibromatosis-like metaplastic carcinoma on core needle biopsy showing heterogeneity across the cores. The core on the right has an area of increased cellularity while the remaining two cores appear largely fibrotic

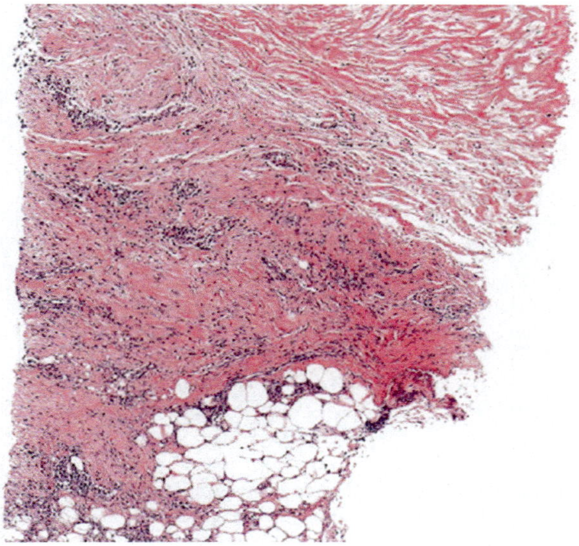

**Fig. 1.8** Fibromatosis-like metaplastic carcinoma on core needle biopsy depicting a focal area of increased stromal cellularity. The cellularity is due to an unassuming spindle cell population that has small hyperchromatic nuclei

**Fig. 1.9** Higher-power image of fibromatosis-like metaplastic carcinoma; note the absence of atypia or mitotic activity

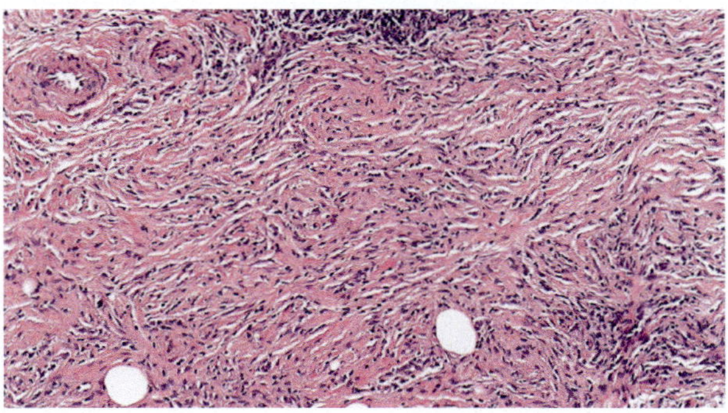

## Immunohistochemistry

A panel of cytokeratin immunohistochemical stains should be employed as these stains may be expressed only focally, especially when dealing with a core needle biopsy. Use of broad spectrum cytokeratins and high molecular weight cytokeratins (CK5/6 and 34βE12) as well as p63 and p40 is suggested (Fig. 1.10). Focal expression of smooth muscle actin is also frequently seen and likely related to myoepithelial differentiation.

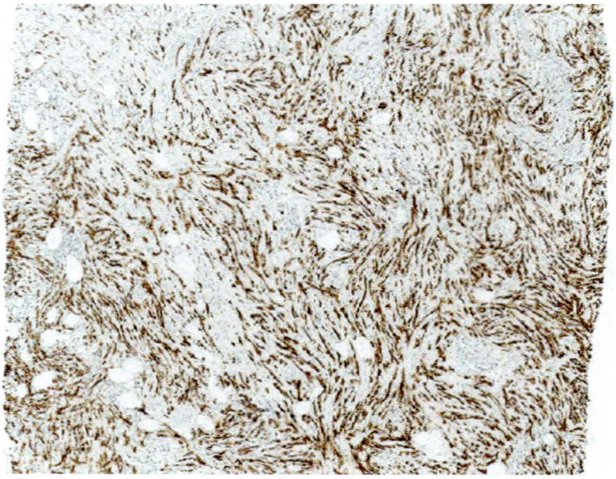

**Fig. 1.10** This stromal cell population showed expression of p63, cytokeratin 5/6, and CAM5.2 confirming the diagnosis of metaplastic carcinoma. Image shows CAM5.2 immunostain

### Differential Diagnosis

As the name implies, fibromatosis-like metaplastic carcinoma shares significant histologic overlap with fibromatosis (described in detail in the chapter entitled "Mesenchymal Breast Tumors with Fibroblastic and Myofibroblastic Differentiation"). The use of a panel of cytokeratins and p63 as described above should allow for distinction between these two lesions as fibromatosis should be negative for cytokeratins and p63 expression. Nuclear β catenin expression is frequently discussed in the literature as a means to identify fibromatosis. A potential immunohistochemistry pitfall is worth noting, identified by Lacroix-Triki et al., wherein they described finding nuclear β catenin in 22% of spindle cell carcinomas of the breast (using two different antibody clones). The spindle cell carcinomas had variable intensity staining with <33% of cells staining, while fibromatosis had diffuse staining. Given this immunophenotypic overlap, the use of a panel is highly encouraged in this differential especially in limited tissue samples.

## Squamous Cell Carcinoma

### Microscopic

Pure squamous cell carcinoma of the breast is often accompanied by cystic degeneration (Fig. 1.11). This can lead to the appearance of squamous lined cysts with squamous epithelium that can range from bland and composed of small uniform cells with ample cytoplasm to poorly differentiated with hyperchromatic pleomorphic nuclei with irregular nuclear contours and prominent nucleoli. The neoplastic squamous cells will infiltrate the adjacent stroma in cords and nests while inciting a fibroinflammatory response (Figs. 1.12 and 1.13). In order to establish a diagnosis

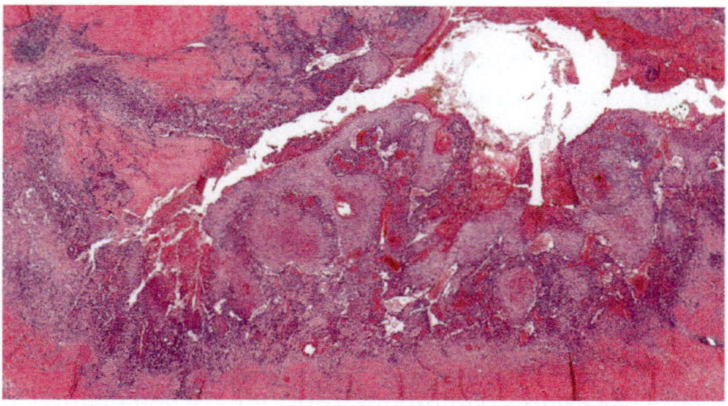

**Fig. 1.11** Low-power image of a metaplastic carcinoma with prominent squamous differentiation. Note the central cystic area that is lined by neoplastic squamous cells

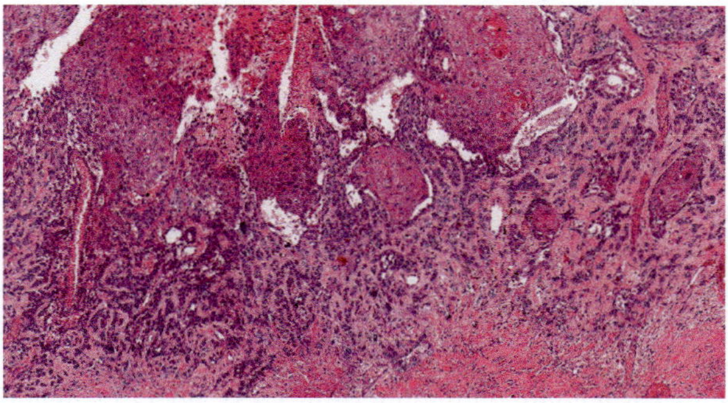

**Fig. 1.12** This image shows the neoplastic squamous epithelium that has prominent eosinophilic cytoplasm, appreciable intercellular bridges, and hyperchromatic nuclei with nuclear membrane irregularities. Seeming to spin off the squamous epithelium are infiltrative malignant cells that are arranged in linear arrays and small clusters

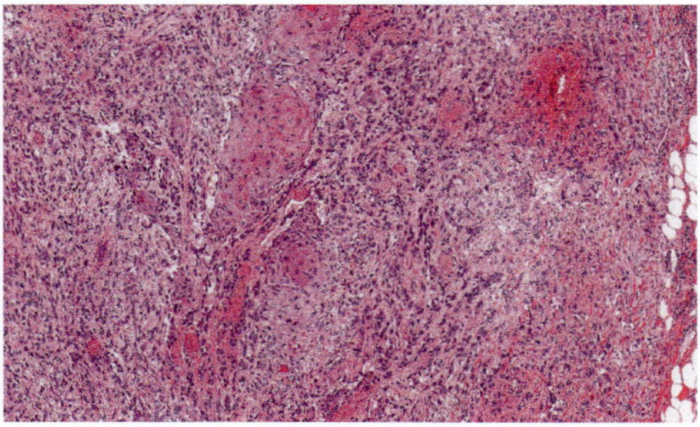

**Fig. 1.13** This metaplastic carcinoma with prominent squamous differentiation has also developed a spindle cell appearance to the cells surrounding the more recognizable squamous nests

of pure squamous cell carcinoma of the breast, a metastasis from a distant site or a cutaneous primary involving the breast has to be excluded. An acantholytic pattern has been described in squamous cell carcinoma in the breast, where atypical squamous cells line irregular spaces creating a pseudoangiosarcomatous morphology.

### Immunohistochemistry

Although not typically required, save for the acantholytic morphology, a similar broad panel of cytokeratins and p63 as described above could be employed to establish the diagnosis.

### Differential Diagnosis

As stated above, in order to establish a diagnosis of pure squamous cell carcinoma of the breast, metastases from other primary sites as well as a cutaneous primary with involvement of the breast parenchyma should be excluded. Unfortunately there are no specific immunostains that will help differentiate these possibilities. Clinical history becomes paramount, especially when dealing with a core needle biopsy that will guide treatment. In larger specimens, finding an in situ component can solidify a breast primary.

## Spindle Cell Carcinoma

### Microscopic

Spindle cell carcinoma is typically composed of atypical spindle cells arranged in a variety of patterns including intersecting and overlapping fascicles, storiform, herringbone, or a random pattern (Fig. 1.14). The cells have vesicular nuclei with coarse chromatin and typically prominent nucleoli. Mitotic activity is often brisk and tumor necrosis is a common finding (Fig. 1.15). Foci of squamous differentiation may be seen. The lesion typically has an infiltrative leading border with

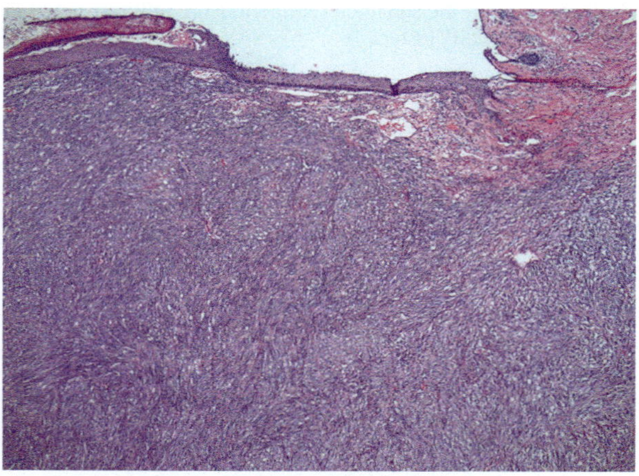

**Fig. 1.14** This low-power image shows a hypercellular spindle cell malignancy that abuts and ulcerates the overlying skin in this 82-year-old female. The cells are arranged in vague intersecting fascicles. The histologic differential includes metaplastic carcinoma (spindle cell type), melanoma, spindle squamous cell carcinoma (skin primary), the sarcomatous component of a malignant phyllodes, and a primary or metastatic sarcoma involving the breast. The most common entity in this differential is by far metaplastic carcinoma

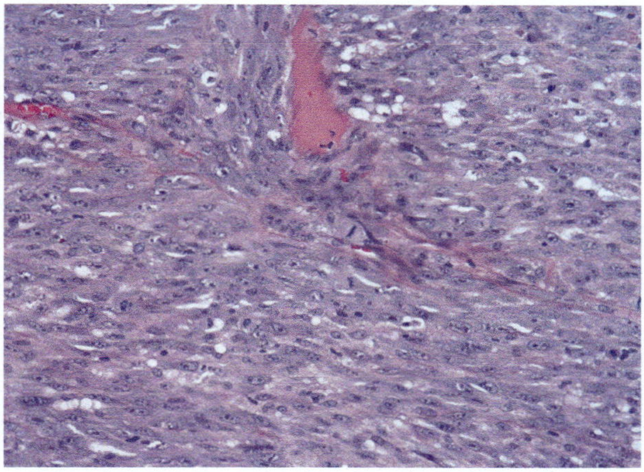

**Fig. 1.15** High-power image of this hypercellular spindle cell malignancy that was cytokeratin 5/6, CAM5.2, and p63 immunoreactive. Given that no other metaplastic elements were identified after thorough sampling, this is consistent with a metaplastic carcinoma, spindle cell type. Note the vesicular chromatin, prominent nucleoli, and brisk mitotic activity

obliteration of the normal breast epithelial elements within the lesion. Ductal carcinoma in situ or conventional invasive mammary carcinoma may be focal and if present support the epithelial make-up of the lesion.

### Immunohistochemistry

When ductal carcinoma in situ or conventional invasive mammary carcinoma is not associated with the spindle cell malignancy, a panel of cytokeratin immunohistochemical stains should be employed as these stains may be expressed only focally, especially when dealing with a core needle biopsy. Use of broad spectrum cytokeratins and high molecular weight cytokeratins (CK5/6 and 34βE12) as well as p63 is most useful. Focal expression of smooth muscle actin is also frequently seen and likely related to myoepithelial differentiation.

### Differential Diagnosis

The differential for spindle cell carcinoma includes phyllodes tumor (PT), primary or metastatic sarcoma to the breast, as well as melanoma. Particularly on core needle biopsies and even in some resection specimens, the stromal component of a phyllodes tumor can become so prominent as to obscure the telltale leaf-like architecture. Spindle cell carcinoma should show immunoreactivity to cytokeratins and p63, while phyllodes tumors historically have not. A pitfall to be mindful of, especially in limited samples, is that Cimino-Mathews et al. identified expression of focal p63, p40, and cytokeratin (AE1/AE3, Cam5.2, 34βE12) in the stroma of malignant PT but not in borderline or benign PT. A CD34 may help in this distinction as the stromal cells of PT are typically immunoreactive for CD34, while a spindle cell carcinoma is not. Primary sarcomas of the breast, outside of angiosarcoma, are exceptionally rare and discussed in detail in the chapter entitled "Miscellaneous Mesenchymal Tumors of the Breast." Melanoma should be remembered as a lesion that can certainly have a spindled appearance and is one of the more common malignancies to metastasize to the breast. In this scenario, clinical history is important and the addition of melanocytic lineage immunostains can be helpful in the distinction. In the differential of breast from melanoma, it is important to remember that S100 and SOX10 may stain both of these entities, so using a melanocytic marker like HMB45 or melan-A may be helpful given that these immunostains are not expressed in breast primaries.

## Metaplastic Carcinoma with Heterologous Mesenchymal Differentiation

### Microscopic

These lesions typically show a component of recognizable carcinomatous differentiation that may be glandular or squamous along with mesenchymal elements that could include chondroid, osseous, or rhabdoid (Figs. 1.16 and 1.17, historically known as matrix-producing metaplastic carcinoma). The mesenchymal elements range from well-differentiated components to overtly malignant and reminiscent of those correlative morphologies found in somatic soft tissue sarcomas. Although chondroid and osseous differentiation is most commonly seen, rare examples of carcinoma with osteoclast like giant cells have been described (Figs. 1.18 and 1.19).

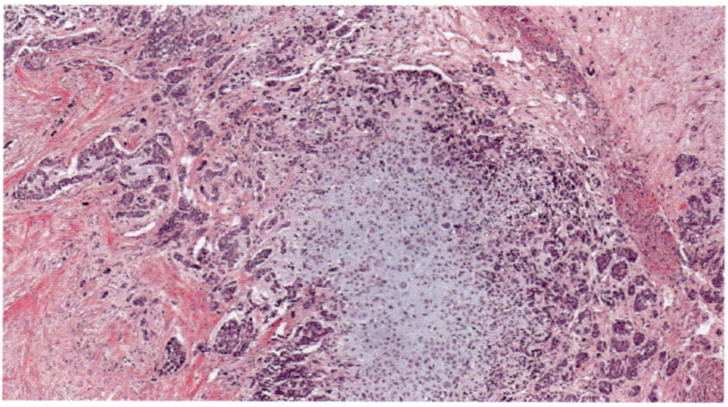

**Fig. 1.16** Metaplastic carcinoma with heterologous mesenchymal differentiation where a carcinomatous component surrounds a central area of chondromyxoid matrix

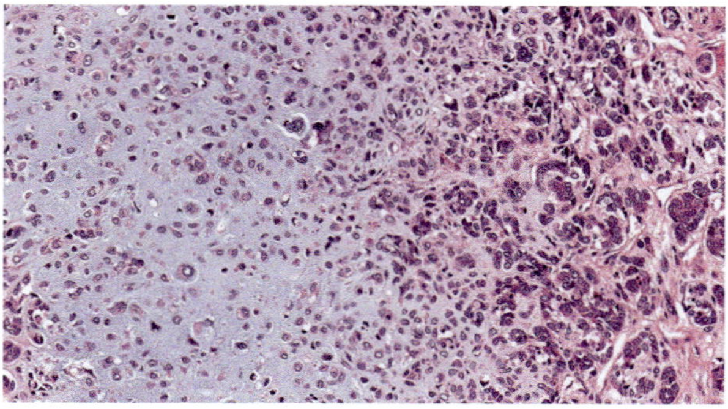

**Fig. 1.17** Higher-power image to illustrate the cohesive high-grade carcinoma composed of cells with high nuclear to cytoplasmic ratios on the right side of the frame while the central aspect shows a chondromyxoid matrix containing single cells with similar high-grade nuclei

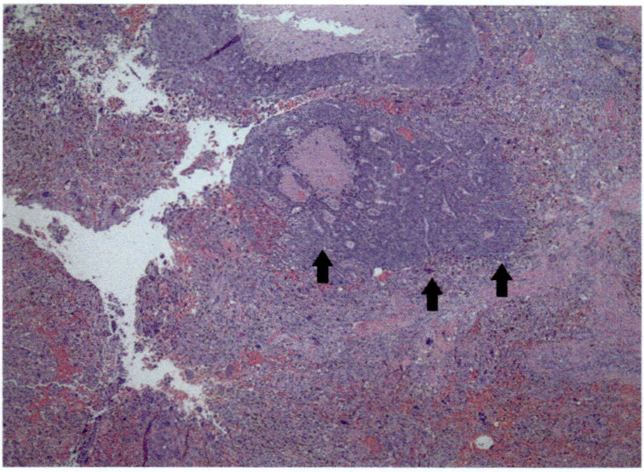

**Fig. 1.18** Rare example of a heterologous mesenchymal differentiation that resembles undifferentiated pleomorphic sarcoma with giant cells. A conventional component of high-grade invasive ductal carcinoma is present (arrows), while the remainder shows prominent hemorrhage, spindle cells, and multinucleated giant cells

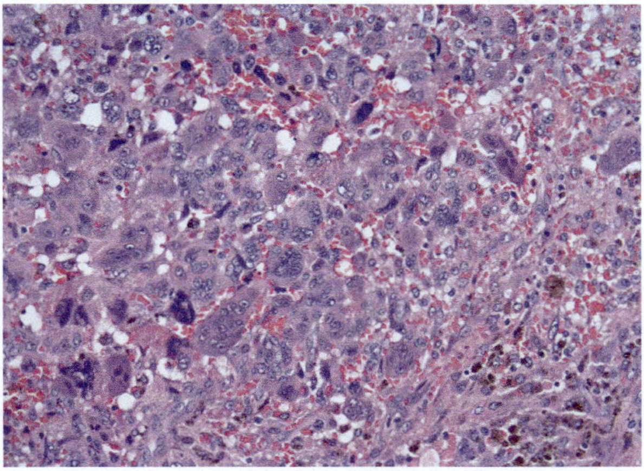

**Fig. 1.19** High-power image of a heterologous component that resembles undifferentiated pleomorphic sarcoma with osteoclast-like giant cells and multinucleated tumor giant cells with hyperchromatic nuclei and an admixed malignant spindle cell component

## Immunohistochemistry

If a definitive epithelial component is identified (either in situ disease or conventional invasive mammary carcinoma), the diagnosis is essentially established as evidence of epithelial differentiation allows for the diagnosis of metaplastic carcinoma with heterologous mesenchymal differentiation. On limited samples where epithelial differentiation may not be evident histologically, employment of a panel of cytokeratins and a p63 can be useful in establishing the diagnosis.

## Differential Diagnosis

The differential diagnosis is somewhat dependent on the mesenchymal components identified. Phyllodes tumor again enters this differential as heterologous elements in a malignant PT may include osseous or chondroid differentiation. If faced with this differential on a core needle biopsy, employing the cytokeratin panel, p63, and CD34 as described above should differentiate between these two processes. If a resection specimen is available, thorough sampling to identify an epithelial component to establish a metaplastic carcinoma diagnosis is warranted along with the use of immunostains if there is lingering uncertainty. Primary sarcoma of the breast again enters this differential and is discussed in detail in the chapter entitled "Miscellaneous Mesenchymal Tumors of the Breast."

## Mixed Metaplastic Carcinoma

### Microscopic

These lesions show a malignant glandular or epithelial component as well as more than one metaplastic element (Figs. 1.20 and 1.21). It is suggested that these lesions be designated as a metaplastic carcinoma and that the metaplastic elements present be specifically delineated in the surgical pathology report.

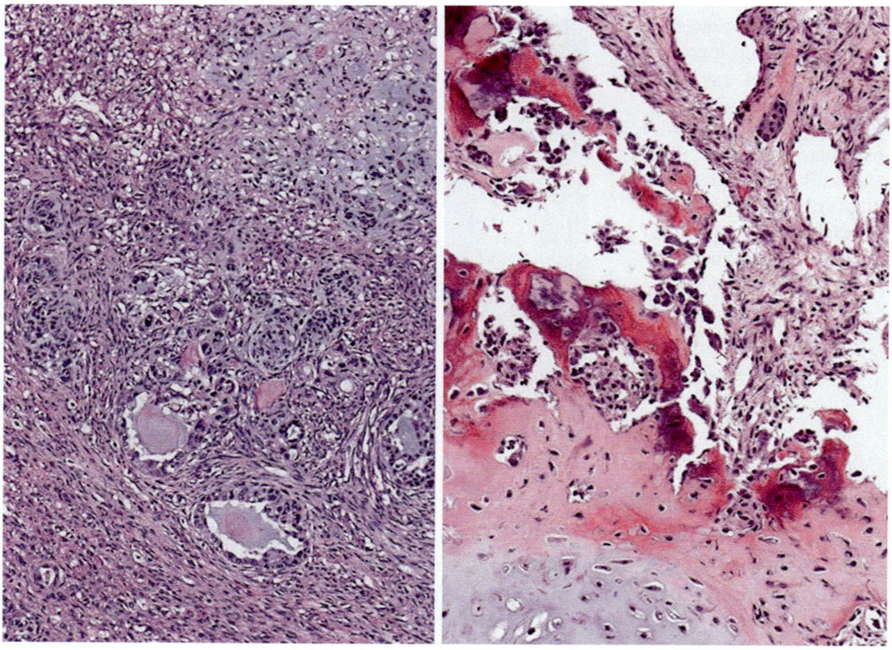

**Fig. 1.20** Mixed metaplastic carcinoma with each panel representing a different morphology identified in this lesion (same lesion is illustrated in Figs. 1.20 and 1.21). The panel on the left shows a focal glandular component as well as a spindle cell component and chondromyxoid matrix. The panel on the right shows osseocartilaginous differentiation

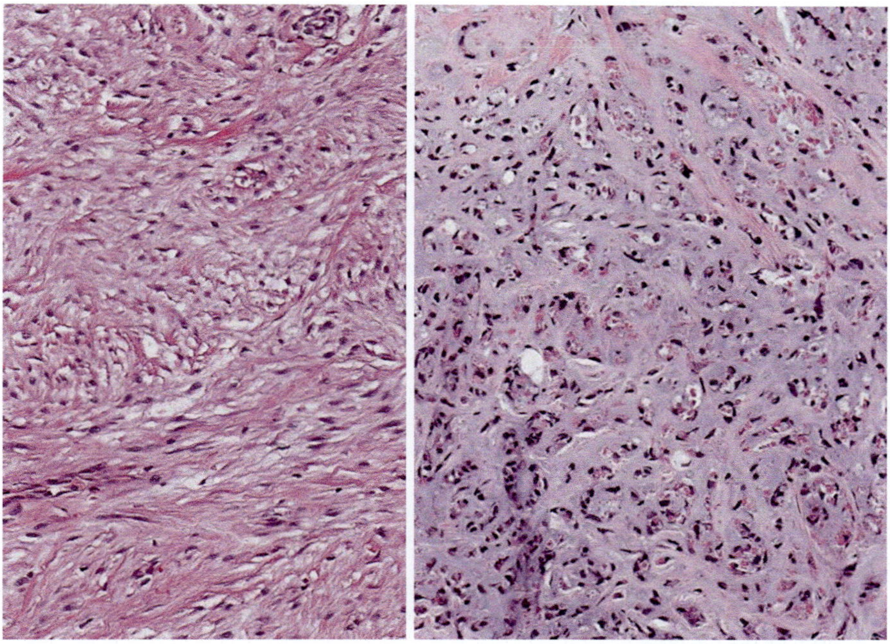

**Fig. 1.21** Mixed metaplastic carcinoma with the left panel showing a low-grade spindle cell component and the right panel showing chondromyxoid matrix infiltrated by hyperchromatic epithelioid cells

## Molecular

Studies have shown clonality in the epithelial and metaplastic elements, supporting the theory of a common precursor for both elements. There are some molecular changes that appear more commonly in certain morphologies. For example, low-grade adenosquamous carcinoma has been found to frequently have *PIK3CA* mutations while they lack the *TP53* mutations commonly identified in other MC. *TP53* mutations have been found across non-metaplastic triple-negative breast cancer (TNBC) and MC other than low-grade adenosquamous carcinoma. *TERT* promoter mutations were identified more commonly in spindle cell carcinoma and squamous cell carcinoma but were not found in those cases with chondroid differentiation. *WNT* pathway mutations have been found more commonly in MC than in non-metaplastic TNBC. From these studies, it appears that metaplastic carcinoma is distinct from TNBC and that different metaplastic morphologies may have differing genetic alterations.

## Treatment and Prognosis

In this heterogenous mix of tumors, prognosis is tied to phenotype. Low-grade adenosquamous carcinoma is known for local recurrence but appears to lack metastatic potential. Fibromatosis-like metaplastic carcinoma is also considered to have a more indolent course although rare examples of axillary and lung metastases have been reported. The other morphologies (spindle cell carcinoma, squamous cell carcinoma, metaplastic carcinoma with heterologous mesenchymal differentiation, and mixed metaplastic carcinoma) are aggressive tumors that have higher rates of distant metastases (brain and lung) than non-metaplastic TNBC. In mixed metaplastic carcinoma, the greater the number of metaplastic morphologies present, appears to correlate with a worse outcome.

## Selected References

1. Carter MR, Hornick JL, Lester S, et al. Spindle cell (sarcomatoid) carcinoma of the breast: a clinicopathologic and immunohistochemical analysis of 29 cases. Am J Surg Pathol. 2006;30(3):300–9.
2. Cimino-Mathews A, Sharma R, Illei PB, et al. A subset of malignant phyllodes tumors express p63 and p40: a diagnostic pitfall in breast core needle biopsies. Am J Surg Pathol. 2014;38(12):1689–96.
3. Cooper CL, Karim RZ, Selinger C, et al. Molecular alterations in metaplastic breast carcinoma. J Clin Pathol. 2013;66(6):522–8.
4. Davis WG, Hennessy B, Babiera G, et al. Metaplastic sarcomatoid carcinoma of the breast with absent or minimal overt invasive carcinomatous component: a misnomer. Am J Surg Pathol. 2005;29(11):1456–63.
5. Drekolias D, Mamounas EP. Metaplastic breast carcinoma: current therapeutic approaches and novel targeted therapies. Breast J. 2019;25(6):1192–7.
6. El Zein D, Hughes M, Kumar S, et al. Metaplastic carcinoma of the breast is more aggressive than triple-negative breast cancer: a study from a single institution and review of literature. Clin Breast Cancer. 2017;17(5):382–91.
7. Gobbi H, Simpson JF, Borowsky A, et al. Metaplastic breast tumors with a dominant fibromatosis-like phenotype have a high risk of local recurrence. Cancer. 1999;85(10):2170–82.
8. Gobbi H, Simpson JF, Jensen RA, et al. Metaplastic spindle cell breast tumors arising within papillomas, complex sclerosing lesions, and nipple adenomas. Mod Pathol. 2003;16(9):893–901.
9. Han M, Salamat A, Zhu L, et al. Metaplastic breast carcinoma: a clinical-pathologic study of 97 cases with subset analysis of response to neoadjuvant chemotherapy. Mod Pathol. 2019;32(6):807–16.
10. Kawaguchi K, Shin SJ. Immunohistochemical staining characteristics of low-grade adenosquamous carcinoma of the breast. Am J Surg Pathol. 2012;36(7):1009–20.
11. Lacroix-Triki M, Geyer FC, Lambros MB, et al. β-Catenin/Wnt signaling pathway in fibromatosis, metaplastic carcinomas and phyllodes tumours of the breast. Mod Pathol. 2010;23(11):1438–48.
12. McCart Reed AE, Kalaw E, Nones K, et al. Phenotypic and molecular dissection of metaplastic breast cancer and the prognostic implications. J Pathol. 2019;247(2):214–27.
13. McMullen ER, Zoumberos NA, Kleer CG. Metaplastic breast carcinoma: update on histopathology and molecular alterations. Arch Pathol Lab Med. 2019;143(12):1492–6.
14. Ng CKY, Piscuoglio S, Geyer FC, et al. The landscape of somatic genetic alterations in metaplastic breast carcinomas. Clin Cancer Res. 2017;23(14):3859–70.

15. Reis-Filho J, Gobbi H, McCart Reed AE, et al. Metaplastic carcinoma. In: Allison KH, Brogi E, Ellis IO et al. eds. *Who Classification of Tumors Editorial Board. Breast Tumors*. Lyon, France: IARC Press; 2019.
16. Rosen PP, Ernsberger D. Low-grade adenosquamous carcinoma. A variant of metaplastic mammary carcinoma. Am J Surg Pathol. 1987;11(5):351–8.
17. Sneige N, Yaziji H, Mandavilli SR, et al. Low-grade (fibromatosis-like) spindle cell carcinoma of the breast. Am J Surg Pathol. 2001;25(8):1009–16.
18. Yang WT, Hennessy B, Broglio K, et al. Imaging differences in metaplastic and invasive ductal carcinomas of the breast. AJR Am J Roentgenol. 2007;189(6):1288–93.

# Phyllodes Tumors

# 2

J. Jordi Rowe

## Contents



## Clinical Features

Phyllodes tumors present as unilateral, lobulated, painless masses that mimic fibroadenoma. All subtypes of phyllodes tumors are seen in a wide age range, 12 to >85 years old. They have a broad range in size, 2–10 cm, with malignant phyllodes tumors often exceeding 10 cm.

J. J. Rowe (✉)
Cleveland Clinic, Department of Pathology, Robert J. Tomsich Pathology and Laboratory Medicine Institute, Cleveland, OH, USA
e-mail: rowej@ccf.org


J. J. Rowe, E. Downs-Kelly (eds.), *Mesenchymal Tumors of the Breast and Their Mimics*, https://doi.org/10.1007/978-3-030-74474-8_2

## Imaging

Phyllodes tumors are seen as opaque, well-circumscribed masses, sometimes with clefting and coarse calcification. On ultrasound, they are described as oval to round, hypoechoic masses. Magnetic resonance imaging highlights the central septated clefts with increasing heterogeneity with increasing tumor grade.

## Pathologic Features

### Gross Features

Phyllodes tumors are delineated, tan to pink fleshy masses with central clefting and coarse stromal calcifications. As the grade of phyllodes increases, so does the size of the lesion and the infiltration into the adjacent breast tissue.

### Microscopic Features

Phyllodes tumors are biphasic fibroepithelial tumors with at least atypical proliferative stroma forming fronds lined by benign epithelium. As their name implies, the stroma is expanded causing leaf-like projections into the ductal lumens. These projections are characteristically rigid, forming squared off or triangular leaves (Fig. 2.1). The "fit" of the leaves in the lumens, or rather the tightness of that fit, varies from benign to malignant phyllodes with malignant tumors having the loosest of "fits." Benign phyllodes have symmetric luminal spaces with very little space seen, reminiscent of the lack of lumens in intracanalicular fibroadenomas. Phyllodes tumors have stromal expansion, creating leaves that project into lumens. These leaf projections distort the lumens and thus the "fit" of the leaves, leaving asymmetric luminal spaces (Fig. 2.2).

The epithelial component of a phyllodes tumor is comprised of an intact myoepithelial cell layer with overlying ductal cells. Usual ductal hyperplasia and apocrine metaplasia may be present. The stroma, or mesenchymal component, of a phyllodes

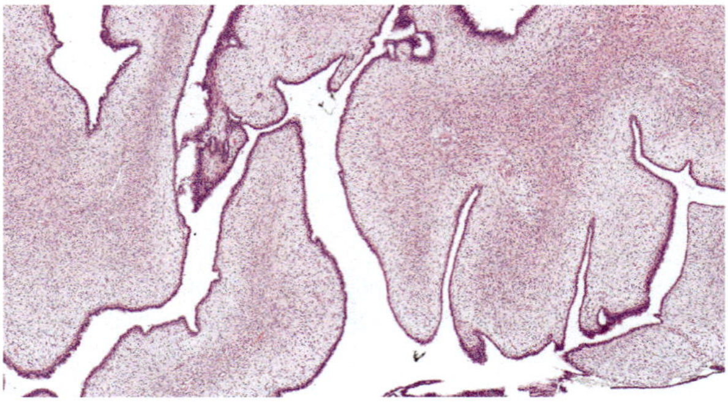

**Fig. 2.1** Phyllodes tumor with stromal projection into the lumen creating the eponymous leaf-like architecture. As this is a benign phyllodes tumor, the fit of the leaves is tight with very little luminal space remaining. H&E 40×

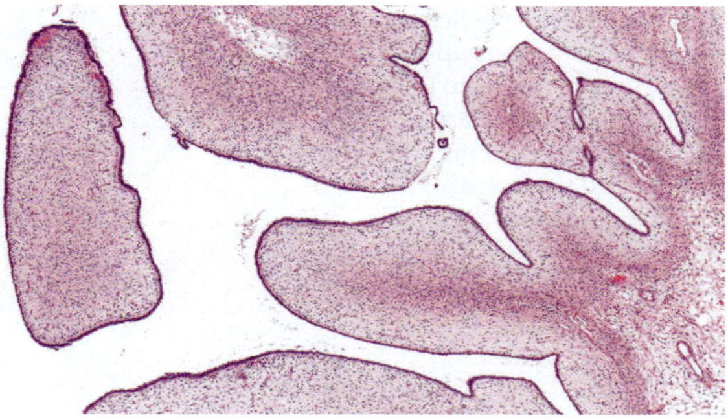

**Fig. 2.2** Asymmetric luminal spaces seen in phyllodes tumor. H&E 40×

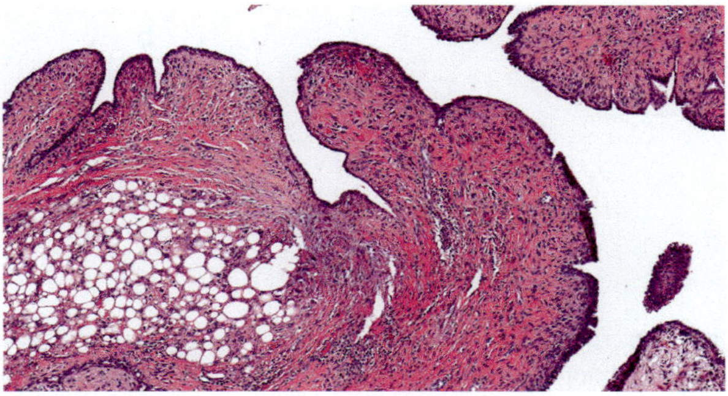

**Fig. 2.3** Well-differentiated liposarcoma arising within a malignant phyllodes tumor. H&E 100×

tumors is evaluated on cellularity, atypia, subepithelial condensation, heterogeneity, overgrowth, and mitotic count. Heterologous differentiation of the stroma can be seen with the most frequent being benign (smooth muscle, adipose tissue, cartilage) and less frequently their sarcomatous counterparts (Fig. 2.3). If sarcomatous differentiation is noted, the tumor is classified as a malignant phyllodes tumor. The one exception to this is the presence of well-differentiated liposarcoma. When present as the sole heterologous component, well-differentiated liposarcoma appears to have a low risk of metastasis. In this setting, grading as a malignant phyllodes tumor would require additional stromal features (see below). As phyllodes tumors are difficult to classify, the World Health Organization (WHO) has proposed criteria, based predominantly on stromal factors, to categorize phyllodes tumors by risk. Benign phyllodes have mild stromal atypia, little stromal expansion, the beginnings of stromal condensation, increased cellularity, and less than 5 mitotic figures (MFs) per 10 high power fields (HPFs) (Fig. 2.4). Borderline phyllodes tumors have more atypia, stromal condensation, and stromal expansion than benign tumors. One of the most helpful features of a borderline phyllodes tumor is the heterogeneity of their stroma, seen as marbling of more cellular to less cellular stroma, often seen within the same tumor and even on the same slide (Fig. 2.5). Varying degrees of stromal cellularity and expansion, within one section of tumor, favor classification of the tumor as borderline. The mitotic count in borderline phyllodes is $\geq 5$ and $< 10$ MFs per 10 HPFs, according to the current WHO criteria. Malignant phyllodes tumors are all

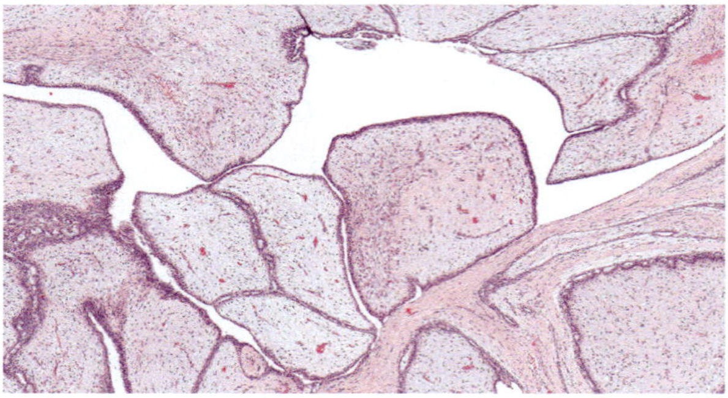

**Fig. 2.4** Benign phyllodes tumor. Note the squared-off leaf projections into the lumen, the low cellularity and homogeneity of the stroma, and the lack of stromal expansion. H&E 40×

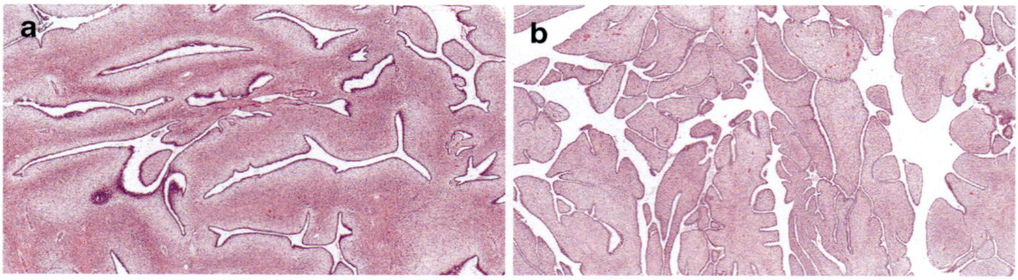

**Fig. 2.5** Borderline phyllodes tumor. (**a**) The stroma is condensed underneath the ductal epithelium. Additional stromal marbling, seen as increased stromal cellularity, is centrally located within the leaves. Contrast with (**b**) where the stroma is not marbled, it lacks condensation, nor does it display central stromal cellularity. H&E 20×, and 40×

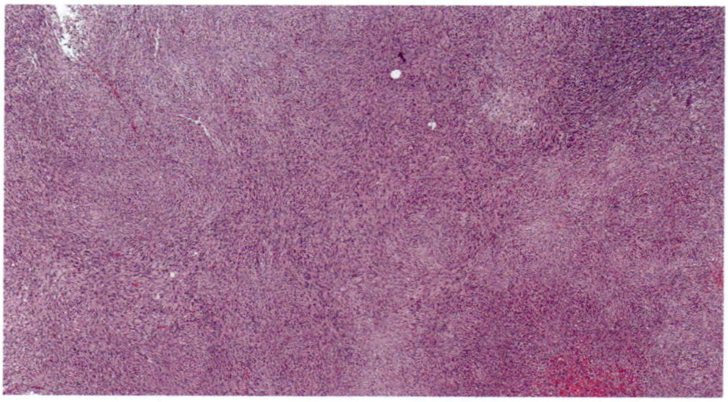

**Fig. 2.6** Malignant phyllodes tumor. Stromal overgrowth defined as a single 4× field without an epithelial component seen within the field. H&E 40×

phyllodes that contain sarcomatous stromal differentiation, stromal overgrowth, and greater than 10 MFs per 10 HPFs. Of note, the definition of stromal overgrowth is one 4x field without an epithelial component present (Fig. 2.6). Finally, the margin of a phyllodes tumor only has significance if it becomes infiltrative into the surrounding breast tissue. Unfortunately, the amount of infiltrate or the percent of tumor border that needs to be involved is not well delineated; no infiltration suggests benign phyllodes, marked infiltration malignant phyllodes, and everything in between, borderline phyllodes (Fig. 2.7).

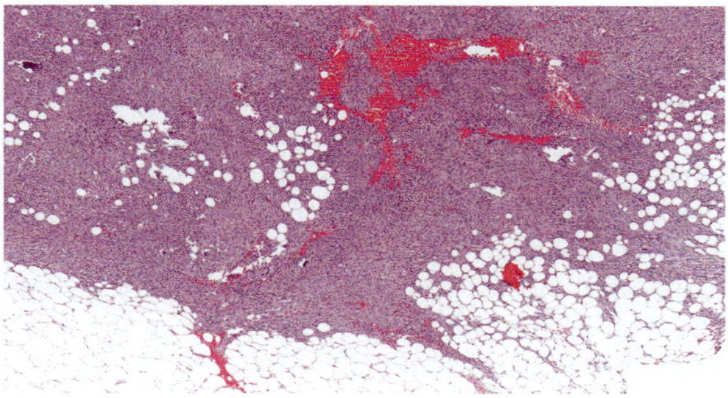

**Fig. 2.7** Malignant phyllodes tumor. Lace like infiltration of the stroma into the adjacent adipose tissue. H&E 40×

## Immunohistochemistry

The majority of phyllodes tumors are diagnosed on hematoxylin and eosin-stained sections, and few, if any, immunohistochemical stains are helpful. The utility of immunohistochemistry is highlighted when the pathologist is presented with a small sample size such as a needle core biopsy. In this instance, immunostains may help categorize a core of spindled stroma toward a particular diagnosis, with the caveat that definitive classification should be performed on the excision specimen.

A CD34 stains highlight the stroma of phyllodes tumors preferentially, as compared with metaplastic carcinoma. A pitfall to note is that as phyllodes tumors increase in grade, they are more apt to lose expression of CD34. In addition, focal nuclear p63 expression has been reported in phyllodes tumor stroma, further muddying the diagnosis. Care should be taken when ordering beta-catenin, as it too has been shown to stain the stroma of phyllodes tumors and should not be used as the sole criteria for a diagnosis of fibromatosis. Estrogen and progesterone receptor staining is consistently positive in the epithelium and typically negative in the stroma of phyllodes tumors.

## Molecular

Currently, there are no molecular findings in phyllodes tumor that have clinical significance or diagnostic utility; however, *MED12* mutations have been found in both phyllodes and fibroadenomas, suggesting a close relationship between entities. Mutations in *MAP3K1, BCOR*, *SETD2*, *KMT2D*, and *FLNA* have been identified predominantly in phyllodes tumors over fibroadenomas, suggesting that multiple additional mutated genes are needed for phyllodes tumor pathogenesis. Additionally, known cancer driver genes and the *WNT* pathway have been shown to be important in the malignant progression of phyllodes tumors. Of note, *MDM2* or *CDK4* amplification has not been identified within liposarcomatous foci in phyllodes tumors.

For difficult cases, it would be helpful if the pathologist could rely on molecular studies. Unfortunately, molecular tests currently offer no diagnostic value for the practicing pathologist.

## Differential Diagnosis

The differential diagnosis of phyllodes tumor is dependent on the specimen received. A core biopsy has the differential of fibroadenoma, fibromatosis, metaplastic carcinoma, periductal stromal tumor, and sarcoma, to name but a few. While an excision, with the benefit of more lesion to peruse, has a more limited differential based on risk stratification of phyllodes. Benign phyllodes is challenging to differentiate from cellular fibroadenoma, and based on the WHO criteria, there is often significant overlap between the two entities. A phyllodes tumor consensus review, published by Tan et al. in 2015, states that, since cellular fibroadenoma and benign phyllodes tumor have similar recurrence rates, the term "benign fibroepithelial lesion" can be used in cases in which it is difficult to discriminate between the two entities (Fig. 2.8). If at all possible, the authors feel that the diagnoses of fibroadenoma and benign phyllodes should be attempted, with this descriptive category used sparingly.

Features of phyllodes tumor include the fit of the leaves with a tight fit favoring fibroadenoma and a looser fit, or asymmetrical lumen, favoring phyllodes tumor.

Metaplastic carcinoma can be a difficult differential, but a selection of keratins and p63 on multiple blocks demonstrating immunoreactivity can confirm the diagnosis of metaplastic carcinoma, with the caveat that focal expression of p63 may be seen in phyllodes tumor as described above. Primary sarcoma is a diagnosis of exclusion and should only be made on excision specimens with the more descriptive diagnosis of malignant spindle cell lesion employed for core biopsies. Periductal stromal tumor lacks the pathognomonic leaf-like architecture. All of these lesions are further discussed in their appropriate chapters.

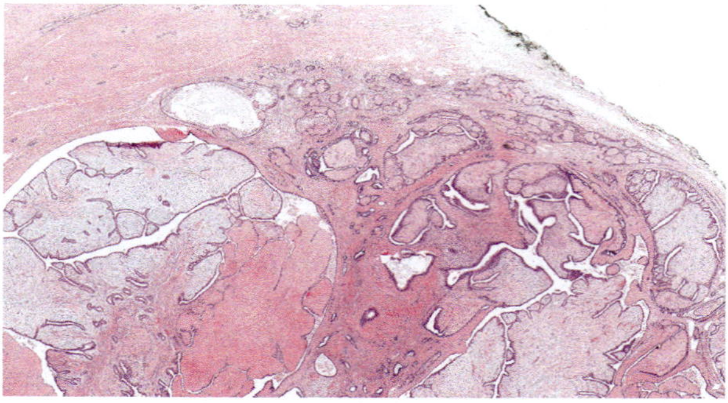

**Fig. 2.8** Fibroepithelial neoplasm (FEN). Note the admixture of conventional fibroadenoma architecture centrally, flanked by the hallmark leaves of phyllodes tumor. As this lesion straddles the diagnostic criteria of cellular fibroadenoma and benign phyllodes tumor, designation as FEN is appropriate. H&E 10×

## Treatment and Prognosis

Historically, the widely accepted treatment for phyllodes tumors was complete excision with negative margins. Complete resection should be considered for large tumors, malignant phyllodes, or recurrent tumors. As axillary metastases are infrequent, sentinel lymph node biopsy and/or axillary dissection is not routine. Radiotherapy has been shown to reduce local recurrence of phyllodes tumors, but has been unable to affect overall or disease-free survival; thus, its role remains undefined. As adjuvant chemotherapy has failed to show a remarkable effect on phyllodes tumor, it should be considered on a case-by-case basis and in the situation of metastatic disease.

The most frequent sites of metastasis are lung and bone. Malignant phyllodes tumors have a metastatic rate of 20–25%, with sarcomatous features and stromal overgrowth acting as loose predictors.

In one large series, the recurrence rate, after local excision, has been reported at 21%, 45%, and 65% for benign, borderline, and malignant phyllodes tumors, respectively. As an increase in local recurrence is primarily associated with a positive margin, wide excision has historically been the treatment of choice. Tan et al., in their consensus review paper, demonstrated that the published rates of recurrence in the literature of fibroadenoma and benign phyllodes tumor show significant overlap, and that watchful waiting could be an acceptable treatment for this category. Local recurrence is primarily related to margin status, while metastatic potential is related to the histologic classification. Malignant heterologous elements impart a worse prognosis.

## Selected References

1. Barth RJ Jr. Histologic features predict local recurrence after breast conserving therapy of phyllodes tumors. Breast Cancer Res Treat. 1999;57:291–5.
2. Cheah AL, Billings SD, Rowe JJ. Mesenchymal tumours of the breast and their mimics: a review with approach to diagnosis. Pathology. 2016 Aug;48(5):406–24.
3. Jones AM, Mitter R, Springall R, et al. A comprehensive genetic profile of phyllodes tumours of the breast detects important mutations, intra-tumoral genetic heterogeneity and new genetic changes on recurrence. J Pathol. 2008;214:533–44.
4. Kersting C, Kuijper A, Schmidt H, et al. Amplifications of the epidermal growth factor receptor gene (egfr) are common in phyllodes tumors of the breast and are associated with tumor progression. Lab Investig. 2006;86:54–61.
5. Lae M, Vincent-Salomon A, Savignoni A, et al. Phyllodes tumors of the breast segregate in two groups according to genetic criteria. Mod Pathol. 2007;20:435–44.
6. Ng CC, Tan J, Ong CK, et al. MED12 is frequently mutated in breast phyllodes tumours: a study of 112 cases. J Clin Pathol. 2015;68:685–91.
7. Pfarr N, Kriegsmann M, Sinn P, et al. Distribution of MED12 mutations in fibroadenomas and phyllodes tumors of the breast—implications for tumor biology and pathological diagnosis. Genes Chromosomes Cancer. 2015;54:444–52.

8. Rodrigues MF, et al. Phyllodes tumors of the breast: the British Columbia Cancer Agency experience. Tumeur phyllodes du sein : l'expérience de l'Agence du cancer de la Cancer/Radiothérapie. 2018;22:112–9.
9. Sawyer EJ, Hanby AM, Rowan AJ, et al. The wnt pathway, epithelial stromal interactions, and malignant progression in phyllodes tumours. J Pathol. 2002;196:437–44.
10. Tan J, Ong CK, Lim WK, et al. Genomic landscapes of breast fibroepithelial tumors. Nat Genet. 2015;47:1341–5.
11. Tan BY, et al. Phyllodes tumours of the breast: a consensus review. Histopathology. 2016;68:5–21. https://doi.org/10.1111/his.12876.
12. WHO Classification of Tumours of the Breast, 5th. Lyon: IARC, 2019.

# Periductal Stromal Hyperplasia and Periductal Stromal Tumor

3

J. Jordi Rowe

## Contents



## Introduction

Periductal stromal tumors (PDST), originally defined by Burga & Tavassoli, are marked by cuffs of spindled, mitotically active stroma encasing open lobules. This group presents a classification challenge. PDST are composed of two entities, the rarer initial presentation of periductal stromal hyperplasia (PDSH) and the more common presentation of periductal stromal sarcoma (PDSS). PDST are uncommon biphasic breast lesions that occur in perimenopausal and postmenopausal women (range: 24–89-years-old). PDST represent <1% of breast neoplasms. Previously thought to be a subcategory of phyllodes tumors, their status as a distinct entity remains unclear.

J. J. Rowe (✉)
Cleveland Clinic, Department of Pathology, Robert J. Tomsich Pathology and Laboratory Medicine Institute, Cleveland, OH, USA
e-mail: rowej@ccf.org





J. J. Rowe, E. Downs-Kelly (eds.), *Mesenchymal Tumors of the Breast and Their Mimics*, https://doi.org/10.1007/978-3-030-74474-8_3

## Clinical Features

Due to the rarity of the lesion, the clinical features are not well characterized. Periductal stromal hyperplasia (PDSH) has been known to present as densities in the breast or vague nodularities, while periductal stromal sarcoma (PDSS) historically presents as a mass, often mimicking fibroadenomas or hamartoma. However, PDSS and PDSH may or may not form masses and vary in size, with a wide range (<1 cm to 24 cm).

## Imaging

Periductal stromal tumors have a range in presentation from densities to mass lesions on mammography, and have been identified on magnetic resonance imaging (MRI). To date, no specific imaging correlate has been identified for PDST.

## Pathologic Features

### Gross Features

Grossly these lesions resemble fibrous tissue or even hamartoma, as they are non-circumscribed vague nodularities, tan to gray, and devoid of obvious clefting.

### Microscopic Features

A study in contradiction, PDST have been shown to be well-circumscribed as well as infiltrative and associated with and without microcalcifications. PDST is thought to arise from the periductal stroma. They encase and entrap adjacent lobules with a proliferation of atypical spindled cells (Fig. 3.1). A pertinent negative would be the absence of clefting, as PDST are devoid of a leaf-like architecture. The mitotic count per 10 high power fields (HPFs) is the determinant between PDSH and

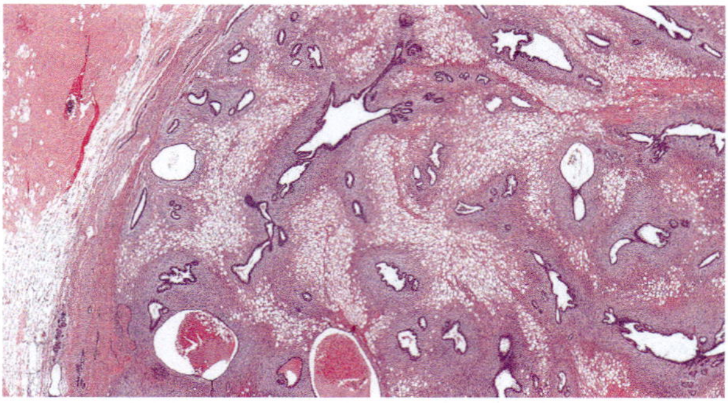

**Fig. 3.1** Low power image of periductal stromal sarcoma. The partially circumscribed border is apparent alongside the lack of a leaf-like architecture. H&E 20x

PDSS. As the stroma expands into the adjacent perilobular adipose tissue, the stromal nodules begin to coalesce into a mass. Recognizing the entrapped fat is paramount in identifying these lesions (Fig. 3.2). Of note, the lobules maintain their architecture and appear, due to their entrapment, to resemble the historically so-called "open lobules" of columnar cell change (Fig. 3.3a,b). Burga and Tavassoli, having the largest series to date, characterized the mitotic count within the cuffs of spindled cells to delineate PDSH with 0–2 mitotic figures per 10 HPFs from PDSS at ≥3 mitoses per 10 HPFs (Fig. 3.4).

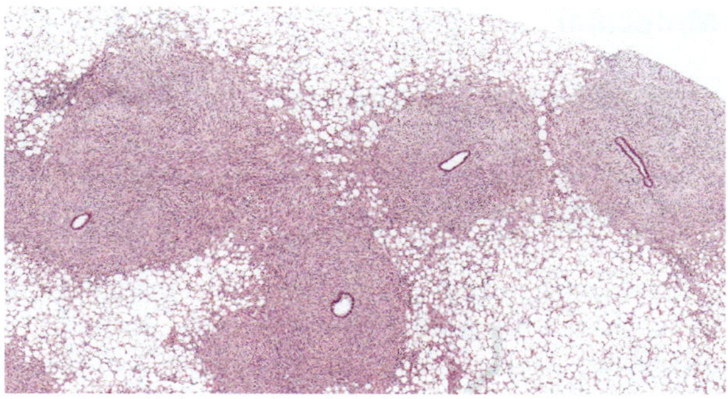

**Fig. 3.2** Periductal stromal sarcoma devoid of a leaf-like architecture and demonstrating the hallmark of coalescing nodules of sarcoma entrapping fat. H&E 40x

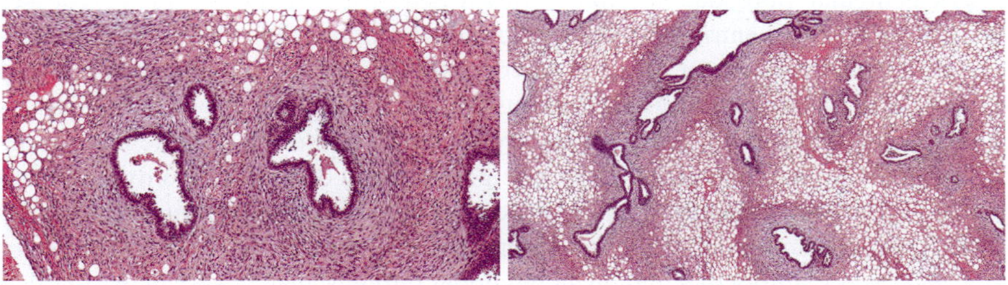

**Fig. 3.3** Periductal stromal sarcoma encasing open lobules. While the stroma is sarcomatous the residual ductal epithelium is benign and is reminiscent of columnar cell change. H&E 4x; H&E 100x

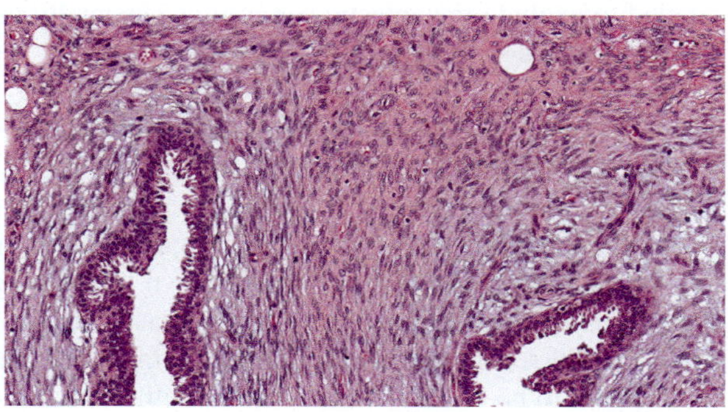

**Fig. 3.4** Higher magnification of the sarcomatous stroma of PDSS where the mitotic count is performed to classify the lesion. H&E 200x

## Immunohistochemistry

Similarly to phyllodes tumors, PDST are negative for estrogen and progesterone receptors, CD117, and cytokeratin 5 within the stroma. In the limited published studies, and by experience, PDST are typically negative for S100 protein, SMA, nuclear beta-catenin, SOX10, p63, and GATA3. A CD34 stain is positive in a high proportion of cases within the stroma, further cementing the similarity between phyllodes tumors and PDST.

## Molecular

There are no molecular signatures for PDST to date.

## Differential Diagnosis

As periductal stromal tumors were once thought to be a type of phyllodes tumor, these should be primarily evaluated by assessing their architecture. Phyllodes tumors are biphasic with an eponymous leaf-like architecture, at least focally demonstrable within the lesion. The circumferential cuffing of open lobules lends a "pericanalicular fibroadenoma-like" growth pattern to PDST. As PDST encases normal lobules and entraps fat, identifying these remnants of normal breast parenchyma is extremely useful. Primary sarcoma, although rare and described in detail under the chapter entitled Miscellaneous Mesenchymal Tumors of the Breast, is also a consideration. A subset of primary sarcomas is lineage-specific and can be confirmed with immunohistochemistry (e.g., SMA and desmin in leiomyosarcoma) while the diagnosis of undifferentiated pleomorphic sarcoma (UPS) is one of exclusion. Thorough sampling of the resection specimen to exclude a leaf-like architecture and the possibility of a malignant phyllodes tumor as well as thorough sampling to exclude either an in situ component or a malignant epithelial process that would support a metaplastic carcinoma is necessary before arriving at a diagnosis of UPS. This differential should be approached through a combination of microscopic features and immunohistochemical stains with a panel of cytokeratins and p63 needed to exclude metaplastic carcinoma, especially in those cases lacking epithelial differentiation by light microscopy.

## Treatment and Prognosis

Currently, PDST are excised with clear margins. Axillary dissection, radiation therapy, or chemotherapy have not been shown to improve outcome. These treatment modalities are limited due to the rarity of cases and limited follow-up. As there is a risk for local recurrence with phyllodes tumors, and presumptive risk of PDST as they appear to be fibroepithelial entities within the same diagnostic spectrum, wide excision is prudently applied to PDST as a precaution.

## Practical Tips

The key criterion for differentiation from phyllodes tumor is the lack of a leaf-like architecture and PDST may or may not form an appreciable mass lesion.

- PDST lack leaf-like architecture of phyllodes tumors.
- PDST encase normal lobules unlike fibroadenoma.
- PDST lacks a specific line of differentiation by immunohistochemistry in contrast to metaplastic carcinoma and specific sarcoma subtypes.
- PDST encase normal lobules unlike diffuse growth pattern of undifferentiated pleomorphic sarcoma.

## Selected References

1. Askan G, Arıbal E, Ak G, Kaya H. Periductal stromal tumor of the breast: a case report and review of the literature. J Breast Health. 2016;12(3):133–6.
2. Burga AM, Tavassoli FA. Periductal stromal tumor: a rare lesion with low-grade sarcomatous behavior. Am J Surg Pathol. 2003;27:343–8.
3. Cheah AL, Billings SD, Rowe JJ. Mesenchymal tumours of the breast and their mimics: a review with approach to diagnosis. Pathology. 2016;48(5):406–24.
4. Cortina CS, et al. An uncommon disease: Periductal stromal tumor of the breast. Breast J. 2018;24(6):1080–1. Epub 2018 Jul 22.
5. Fard EV, et al. Periductal Stromal Tumor of the Breast: Case Report and Literature Review. Ann Clin Lab Sci. 2018;48(6):770–5.
6. Ki SY, et al. Periductal stromal tumor of the breast with synchronous bilateral breast cancer. Anticancer Res. 2014;34(7):3635–9.
7. Lakhani SR, et al. WHO classification of tumours of the breast. 4th ed. Lyon: IARC; 2012. p. 145–6.
8. Tomas D, et al. Low-grade periductal stromal sarcoma of the breast with myxoid features: immunohistochemistry. Pathol Int. 2009;59:588–91.
9. WHO Classification of Tumours. WHO Classification of Tumours of the Breast. 5th ed. Lyon: IARC; 2019.

# Vascular Tumors of the Breast

# 4

Steven D. Billings

## Contents




S. D. Billings (✉)
Cleveland Clinic, Department of Pathology, Robert J. Tomsich Pathology and Laboratory Medicine Institute, Cleveland, OH, USA
e-mail: billins@ccf.org







J. J. Rowe, E. Downs-Kelly (eds.), *Mesenchymal Tumors of the Breast and Their Mimics*, https://doi.org/10.1007/978-3-030-74474-8_4

## Benign Vascular Tumors of the Breast

### Perilobular Hemangioma

#### Clinical Features

Perilobular hemangioma is the most common vascular tumor of the breast, seen in between 1% and 11% of patients. Clinically, they are small, ranging in size from 1 to 3 mm, asymptomatic lesions that are discovered as incidental findings.

### Imaging

They are not typically identified with imaging studies, with rare exceptions.

#### Pathologic Features

**Gross Features** Grossly, they are inconspicuous and not typically recognized.

**Microscopic Features** Histologically, they consist of a lobular proliferation of capillaries. Usually, they are associated with epithelial structures of the terminal

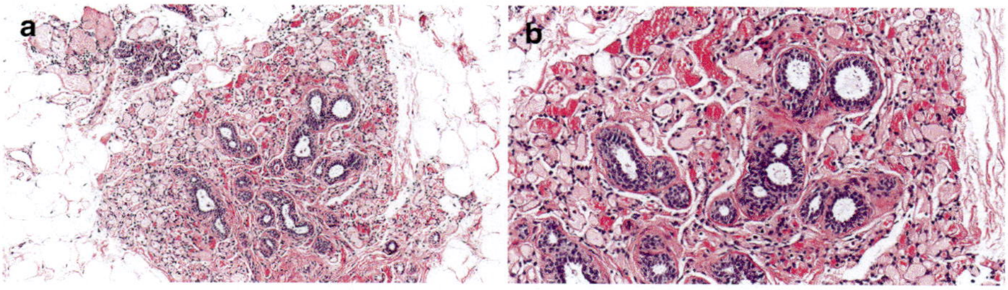


**Fig. 4.1** Perilobular hemangioma (**a**). Medium power image demonstrating a circumscribed proliferation of capillaries associated with a terminal duct lobular unit. (**b**). Higher power image demonstrated small capillaries lined by bland endothelial cells

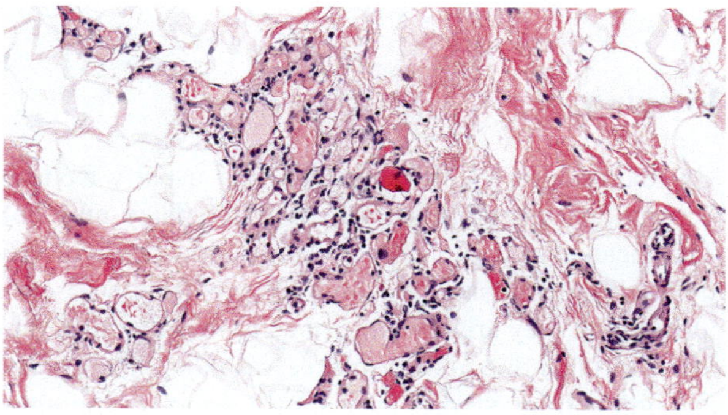

**Fig. 4.2** Perilobular hemangioma. Some perilobular hemangiomas are not associated with a terminal duct lobular unit

lobular duct unit. The vascular proliferation may intimately intercalate around the epithelial structures without disrupting or distorting the overall architecture (Fig. 4.1). Occasional cases are not associated with a breast lobule (Fig. 4.2) and consist of small vascular proliferations in the perilobular stroma. The vessels are typically ectatic, thin-walled, and lined by bland endothelial cells without atypia or multilayering and contain numerous erythrocytes. Rare examples may have nuclear hyperchromasia, and these have been termed "atypical perilobular hemangioma". This so-called atypical perilobular hemangioma still maintains the architecture of a typical perilobular hemangioma.

## Immunohistochemistry

They are positive for vascular markers such as CD31, CD34, and ERG.

## Differential Diagnosis

Given their small size and bland features, perilobular hemangiomas are rarely a diagnostic challenge. They can be confused with other hemangioma subtypes, but their incidental nature, small size, and architecture consisting of clusters of capillaries allow for distinction. A partially sampled, well-differentiated angiosarcoma could be considered in the differential, but angiosarcomas are larger, infiltrative tumors with inter-anastomosing vessels and typically exhibit significant cytologic atypia.

### Treatment and Prognosis

Perilobular hemangiomas are benign and no definitive treatment is necessary.

## Hemangiomas

### Clinical Features

Hemangiomas may be seen at any age and have a mean age at diagnosis of approximately 60 years. Unlike perilobular hemangioma, other hemangiomas may present as palpable masses or be detected by imaging studies. Hemangiomas as a group are more common in women than men. There is at least one report of a cavernous hemangioma associated with a breast implant.

### Imaging

On mammography, hemangiomas are usually isodense, lobular to oval, with circumscribed to microlobulated borders. They may contain rounded calcifications. The mean size is typically ~1 cm with a range of 0.6 cm to 2.5 cm. It should be pointed out that rare cases may be greater than 5 cm in maximum dimension. By ultrasound, they are circumscribed to microlobulated masses. The echo patterns are often variable due to the multiple vascular channels and, in some cases, thrombosis and phleboliths. Studies have shown a good correlation with radiologic diagnosis of hemangiomas and the final pathologic diagnosis.

### Pathologic Features

**Gross Features** They are often red-brown on cut section and those with a cavernous architecture may have a spongy appearance.

**Microscopic Features** Hemangiomas are typically located in the extralobular stroma. Classically, hemangiomas of the breast have been divided into two broad categories: cavernous and capillary hemangiomas. Cavernous hemangioma is the most common clinically detected benign vascular tumor. Microscopically, cavernous hemangiomas are circumscribed and composed of large ectatic vascular spaces, without architectural complexity, lined by bland endothelial cells (Fig. 4.3). Areas of thrombosis with papillary endothelial hyperplasia and calcification may be present (Fig. 4.4). Capillary hemangiomas consist of densely packed, smaller ectatic vessels lined by bland endothelial cells (Fig. 4.5). A given lesion may contain an admixture of cavernous areas and capillary-like areas. Tumors with combined features have been termed complex hemangiomas. Rare cases of breast hemangioma have a sinusoidal appearance (Fig. 4.6), and likely represent a variant of a so-called complex hemangioma.

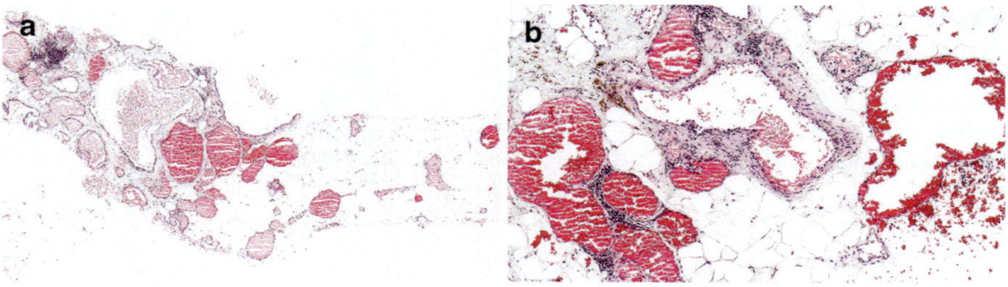


**Fig. 4.3** Cavernous hemangioma. (**a**). Low power image of needle core biopsy of cavernous hemangioma with enlarged, ectatic vascular spaces. (**b**). The vessels are ectatic and lined by bland endothelial cells

**Fig. 4.4** Hemangioma with fibrosis, calcification, and papillary endothelial hyperplasia

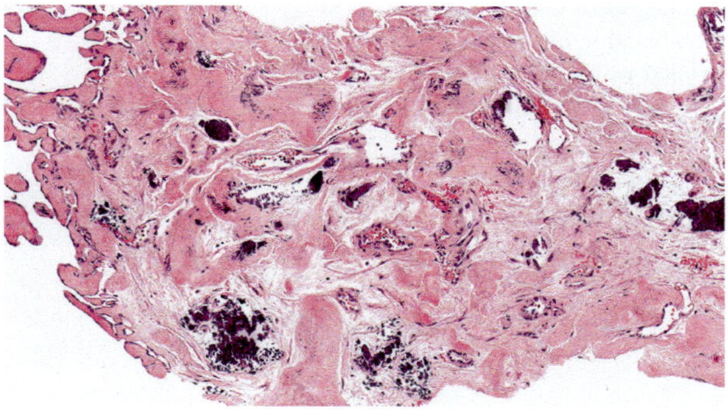

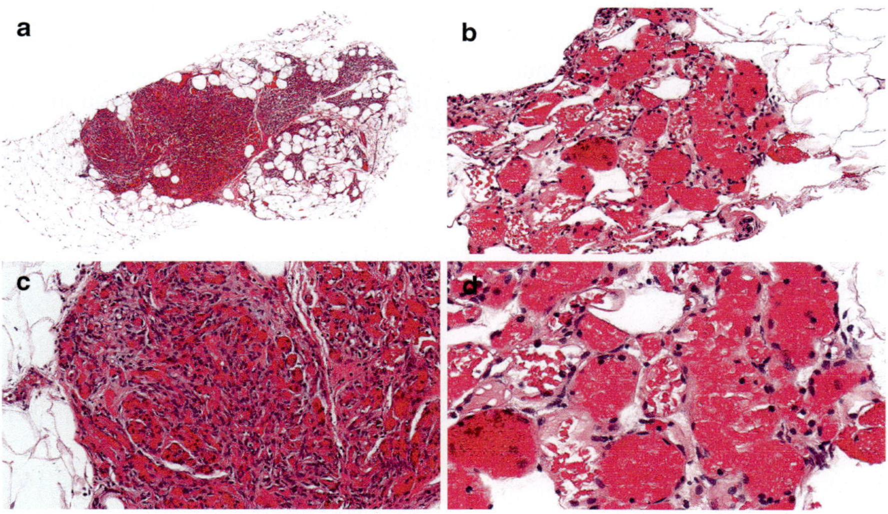


**Fig. 4.5** Capillary hemangioma. (**a**). Needle core biopsy demonstrating the circumscribed proliferation of closely packed capillaries. (**b**). Medium power image demonstrating densely packed, thin-walled capillaries. (**c**). In this capillary hemangioma, the vessels are somewhat compressed. (**d**). High power image demonstrating the bland endothelial cells lining the vessels

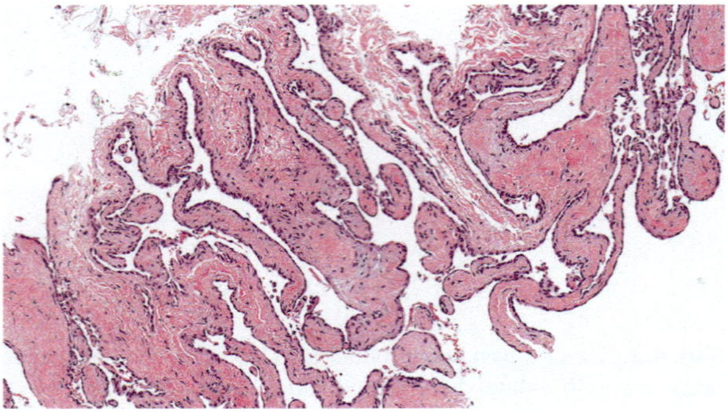

**Fig. 4.6** Sinusoidal hemangioma composed of well-circumscribed but somewhat branching vessels lined by bland endothelial cells

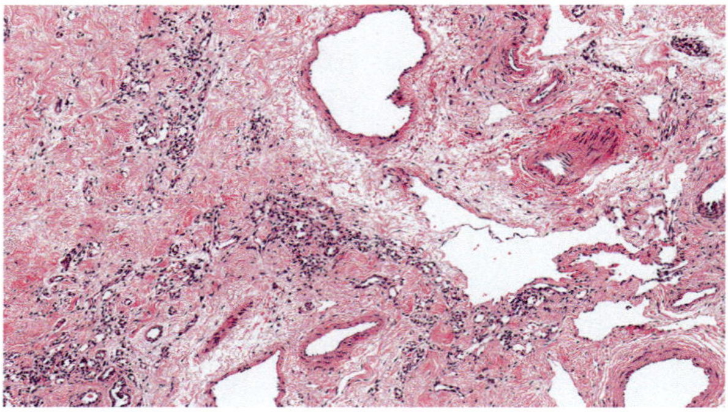

**Fig. 4.7** Venous hemangioma with a combination of thicker-walled vessels centrally and smaller capillaries at the periphery

Atypical hemangioma is a somewhat nebulous category. This designation has been used for vascular tumors with some mild nuclear atypia or focal anastomosing vascular channels in a lesion that otherwise has architectural features of a hemangioma.

A variant, termed venous hemangioma, has also been described. They consist of irregularly shaped dilated vessels lined with a variably developed smooth muscle wall (Fig. 4.7). The endothelial cells are bland without multilayering or atypia. Likely, some venous hemangiomas represent vascular malformations rather than true hemangiomas.

## Immunohistochemistry

The endothelial cells are positive for vascular markers such as CD31, CD34, and ERG. The vessels are often surrounded by a pericyte layer or smooth muscle that can be demonstrated by stains for SMA. Hemangiomas have a low Ki-67 labeling index.

## Differential Diagnosis

The primary differential diagnosis is with well-differentiated angiosarcoma. The circumscribed nature of hemangiomas and the lack of atypia usually allow for distinction. In problematic cases, an immunostain for Ki-67 may be useful, as angiosarcomas typically have a higher labeling index in comparison to hemangiomas. It has been suggested that a cut-off of 150–175 Ki-67-positive cells out of 600 counted nuclei has been proposed as a discriminator of angiosarcoma from hemangiomas, with a sensitivity of 80–91%.

### Treatment and Prognosis

Although hemangiomas are benign, it has traditionally been recommended that all hemangiomas be completely excised given the diagnostic difficulty, especially in the setting of core needle biopsies. A more recent study, however, has challenged that notion, showing high concordance of radiologic diagnosis of hemangioma and final pathologic classification. This of course is dependent on operator experience. Certainly, if there is any doubt, the lesion should be excised. If expectant management is pursued, then the patient should have continued clinical follow-up with the continuation of age-appropriate screening.

## Angiomatosis

### Clinical Features

Angiomatosis of the breast is rare with relatively few cases reported. In one of the largest series, the mean age was 51 years, but there are several case reports of angiomatosis in younger adults. Patients typically present with a palpable mass with a mean size of 3 cm, ranging in size up to 9 cm. Most present in the upper outer quadrant. Patients may also have overlying skin discoloration and may clinically mimic angiosarcoma.

### Imaging

Detailed reports on the imaging characteristics of angiomatosis are limited, owing to the rarity of this entity. On mammography, angiomatosis is less well-defined in comparison to hemangiomas and may also contain calcifications. Ultrasound has shown a macrolobulated, oval, mixed-echogenic mass. MRI is isointense on T1W1 images and hyperintense on T2W1 images.

### Pathologic Features

**Gross Features** Grossly, angiomatosis tends to be hyperemic and less well-defined than hemangiomas.

**Microscopic Features** Angiomatosis is a diffuse vascular proliferation that infiltrates between and around terminal duct lobular units, but not into the intralobular

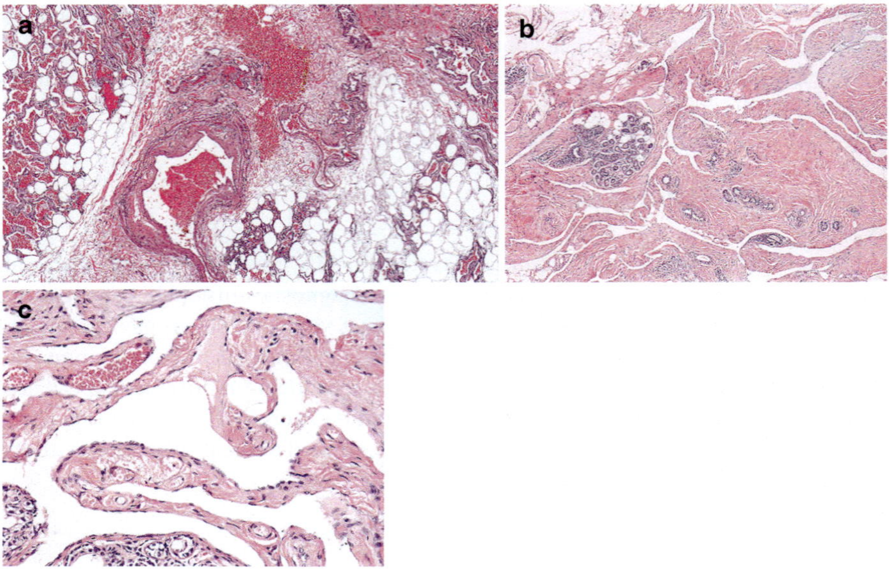

**Fig. 4.8** Angiomatosis. (**a**). There is a diffuse proliferation of vessels that have partially developed muscular walls, capillary-like vessels, and some with an anastomosing pattern at the periphery. (**b**). Angiomatosis with elongated vessels coursing between the breast lobules. (**c**). Higher power image demonstrating bland endothelial cells lining the vascular channels. (**b** & **c**: Images courtesy of Stuart Schnitt, MD, Dana-Farber/Brigham and Women's Cancer Center)

stroma. The border has an infiltrative appearance. The vessels comprising the lesion can range from capillary-like to ectatic, lymphangioma-like, to thicker vessels with muscular walls (Fig. 4.8). Some anastomosing channels may be present, but this finding should be focal. The vessels are lined by bland, flattened endothelial cells. Nuclear atypia and mitotic activity are absent.

## Immunohistochemistry

As expected, angiomatosis is positive for vascular markers, CD31, CD34, and ERG. Vessels resembling lymphatic channels are positive for podoplanin (D2–40). The Ki-67 labeling index is $<1\%$.

## Differential Diagnosis

The primary differential diagnosis is between hemangioma and well-differentiated angiosarcoma. Hemangiomas have a circumscribed border unlike angiomatosis.

Well-differentiated angiosarcomas have more anastomosing channels and typically more cytologic atypia. Growth within the intralobular stroma is also a feature of angiosarcoma. Pseudoangiomatous stromal hyperplasia (PASH) is also in the differential diagnosis. PASH is positive for CD34, but negative for CD31 and ERG.

### Treatment and Prognosis

Angiomatosis is primarily managed with surgery. A case using preoperative radiation therapy, in order to facilitate breast-conserving surgery, has been reported. Local recurrence is a risk, especially in larger tumors.

## Intravascular Papillary Endothelial Hyperplasia

### Clinical Features

Intravascular papillary endothelial hyperplasia (Masson tumor) is much more common in women, with a mean age of ~60 years and range from 13 to 85 years. Most patients present with a palpable mass. A subset is detected by imaging. Cases associated with breast implants have been reported.

### Imaging

Mammography demonstrates a small circumscribed or lobulated mass, usually ranging in size from 0.5 to 1.5 cm. Microcalcifications may be present. It is typically found in the superficial subcutaneous tissue.

### Pathologic Features

**Gross Features** Intravascular papillary endothelial hyperplasia varies from red to tan with a cut surface that ranges from friable to rubbery.

**Microscopic Features** Intravascular papillary endothelial hyperplasia is typically seen in the subcutaneous fibroadipose tissue without breast lobules or ducts in the surrounding tissue, though occasional cases may be intraparenchymal. They are typically well-circumscribed. Papillary areas are seen in the periphery, whereas the central zone is often more collagenized. The papillary areas show small papillae lined by bland endothelial cells and a variably collagenized core (Fig. 4.9). Mitotic activity is typically low (<1 MF/ 10 HPFs). In close to half of cases, there are ectatic

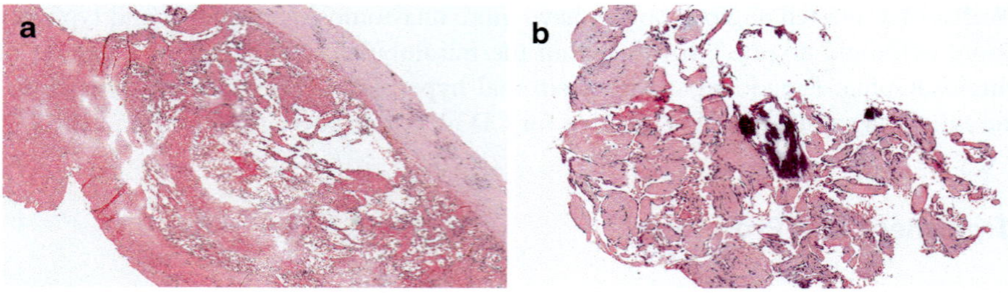

**Fig. 4.9** (**a**). Low power image of papillary endothelial hyperplasia with papillary architecture peripherally, and central collagenous zone. (**b**). Needle core biopsy of papillary endothelial hyperplasia. Note the variably complex papillary structures lined by bland endothelial cells without multilayering. Papillary endothelial hyperplasia may have foci of calcification

vascular spaces at the periphery. Areas of intravascular papillary endothelial hyperplasia may also be seen within cavernous hemangiomas.

### Immunohistochemistry

The endothelial cells are positive for CD31, CD34, and ERG.

### Differential Diagnosis

The primary differential diagnosis is well-differentiated angiosarcoma. Both can have a papillary architecture, but angiosarcoma has more atypia and often demonstrates multilayering of endothelial cells, unlike intravascular papillary endothelial hyperplasia. Angiosarcoma also infiltrates around breast lobules and ducts, unlike intravascular papillary endothelial hyperplasia.

### Treatment and Prognosis

Intravascular papillary endothelial hyperplasia is benign. Definitive treatment is not necessary, with the caveat that any diagnostic uncertainty should result in additional sampling/excision.

## Radiation and Lymphedema-Associated Vascular Tumors

### Atypical Vascular Lesion

#### Clinical Features

Atypical vascular lesion (also called benign lymphangiomatous papule) is a radiation-induced vascular lesion, typically in the setting of breast-conserving surgery for carcinoma. The average latency is between 3 and 5 years from completion of radiation therapy, but lesions can occur as early as 1 year after radiation therapy or many years later. Patients usually present with one or more cutaneous skin-colored to erythematous papules or nodules within the radiation field.

## Imaging

Imaging plays no role, as they are detected on physical examination.

## Pathologic Features

**Gross Features** Grossly, these lesions are relatively unremarkable, given that they are typically received as small skin biopsies.

**Microscopic Features** Atypical vascular lesions are relatively well-circumscribed and symmetrical with a vaguely wedge-shaped silhouette. The well-formed vascular structures comprising the lesion are usually confined to the papillary and superficial-to-mid reticular dermis. In rare cases, the lesion may extend to the subcutis. The superficial portion typically contains more dilated vascular spaces than the deeper aspect. In the deeper component, the vessels are compressed and may show a dissecting pattern between collagen bundles. They have been divided into two histologic subtypes: (1) lymphatic type and (2) vascular type. The former histologically mimics a cutaneous lymphangioma, with ectatic vessels lined by flattened endothelial cells. Some architectural complexity may be present (Fig. 4.10). The vascular type resembles hemangiomas (Fig. 4.11) and may resemble a hobnail hemangioma with hobnail endothelial cells. Neither subtype has multi-layering of endo-

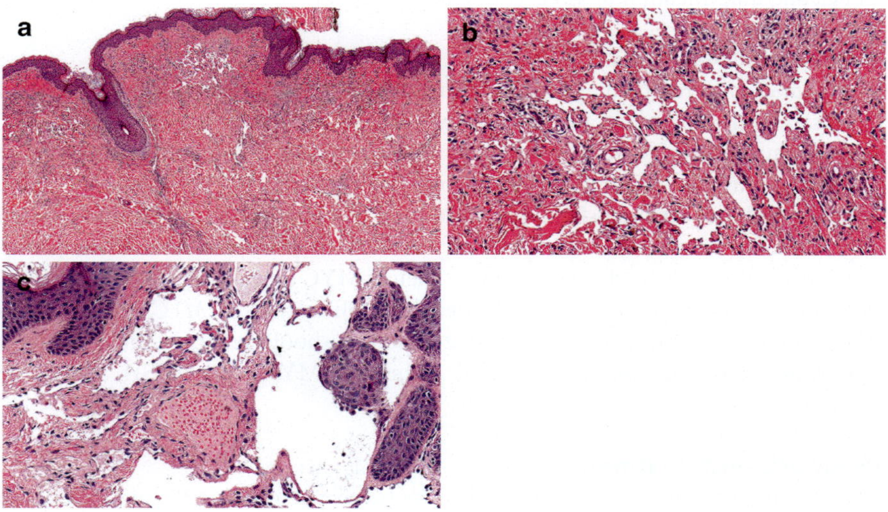


**Fig. 4.10** Lymphatic type atypical vascular lesion. (**a**). Low power image demonstrating ectatic vessels of lymphatic type atypical vascular lesion in the superficial dermis. (**b**). The vessels of lymphatic type atypical vascular lesion can be somewhat architecturally complex, but the vessels are lined by bland endothelial cells without multilayering. (**c**). Valve-like structures are often present in the ectatic vessels

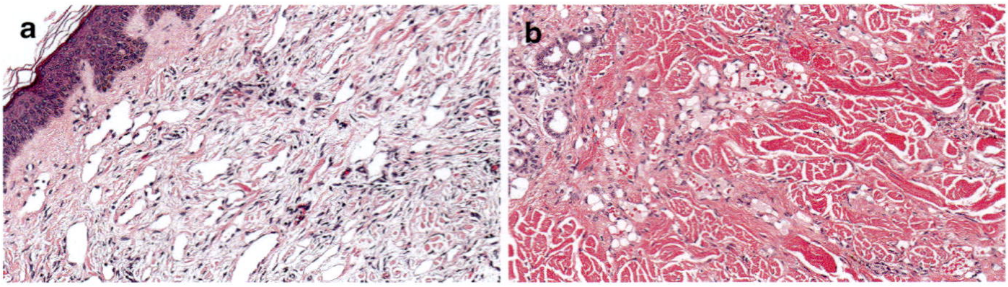


**Fig. 4.11** Vascular type atypical vascular lesion. (**a**). In the vascular type, the vessels often resemble those of a capillary hemangioma, lacking the complexity seen in the lymphatic type atypical vascular lesion or angiosarcoma. (**b**). The endothelial cells may have slightly enlarged nuclei, but true atypia and multilayering is absent

thelial cells, and show only mild, if any, cytologic atypia in the form of nuclear hyperchromasia and hobnailing. Mitotic activity is absent. In a given case, it may not be possible to subclassify the lesion into lymphatic type or vascular type atypical vascular lesion. The distinction is largely academic. The main diagnostic goal is to diagnose them as atypical vascular lesion, and to not misdiagnose them as angiosarcoma (see below).

## Immunohistochemistry

Atypical vascular lesion is positive for CD31, CD34, and ERG. The lymphatic subtype may be positive for podoplanin. The vascular type will have an SMA-positive pericyte layer. Atypical vascular lesion is negative, or rarely focally positive, for MYC, and amplification of *MYC* is absent.

## Differential Diagnosis

The primary differential diagnosis is with a well-differentiated radiation-associated angiosarcoma. Angiosarcomas clinically tend to be larger, violaceous lesions. Angiosarcoma usually is more infiltrative with greater cytologic atypia in most cases. Multilayering of endothelial cells is often present. That being said, it can be very difficult to distinguish atypical vascular lesion from a well-differentiated angiosarcoma in selected cases, especially in small biopsy specimens. In that situation either immunohistochemical stains to detect MYC expression (positive in post-radiation angiosarcoma) or FISH to detect amplification of *MYC* (amplified in post-radiation angiosarcoma) allows distinction. It should be noted that if there is any doubt with immunohistochemical stains for MYC, then FISH should be performed.

## Prognosis and Treatment

The vast majority of atypical vascular lesions behave in a benign fashion. There are isolated cases documented that have transformed into angiosarcoma, but this seems to be a rare event, and atypical vascular lesion is not considered an obligate precursor to post-radiation angiosarcoma. However, given the theoretic risk, conservative but complete excision is recommended if clinically feasible. In a patient with numerous atypical vascular lesions when multiple complete excision become impractical, then very close clinical monitoring is another approach that can be considered.

## Post-Radiation and Lymphedema-Associated Angiosarcoma

### Clinical Features

This group of tumors is seen in the setting of breast cancer. Therefore, patients are typically older, post-menopausal women. In the past when radical mastectomy was the mainstay of surgical treatment, lymphedema-induced angiosarcoma (Stewart-Treves syndrome) was a late complication. Patients developed angiosarcoma on the ipsilateral arm or chest wall of the prior mastectomy site, typically with an average latency of 10 years or more. In post-radiation angiosarcoma, the clinical setting is in patients with lumpectomy and adjuvant radiation therapy. In this setting, the average latency is only 5 years, and cases can develop in as little as 1–2 years after radiation therapy. In both settings, the tumors usually present as erythematous to violaceous nodules to plaques. Occasional cases present as diffuse erythema and rarely as subtle induration.

### Imaging

Imaging does not typically play a role in this setting.

### Pathologic Features

**Gross Features** The tumors often present as ill-defined erythematous to hemorrhagic masses. Occasional cases can be very subtle and the tumor inapparent, at least in some areas.

**Microscopic Features** Post-radiation angiosarcomas have a wide range of patterns. They can be well-differentiated and composed of anastomosing vessels lined by hyperchromatic endothelial cells (Fig. 4.12). Some cases have a prominent papillary architecture (Fig. 4.13). They can also have a sieve-like pattern of back to back vessels (Fig. 4.14), a solid sheet-like growth pattern of atypical spindled cells with admixed erythrocytes (Fig. 4.15), and epithelioid morphology (Fig. 4.16). A given tumor may have more than one pattern within a single lesion. Two unusual histologic patterns have been described: the capillary lobule pattern and the so-called radiation dermatitis-like pattern. In the capillary lobule pattern, there are distinct nodules of atypical vessels somewhat reminiscent of a hemangioma or tufted angioma (Fig. 4.17). In the radiation dermatitis-like pattern there are individual atypical cells and non-complex worm-like vessels lined by atypical endothelial cells (Fig. 4.18).

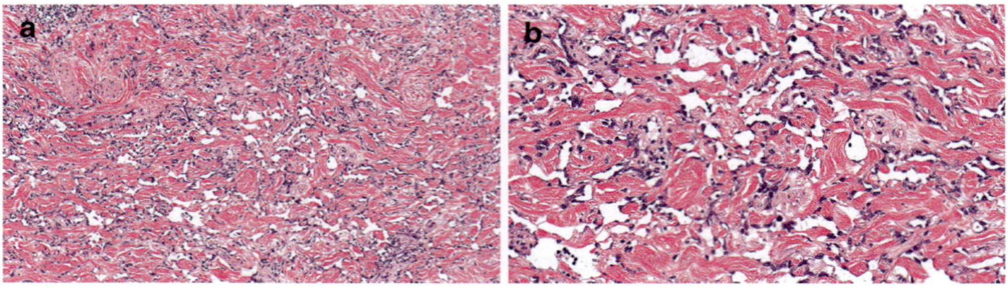


**Fig. 4.12** Well-differentiated post-radiation angiosarcoma. (**a**). The tumor is composed of anastomosing vessels with an infiltrative growth pattern. (**b**). In well-differentiated tumors, the endothelial cells may not show prominent atypia or multilayering

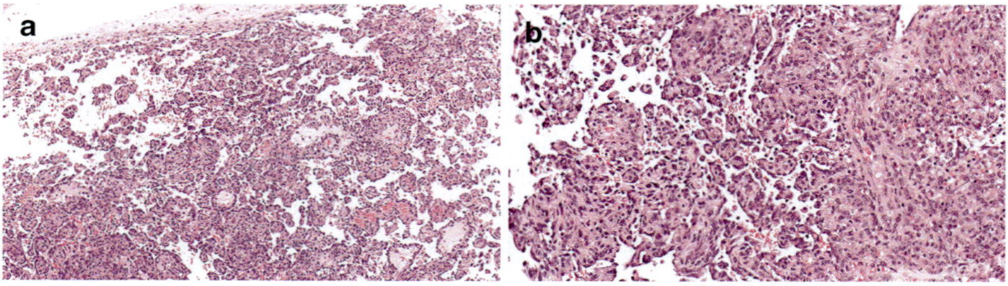


**Fig. 4.13** Post-radiation angiosarcoma. (**a**). Individual tumors may have a combination of solid areas as well as vasoformative areas. (**b**). Higher power view demonstrating the complex papillary architecture and more solid areas

**Fig. 4.14** Post-radiation angiosarcoma with sieve-like pattern of back to back neoplastic vessels

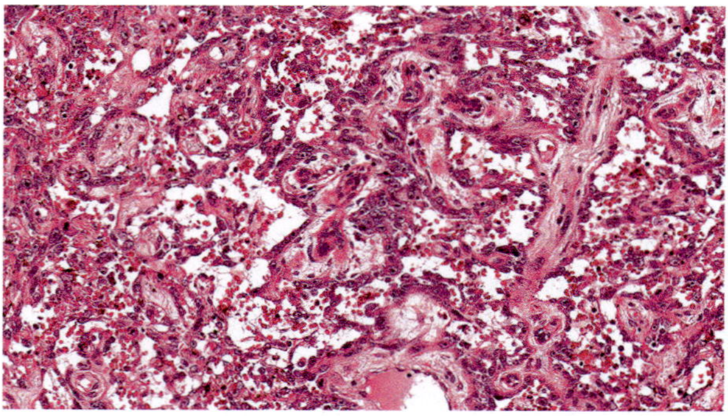

**Fig. 4.15** Post-radiation angiosarcoma composed of solid sheets of atypical spindled cells associated with intratumoral hemorrhage

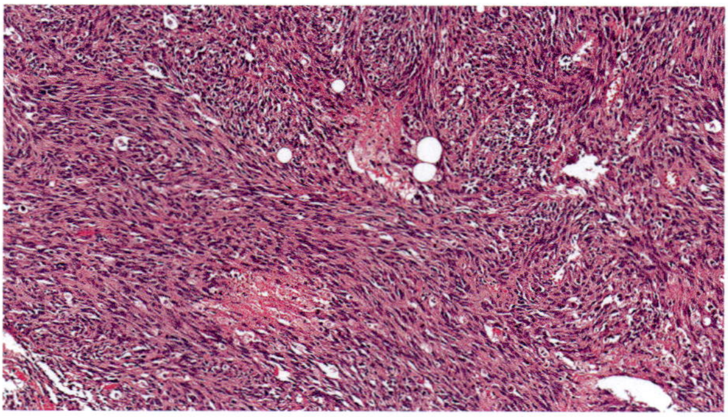

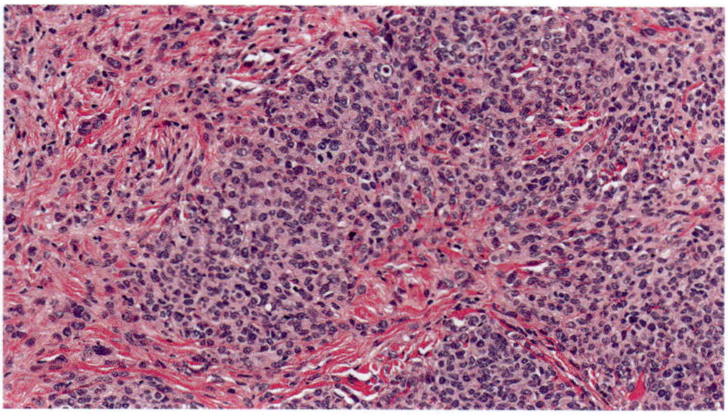

**Fig. 4.16** Post-radiation angiosarcoma with an epithelioid morphology

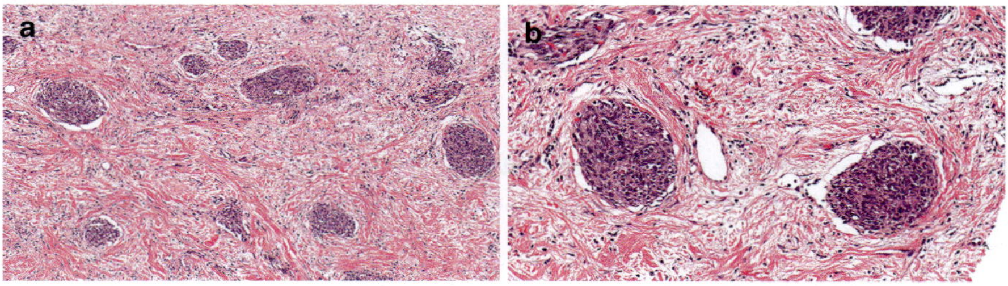

**Fig. 4.17** Post-radiation angiosarcoma, capillary lobule pattern. (**a**). In this rare variant, the tumor is composed of discrete solid nodules within the dermis. (**b**). Higher power image demonstrating discrete nodules of atypical endothelial cells

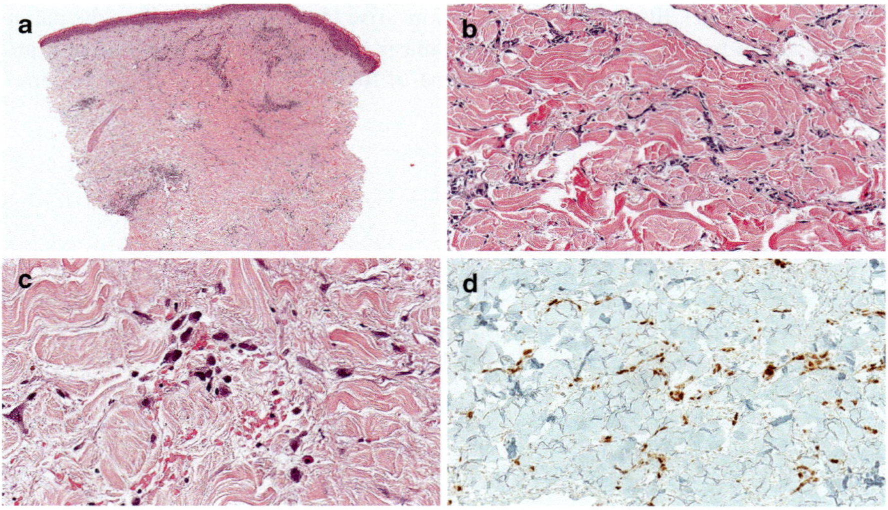

**Fig. 4.18** Post-radiation angiosarcoma, radiation dermatitis-like pattern. (**a**). In this histologic variant, the tumor is typically inapparent at scanning magnification and may be confused with radiation dermatitis. (**b**). This pattern often has compressed, worm-like vascular channels lined by hyperchromatic endothelial cells. (**c**). The atypical cells are often associated with extravasated erythrocytes. (**d**). Typical of post-radiation angiosarcoma, the tumor cells have nuclear immunoreactivity for MYC

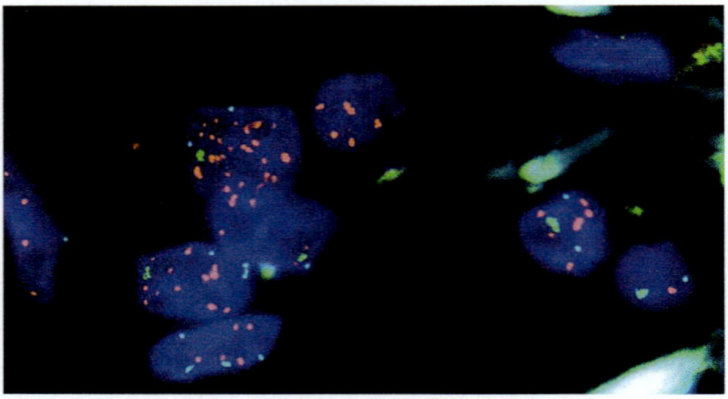

**Fig. 4.19** Post-radiation and lymphedema-associated angiosarcoma of the breast has amplification of *MYC* in close to 100% of cases. There are numerous copies of the red signal for *MYC* in comparison to the blue centromere control probe (Courtesy Caroline Astbury, PhD, Cleveland Clinic)

## Immunohistochemistry

The tumors are positive for vascular markers CD31, CD34, and ERG. Greater than 90% are positive for MYC by immunohistochemistry (Fig. 4.18) or *MYC* amplification by FISH (Fig. 4.19).

## Differential Diagnosis

The differential diagnosis with atypical vascular lesion is outlined above. Histologically, post-radiation angiosarcoma and primary angiosarcoma may be identical. However, the post-radiation tumors arise in the skin rather than the parenchyma of the breast. Primary angiosarcoma is negative for MYC expression and *MYC* amplification. Primary angiosarcoma of the breast also has different demographic features (see below).

## Prognosis and Treatment

Post-radiation angiosarcoma has a high rate of local recurrence. The lungs are the most common site of metastasis, but metastases may involve lymph nodes, bone, and the contralateral breast. Mastectomy is the primary treatment but adjuvant radiation therapy or chemotherapy may also be employed.

## Primary Angiosarcoma

### Clinical Features

Primary angiosarcoma typically arises in the third to fourth decades. Most patients present with a painless mass. In some patients, the overlying skin may be erythematous or violaceous if there is extension into the overlying skin.

## Imaging

Mammography usually reveals a noncalcified mass, but mammography may be negative in close to one third of cases. Ultrasound may be hyperechoic or mixed. MRI is usually heterogenous with variable intensity.

## Pathologic Features

**Gross Features** Primary angiosarcomas are usually large, ill-defined masses (mean size ~7 cm) with the tumor larger than what is grossly apparent. They may be erythematous to violaceous on the cut surface. The tumor can consist of punctate areas of hemorrhage or large and spongy masses.

**Microscopic Features** Primary angiosarcoma has a range of appearances as described above for post-radiation angiosarcoma (Fig. 4.20). They can be well-differentiated tumors composed of anastomosing channels dissecting through the breast parenchyma to more solid sheet-like patterns of atypical endothelial cells. The endothelial cells may be relatively small and hyperchromatic, hobnailed, epithelioid, or spindled. Mitotic activity is frequently conspicuous. An important feature that is a clue to the diagnosis is the presence of the tumor within the intralobular stroma. Areas where the tumor infiltrates fat can sometimes be very subtle.

## Immunohistochemistry

Primary angiosarcomas of the breast are positive for vascular markers CD31, CD34, and ERG. They typically have an elevated Ki-67 labeling index as previously mentioned. They are negative for MYC expression and *MYC* amplification.

## Differential Diagnosis

Well-differentiated angiosarcomas must be distinguished from hemangioma, angiomatosis, and intravascular papillary endothelial hyperplasia. This has been discussed previously in the above sections. Briefly, infiltrative borders, infiltration within lobular parenchyma, anastomosing vascular channels, and cytologic atypia all point to the diagnosis of angiosarcoma. Pseudoangiomatous stromal hyperplasia (PASH) has a collagenous stroma in contrast to angiosarcoma which infiltrates normal breast parenchyma and lacks cytologic atypia or multilayering. PASH is positive for CD34, but negative for CD31 and ERG.

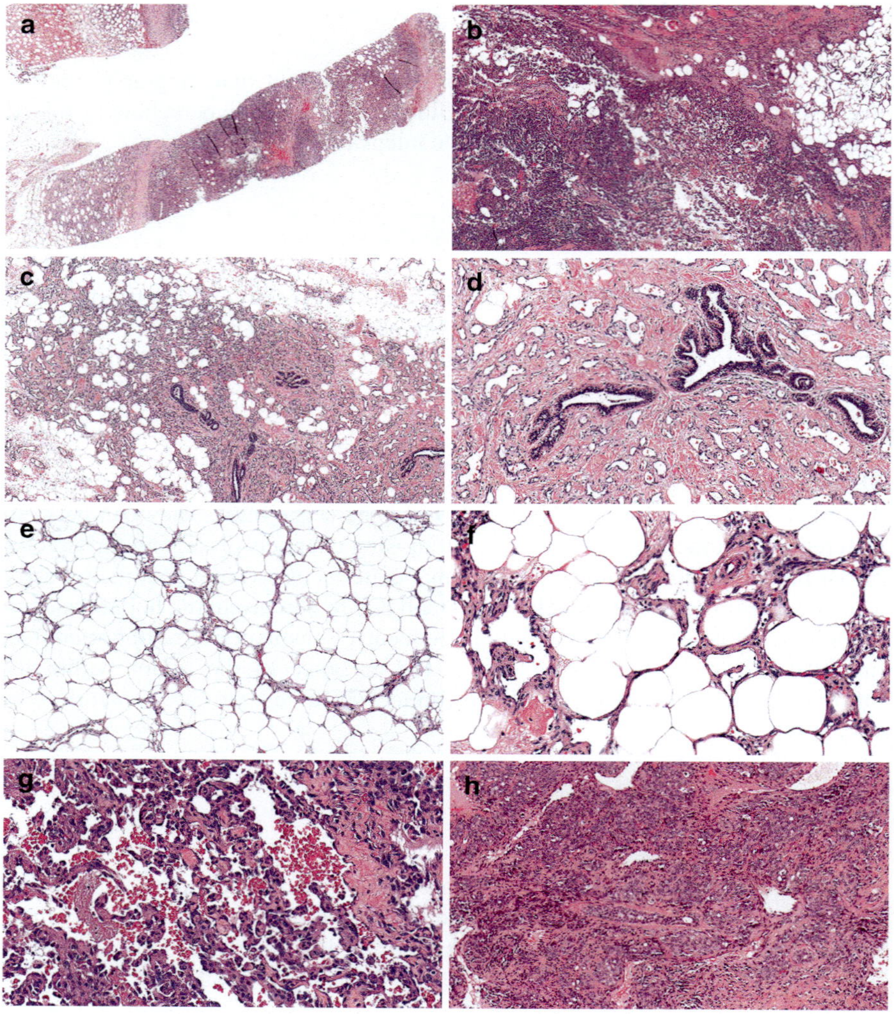


**Fig. 4.20** Primary angiosarcoma. (**a**). Scanning image of needle core biopsy that demonstrates solid growth pattern centrally and vasoformation peripherally. (**b**). Low power image demonstrating both complex vasoformative and solid areas. (**c**). Well-differentiated angiosarcoma infiltrating within the lobular parenchyma. (**d**). Higher power image of architecturally complex vessels lined by atypical endothelial cells infiltrating lobular parenchyma. (**e**). Well-differentiated tumors intercalating between fat can be histologically subtle. (**f**). Higher power image of subtle well-differentiated angiosarcoma infiltrating fat. Note the hyperchromatic endothelial cells and anastomosing vascular architecture. (**g**). Angiosarcoma with complex vasoformative channels with papillary architecture. (**h**). Epithelioid angiosarcoma with a largely solid growth pattern

## Prognosis and Treatment

Primary angiosarcomas are aggressive tumors with a high risk of recurrence and mortality. Previous studies suggested that histologic grade was associated with prognosis. However, other studies have shown no difference in outcome related to grade. So-called low-grade tumors may behave equally as aggressively as intermediate to high-grade tumors. Therefore, we do not recommend grading primary (or secondary) angiosarcoma of the breast.

Mastectomy is the primary treatment modality. Radiation therapy and chemotherapy may also be used, but the literature regarding their efficacy is thin. Despite aggressive treatment, overall survival is approximately 5 years or less.

## Selected References

1. Adwani A, Bees N, Arnaout A, Lanaspre E. Hemangioma of the breast: clinical, mammographic, and ultrasound features. Breast J. 2006;12(3):271.
2. Aydın OU, Soylu L, Ercan Aİ, Bilezikçi B, Özbaş S. Cavernous hemangioma in the breast. J Breast Health. 2015;11(4):199–201.
3. Baker GM, Schnitt SJ. Vascular lesions of the breast. Semin Diagn Pathol. 2017;34(5):410–9.
4. Billings SD, McKenney JK, Folpe AL, Hardacre MC, Weiss SW. Cutaneous angiosarcoma following breast-conserving surgery and radiation: an analysis of 27 cases. Am J Surg Pathol. 2004;28(6):781–8.
5. Branton PA, Lininger R, Tavassoli FA. Papillary endothelial hyperplasia of the breast: the great impostor for angiosarcoma: a clinicopathologic review of 17 cases. Int J Surg Pathol. 2003;11(2):83–7.
6. Brenn T, Fletcher CD. Radiation-associated cutaneous atypical vascular lesions and angiosarcoma: clinicopathologic analysis of 42 cases. Am J Surg Pathol. 2005;29(8):983–96.
7. Brodie C, Provenzano E. Vascular proliferations of the breast. Histopathology. 2008;52(1):30–44.
8. Chulakadabba A, Denariyakoon S, Chakkabat P, et al. Preoperative radiation in large angiomatosis of the breast, attempting breast conserving surgery: multidisciplinary approach. J Surg Case Rep. 2018;2018(2):rjy024.
9. Cui L, Zhang J, Zhang X, et al. Angiosarcoma (Stewart-Treves syndrome) in postmastectomy patients: report of 10 cases and review of literature. Int J Clin Exp Pathol. 2015;8(9): 11108–15.
10. Daniels BH, Ko JS, Rowe JJ, Downs-Kelly E, Billings SD. Radiation-associated angiosarcoma in the setting of breast cancer mimicking radiation dermatitis: a diagnostic pitfall. J Cutan Pathol. 2017;44(5):456–61.
11. de Mello Tucunduvà TC, Gaziero A, Tostes VS, et al. Cavernous hemangioma between the elastomer and fibrous capsule of a breast implant. Aesthet Plast Surg. 2018;42(5):1257–60.
12. Di Tommaso L, Rosai J. The capillary lobule: a deceptively benign feature of post-radiation angiosarcoma of the skin: report of three cases. Am J Dermatopathol. 2005;27(4):301–5.
13. Diaz-Cascajo C, Borghi S, Weyers W, Retzlaff H, Requena L, Metze D. Benign lymphangiomatous papules of the skin following radiotherapy: a report of five new cases and review of the literature. Histopathology. 1999;35(4):319–27.

14. Donnell RM, Rosen PP, Lieberman PH, et al. Angiosarcoma and other vascular tumors of the breast. Am J Surg Pathol. 1981;5(7):629–42.
15. Fernandez AP, Sun Y, Tubbs RR, Goldblum JR, Billings SD. FISH for MYC amplification and anti-MYC immunohistochemistry: useful diagnostic tools in the assessment of secondary angiosarcoma and atypical vascular proliferations. J Cutan Pathol. 2012;39(2):234–42.
16. Fineberg S, Rosen PP. Cutaneous angiosarcoma and atypical vascular lesions of the skin and breast after radiation therapy for breast carcinoma. Am J Clin Pathol. 1994;102(6):757–63.
17. Fraga-Guedes C, Gobbi H, Mastropasqua MG, et al. Clinicopathological and immunohistochemical study of 30 cases of post-radiation atypical vascular lesion of the breast. Breast Cancer Res Treat. 2014;146(2):347–54.
18. Ginter PS, McIntire PJ, Irshaid L, Liu YF, Shin SJ. Angiomatosis of the breast: a clinicopathological and immunophenotypical characterisation of seven cases. J Clin Pathol. 2019;72(9):597–602.
19. Guilbert MC, Frost EP, Brock JE, Lester SC. Distinguishing papillary endothelial hyperplasia and angiosarcoma on core needle biopsy of the breast: the importance of clinical and radiologic correlation. Breast J. 2018;24(4):487–92.
20. Hoda SA, Cranor ML, Rosen PP. Hemangiomas of the breast with atypical histological features. Further analysis of histological subtypes confirming their benign character. Am J Surg Pathol. 1992;16(6):553–60.
21. Jesinger RA, Lattin GE Jr, Ballard EA, Zelasko SM, Glassman LM. Vascular abnormalities of the breast: arterial and venous disorders, vascular masses, and mimic lesions with radiologic-pathologic correlation. Radiographics. 2011;31(7):E117–36.
22. Jozefczyk MA, Rosen PP. Vascular tumors of the breast. II. Perilobular hemangiomas and hemangiomas. Am J Surg Pathol. 1985;9(7):491–503.
23. Lesueur GC, Brown RW, Bhathal PS. Incidence of perilobular hemangioma in the female breast. Arch Pathol Lab Med. 1983;107(6):308–10.
24. Lorente-Ramos RM, Azpeitia Armán J, Martínez Izquierdo MA, Pérez QA. Papillary endothelial hyperplasia (Masson's tumor) developed in the capsule of the implant in a breast cancer patient treated with mastectomy and radiation therapy. J Clin Ultrasound. 2020; 48(4):222–6.
25. Ma W, Jin F, Wu Y. Capillary hemangioma of the breast-a rare type of benign breast tumor. Breast J. 2016;22(3):355–6.
26. Mantilla JG, Koenigsberg T, Reig B, Shapiro N, Villanueva-Siles E, Fineberg S. Core biopsy of vascular neoplasms of the breast: pathologic features, imaging, and clinical findings. Am J Surg Pathol. 2016;40(10):1424–34.
27. Mentzel T, Schildhaus HU, Palmedo G, Büttner R, Kutzner H. Postradiation cutaneous angiosarcoma after treatment of breast carcinoma is characterized by MYC amplification in contrast to atypical vascular lesions after radiotherapy and control cases: clinicopathological, immunohistochemical and molecular analysis of 66 cases. Mod Pathol. 2012;25(1):75–85.
28. Nascimento AF, Raut CP, Fletcher CD. Primary angiosarcoma of the breast: clinicopathologic analysis of 49 cases, suggesting that grade is not prognostic. Am J Surg Pathol. 2008;32(12):1896–904.
29. Patton KT, Deyrup AT, Weiss SW. Atypical vascular lesions after surgery and radiation of the breast: a clinicopathologic study of 32 cases analyzing histologic heterogeneity and association with angiosarcoma. Am J Surg Pathol. 2008;32(6):943–50.
30. Rosen PP, Jozefczyk MA, Boram LH. Vascular tumors of the breast. IV. The venous hemangioma. Am J Surg Pathol. 1985;9(9):659–65.
31. Rosen PP, Kimmel M, Ernsberger D. Mammary angiosarcoma. The prognostic significance of tumor differentiation. Cancer. 1988;62(10):2145–51.

32. Rosen PP, Ridolfi RL. The perilobular hemangioma. A benign microscopic vascular lesion of the breast. Am J Clin Pathol. 1977;68(1):21–3.
33. Rosen PP. Vascular tumors of the breast. III Angiomatosis. Am J Surg Pathol. 1985;9(9):652–8.
34. Shin SJ, Lesser M, Rosen PP. Hemangiomas and angiosarcomas of the breast: diagnostic utility of cell cycle markers with emphasis on Ki-67. Arch Pathol Lab Med. 2007;131(4):538–44.
35. Stewart FW, Treves N. Lymphangiosarcoma in postmastectomy lymphedema; a report of six cases in elephantiasis chirurgica. Cancer. 1948;1(1):64–81.
36. Tilve A, Mallo R, Pérez A, Santiago P. Breast hemangiomas: correlation between imaging and pathologic findings. J Clin Ultrasound. 2012;40(8):512–7.

# Mesenchymal Breast Tumors with Fibroblastic and Myofibroblastic Differentiation

# 5

Paul Weisman and Darya Buehler

## Contents




P. Weisman · D. Buehler (✉)
Department of Pathology and Laboratory Medicine, School of Medicine and Public Health, University of Wisconsin-Madison, Madison, WI, USA
e-mail: buehler2@wisc.edu





J. J. Rowe, E. Downs-Kelly (eds.), *Mesenchymal Tumors of the Breast and Their Mimics*, https://doi.org/10.1007/978-3-030-74474-8_5

## Myofibroblastoma

### Clinical Features

Mammary myofibroblastoma (MM) is a benign tumor seen predominantly in middle-aged to elderly patients with a roughly equal incidence in males and females. MM presents as a painless, slowly growing mobile mass. In breast, myofibroblastomas rarely grow larger than 4 cm in size, with most examples measuring approximately 2 cm. While it was originally thought that these tumors were related to solitary fibrous tumors, the lack of *STAT6* rearrangements and/or STAT6 overexpression by immunohistochemistry (IHC) and the presence of chromosomal deletions of the 13q14 region, which includes the *RB1* and *FOXO1A* genes, subsequently revealed a close relationship to spindle cell lipomas and vulvovaginal cellular angiofibromas. Morphologically and genetically identical lesions that occur outside of the breast parenchyma (in the inguinal region and groin, axilla, trunk and, rarely, the extremities or retroperitoneum) are often referred to as mammary-type myofibroblastomas.

### Imaging

Well-circumscribed, homogenous non-calcified solid mass that closely mimics fibroadenoma.

### Pathologic Features

#### Gross Features

Well-circumscribed, firm, white or yellow (depending on the amount of the adipocytic component) fibrous-appearing mass.

## Microscopic Features

Myofibroblastoma typically exhibits a well-circumscribed pushing border with the uninvolved breast parenchyma. In contrast to other lesions arising from specialized breast stroma (fibroepithelial tumors, pseudoangiomatous stromal hyperplasia, hamartoma), myofibroblastoma lacks epithelial elements except for occasional entrapped breast glands at the periphery. Myofibroblastomas are composed of short spindle cells arranged in somewhat parallel fascicles and interspersed with brightly eosinophilic collagen. The latter can be broad and keloid-like or thin and "ropey" in quality, reminiscent of their close relative, spindle cell lipoma. The lesional spindle cells show ovoid nuclei and pale eosinophilic cytoplasm with indistinct cytoplasmic borders. The vasculature is inconspicuous. Interspersed mast cells are often present, and chondroid, osseous, or smooth muscle metaplasia may occur. There is no appreciable nuclear atypia above and beyond occasional degenerative changes similar to those seen in nerve sheath tumors. Mitotic figures are rare or absent, and there is no necrosis (Figs. 5.1, 5.2, and 5.3).

The adipocytic component is highly variable and can be entirely absent or quite extensive; the latter is often described as the lipomatous variant of myofibroblastoma (Figs. 5.4 and 5.5). The significance of this variant is that the intermingling of the spindle cells and the intralesional adipocytes may produce a false impression of an infiltrative edge and raise the possibility of fibromatosis, fibromatosis-like metaplastic carcinoma, or another infiltrative tumor.

Other notable variant morphologies of myofibroblastoma include epithelioid, deciduoid, myxoid, leiomyomatous, and palisaded variants. These are represented in Figs. 5.6, 5.7, 5.8, and 5.9 and are discussed below under the differential diagnosis section since their mimickers give these variant morphologies their significance.

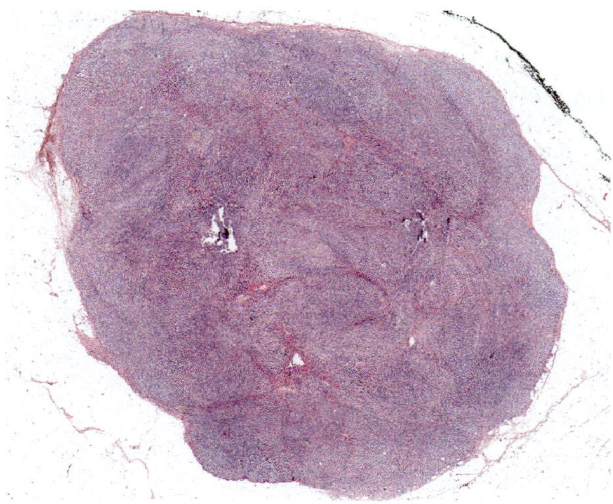

**Fig. 5.1** Myofibroblastoma showing a sharp demarcation from the surrounding tissue

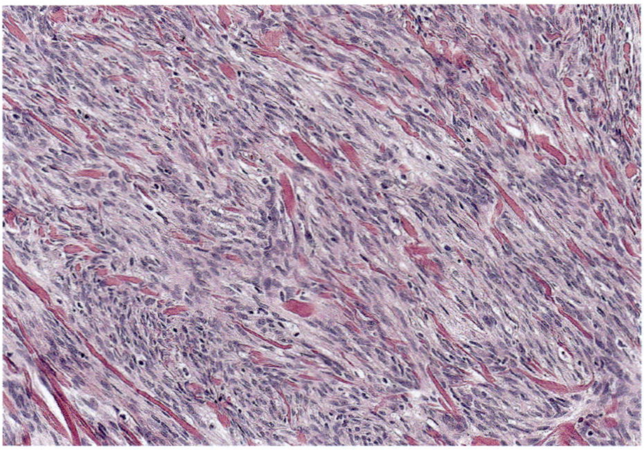

**Fig. 5.2** Myofibroblastoma composed of fascicles of short myofibroblastic spindle cells interspersed with brightly eosinophilic collagen fibers

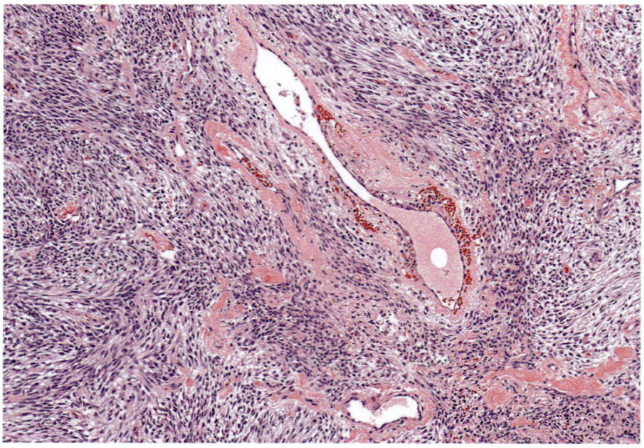

**Fig. 5.3** Another example of myofibroblastoma showing prominent hyalinized vessels

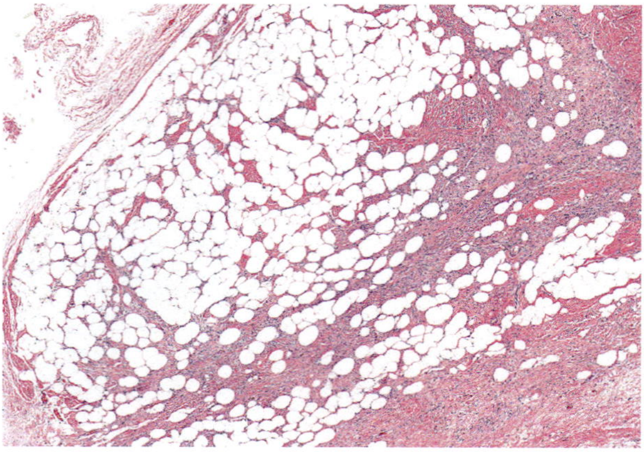

**Fig. 5.4** Lipomatous myofibroblastoma imparting an infiltrative look at low power; however, the border of the lesion is circumscribed

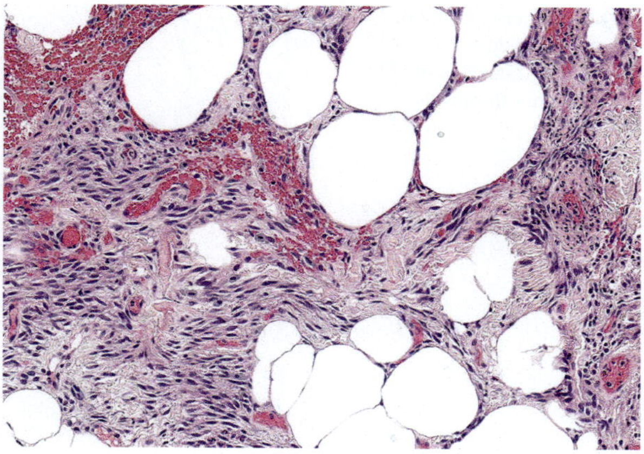

**Fig. 5.5** Lipomatous myofibroblastoma showing short bundles of spindle cells admixed with adipocytes, collagen fibers, and scattered mast cells. This appearance is essentially indistinguishable from spindle cell lipoma

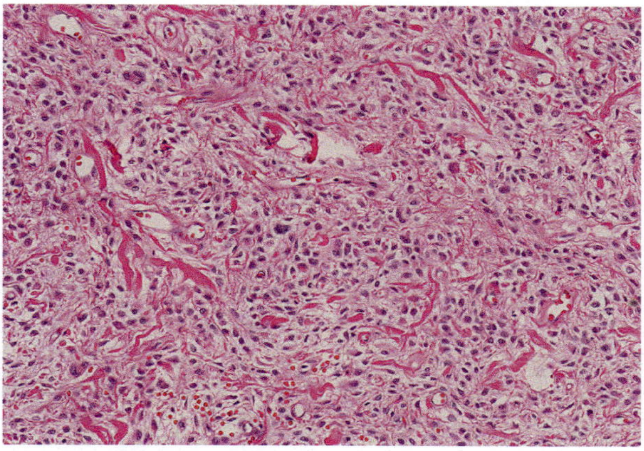

**Fig. 5.6** Epithelioid myofibroblastoma composed of cords, nests, or trabeculae of polygonal fibroblastic cells resembling infiltrating lobular carcinoma of the breast

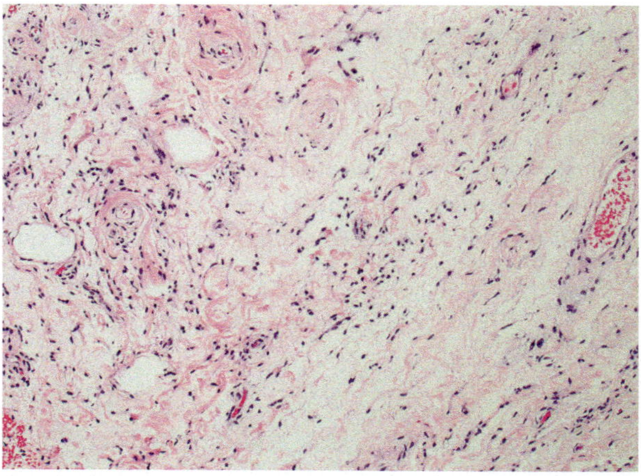

**Fig. 5.7** Myxoid myofibroblastoma showing hypocellular myxoid stroma containing loosely arranged myofibroblasts; collagen fibers can still be appreciated

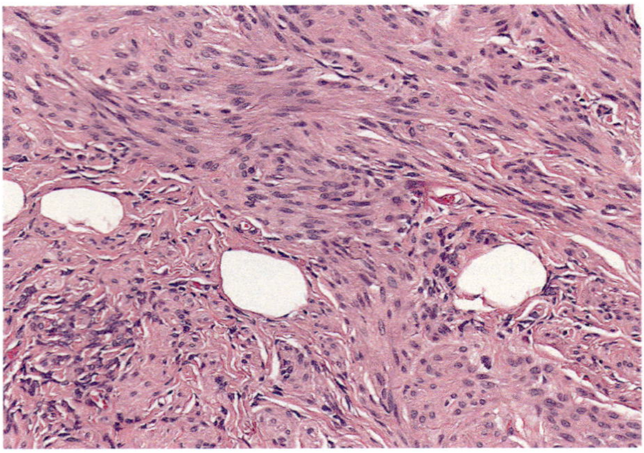

**Fig. 5.8** Leiomyomatous myofibroblastoma containing fascicles of benign smooth muscle cells

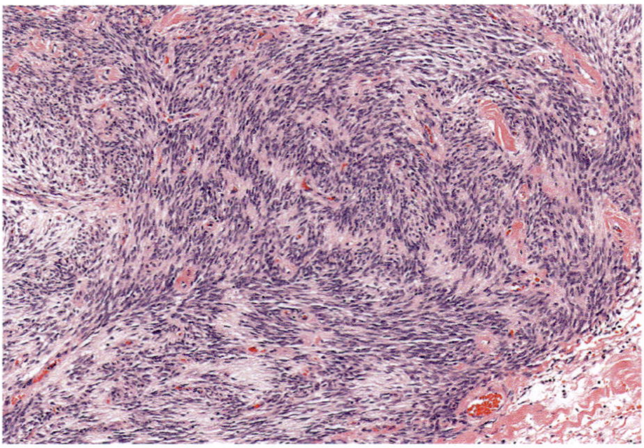

**Fig. 5.9** Palisaded myofibroblastoma resembling schwannoma

## Immunohistochemistry

Myofibroblastoma characteristically expresses CD34, estrogen, progesterone, and androgen receptors and, consistent with its myofibroblastic lineage, desmin, SMA, and calponin (Figs. 5.10 and 5.11). Myofibroblastomas negative for CD34, including the leiomyomatous variant, are rare. Notably, myoribroblastoma is negative for STAT6 and cytokeratins (including the epithelioid variant – discussed below).

## Molecular

Most cases of myofibroblastoma exhibit chromosomal deletions of the 13q14 region, much like the closely related spindle cell lipoma and vulvovaginal cellular angiofibroma. As this region includes the Rb gene, loss of Rb expression by IHC is a supportive adjunctive test in difficult cases; alternatively, fluorescence in situ

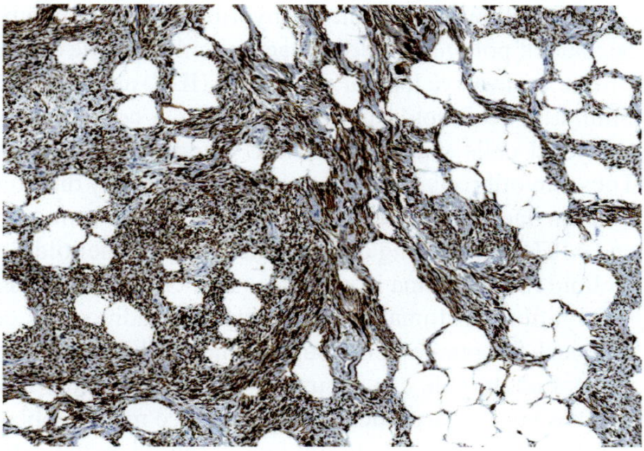

**Fig. 5.10** Robust expression of desmin in myofibroblastoma

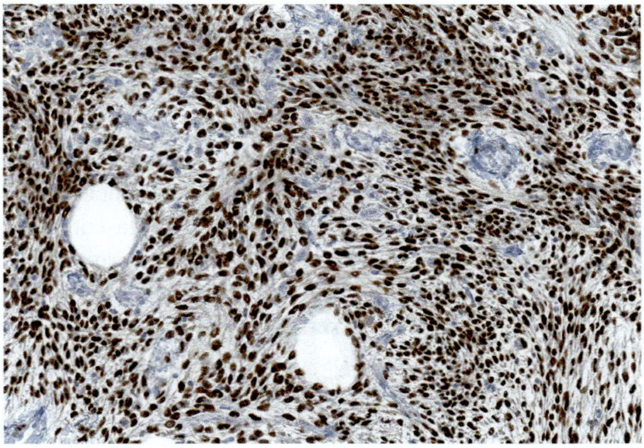

**Fig. 5.11** Myofibroblastomas are usually strongly positive for estrogen (depicted here), progesterone, and androgen receptor expression

hybridization (FISH) studies with probes directed against the *RB1* or *FOXO1* gene, which is also in this region, can be useful in demonstrating the characteristic deletion.

## Differential Diagnosis

Solitary fibrous tumor (discussed elsewhere in this text) can closely resemble myofibroblastoma histologically and by robust CD34 expression. Positive staining for STAT6 by IHC is pathognomonic for solitary fibrous tumor in this setting and STAT6 has been shown to be negative in myofibroblastoma. A more important mimic of classic myofibroblastoma, especially in core needle biopsies, is low-grade fibromatosis-like metaplastic carcinoma. Low-grade fibromatosis-like metaplastic carcinoma is negative for CD34 and strongly positive for cytokeratin, especially high molecular weight cytokeratins, and p63, while myofibroblastoma is reliably negative for these markers.

The epithelioid variant of myofibroblastoma composed of cords, nests, or trabeculae of polygonal or plasmacytoid fibroblastic cells (Fig. 5.6) can be deceptively similar to invasive lobular carcinoma (ILC) and sclerosing epithelioid fibrosarcoma. Similarly, deciduoid myofibroblastoma is composed of larger, polygonal, or plasmacytoid cells with eosinophilic cytoplasm and can mimic apocrine carcinoma. These myofibroblastoma variants can be readily distinguished from their mimickers by their lack of immunoreactivity for cytokeratins (militating against carcinoma) and MUC4 (militating against sclerosing epithelioid fibrosarcoma). Sclerosing epithelioid fibrosarcoma is also discussed elsewhere in this chapter.

Myofibroblastoma with an extensive adipocytic component looks essentially identical to spindle cell lipoma which, while prevalent in the posterior head and neck of adult men, can occur in both genders and at a variety of sites. This distinction has very little clinical relevance since myofibroblastomas and spindle cell lipomas belong to the same tumor family (based on their shared 13q14 region deletions) and, most importantly, are benign and almost never recur.

A more significant problem is that adipocyte-rich myofibroblastoma may appear rather infiltrative and even incorporate mammary glands (unlike most classic examples, which are devoid of mammary glands). Accordingly, this variant can mimic a number of infiltrative spindle cell neoplasms, including desmoid fibromatosis and dermatofibrosarcoma protuberans (DFSP). CD34 may be used to differentiate myofibroblastoma from desmoid fibromatosis, since it is almost always negative in the latter. In contrast, nuclear expression of beta-catenin by IHC is supportive of desmoid fibromatosis, with a few caveats concerning the interpretation of this immunostain (discussed below under "desmoid fibromatosis"). DFSP is also diffusely positive for CD34 but is reliably negative for estrogen and progesterone receptor and does not show Rb loss by IHC. In problematic cases, molecular testing for mutations in exon 3 of CTNNB1 or alterations in APC gene (fibromatosis) or testing for the *COL1A1-PDGFRB* fusion (DFSP) may be performed, but this is usually unnecessary. Both DFSP and desmoid fibromatosis are discussed separately in this chapter.

The myxoid variant of myofibroblastoma, in which myxoid stroma comprises the bulk of the lesion (Fig. 5.7), can mimic nodular fasciitis, myxoma, and superficial angiomyxoma. Fibroepithelial tumors with widespread myxoid change (myxoid fibroadenoma, benign phyllodes tumor) can also resemble myxoid myofibroblastoma in small biopsies as the epithelial component in these lesions is often under-sampled. No single morphologic feature (not even CD34 immunohistochemistry) can reliably separate myxoid myofibroblastoma from the above mimics in small biopsies. When this distinction is relevant, Rb IHC (lost in myofibroblastoma) and molecular or FISH testing for *USP6* gene rearrangement (nodular fasciitis) can provide an objective confirmation of the diagnosis.

Schwartz and colleagues recently described four cases of a benign mammary myxoid lesion that they designated "benign fibromyxoid lesion of the breast", which at least morphologically appears to be very similar to myxoid myofibroblastoma. These occurred in females with mean age of 41 years, and the presenting finding was a well-circumscribed, solid nodule by ultrasound (one case was seen as non-mass-enhancement by MRI). None of the patients in this series had a history of Carney complex and none of the tumors involved the nipple-areola complex, arguing that these lesions did not represent nodular mucinosis of the nipple. Microscopically, these lesions were circumscribed and showed features overlapping with those of myxoid myofibroblastoma, being composed of paucicellular bland spindle cells within an Alcian blue positive myxoid stroma, also containing delicate vessels and dispersed collagen fibers. No epithelial component was seen, militating against the possibility that these lesions represented myxoid fibroadenomas. Like myofibroblastoma, the spindle cells were diffusely and strongly positive for CD34 and SMA, but were negative for desmin, ER, PR, S100, STAT6, and beta-catenin. Rb showed retained expression in all cases of benign fibromyxoid lesion of the breast and FISH for 13q14 (using probes directed against *FOXO1*) was negative. These results argue that these lesions are likely distinct from myxoid myofibroblastoma but their biology and relationship to other myxoid lesions of the breast has yet to be fully elucidated.

On the malignant side, myxoid myofibroblastoma can mimic the rare breast occurrence of low-grade fibromyxoid sarcoma (Evans tumor, discussed below). Similar to the closely related sclerosing epithelioid fibrosarcoma mentioned above, MUC4 would be the most useful stain for differentiating myofibroblastoma from Evans tumor, since it would be negative in the former and positive in the latter. CD34 is also typically negative in low-grade fibromyxoid sarcoma.

Palisaded myofibroblastoma (Fig. 5.8) can mimic schwannomas but can be readily distinguished based on the presence of abundant collagen (collagen is uncommon in schwannomas) and lack of SOX10 expression; it is worth noting that S100 can occasionally be positive in myofibroblastoma. Finally, the uncommon leiomyomatous variant of myofibroblastoma (Fig. 5.9) can mimic myoid hamartoma, myoid stroma in fibroepithelial lesions as well as primary leiomyoma of the breast parenchyma. The epithelial and the stromal components in myoid hamartomas and biphasic fibroepithelial lesions are always intermixed, allowing for an easy separation from myofibroblastoma which, by definition, lacks mammary glands. True smooth muscle tumors are negative for CD34, but the latter is also more variably expressed and can be weak or negative in leiomyomatous myofibroblastoma. In rare problematic cases, one can resort to Rb IHC or *RB1/FOX01* FISH which are expected to show retained expression and no deletions, respectively, in all of the above mimics.

## Prognosis and Treatment

Myofibroblastoma is benign and virtually never recurs, even if treated by simple excision. Increased cellularity or degenerative type atypia have no prognostic relevance. Nevertheless, complete excision is recommended when a myofibroblastoma is diagnosed on a needle core biopsy. Recently, the first example of sarcomatoid transformation of an extramammary leiomyomatous myofibroblastoma was reported showing a transition to areas with increased cellularity, overt nuclear atypia, and mitotic activity accompanied by *TP53* mutation. This phenomenon has also been reported in closely related vulvovaginal cellular angiofibromas, but its clinical significance is unclear as all of these tumors have behaved in an indolent fashion to date and should probably be closely followed clinically rather than treated aggressively in order to avoid overtreatment.

## Desmoid Fibromatosis

### Clinical Features

Fibromatosis of the breast is an infiltrative myofibroblastic proliferation identical to desmoid fibromatosis occurring at other anatomic sites that, despite its bland histologic appearance, has the significant potential for locoregional recurrence. Fibromatosis of the breast occurs over a wide age range with a median age in the mid-forties, and a significant female predominance. Breast parenchyma-based cases comprise less than 10% of all cases of desmoid-type fibromatosis; this process can also involve the subcutaneous tissue of the breast region or the underlying pectoralis fascia/chest wall. Fibromatosis of the breast presents as a palpable yet painless mass that may clinically mimic carcinoma due to its propensity to pucker the overlying skin. Reported median size is 2.5 to 5.5 cm. In approximately one-third of cases, fibromatosis of the breast is associated with antecedent local trauma or operative procedure such as breast reconstruction or augmentation. A subset of cases occurs in familial adenomatous polyposis/Gardner syndrome (approximately 2%).

### Imaging

An ill-defined mass with a stellate radiographic appearance mimicking primary breast carcinoma.

### Pathologic Features

#### Gross Features

An ill-defined, densely fibrous mass or scar-like process; deep-seated chest wall fibromatoses may present as a seemingly circumscribed mass, which will invariably show an infiltrative edge microscopically.

#### Microscopic Features

Similar to desmoid fibromatoses arising at extramammary sites, fibromatosis of the breast is an infiltrative lesion, often enveloping fat, benign glandular elements, and, when located posteriorly in the breast, the skeletal muscle fibers of the pectoralis musculature. It is composed of very bland-appearing myofibroblasts arranged in long, sweeping fascicles. The tumor nuclei are evenly spaced and slender, with tapered ends, and have characteristically pale chromatin to the extent that the nuclei of adjacent endothelial cells may appear dark in comparison. Regularly distributed slit-like or gaping vessels are seen throughout the lesion, and perivascular edema and extravasated red blood cells in the vicinity of these vessels are a common and characteristic feature (Figs. 5.12 and 5.13). Keloid-like collagen deposition is common, and some cases of fibromatosis can be indistinguishable from a scar in limited biopsy material. Peripheral lymphoid aggregates are another common and very helpful feature (Fig. 5.14). Mitotic activity is absent or sparse, and there is no necrosis. Hyalinized areas are strikingly hypocellular and can be difficult to differentiate from normal connective tissue or a scar (Fig. 5.15).

## Immunohistochemistry

Consistent with its myofibroblastic phenotype, fibromatosis of the breast shows variable, typically weak immunoreactivity for SMA and desmin but is almost always negative for CD34, in contrast to mammary stromal fibroblasts. Cytokeratins

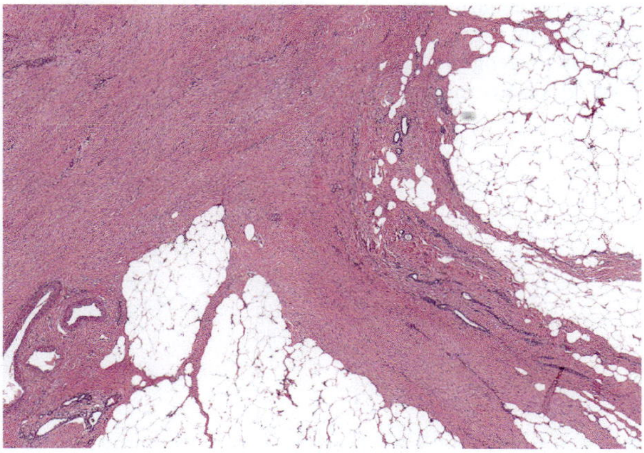

**Fig. 5.12** Desmoid fibromatosis of the breast with a strikingly infiltrative growth pattern enveloping adipose tissue and benign glandular elements

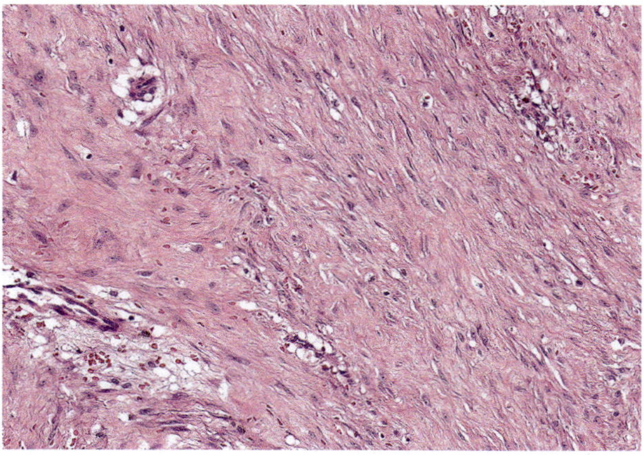

**Fig. 5.13** Desmoid fibromatosis composed of bland, evenly spaced myofibroblasts arranged in long fascicles. Regularly distributed slit-like or gaping vessels with perivascular edema and a sprinkle of extravasated red blood cells are characteristic

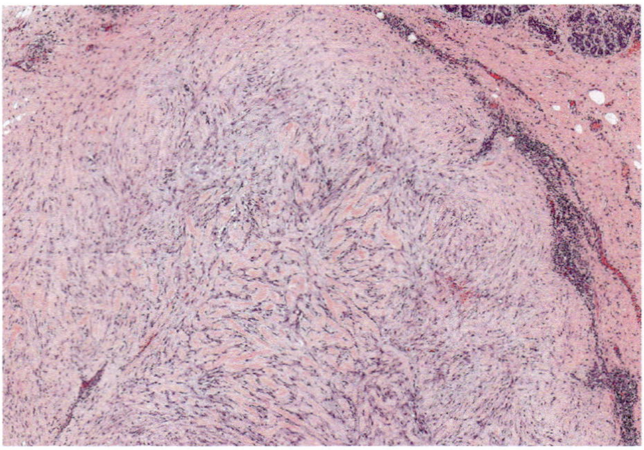

**Fig. 5.14** The presence of lymphoid aggregates at the periphery of fibromatosis is a subtle and helpful feature; keloidal collagen fibers are often present

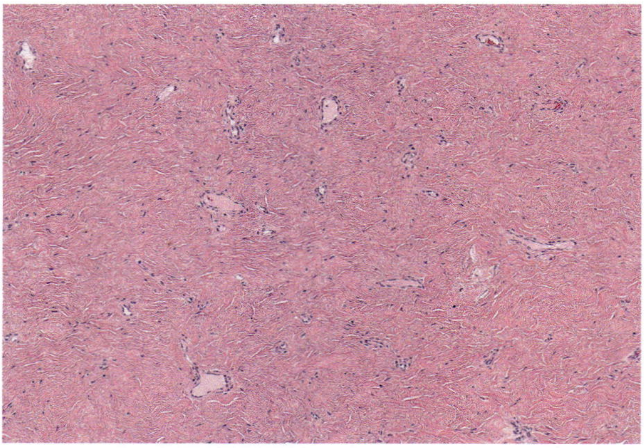

**Fig. 5.15** Hypocellular and heavily collagenized areas in desmoid fibromatosis may be difficult to recognize as such, especially in small samples

are negative, a helpful feature in distinguishing fibromatosis from its most important histologic mimic, low-grade fibromatosis-like metaplastic carcinoma. While nuclear staining for beta-catenin is supportive of a diagnosis of fibromatosis (present in approximately 80% of breast fibromatosis cases), the interpretation of this stain can be problematic, since even a "negative" result retains a considerable level of membranous staining which, in the context of a myofibroblastic tumor with slender spindle cells, can be difficult to distinguish from bona fide nuclear staining. Nuclear expression of beta catenin can also be observed in the stromal component of phyllodes tumors and in metaplastic carcinomas.

## Molecular

At the molecular level, fibromatosis harbors either mutations in exon 3 of *CTNNB1* or inactivating alterations of the *APC* gene, including mutation, chromosome 5q allelic loss, or both. A subset of *CTNNB1* and *APC* wild-type cases have recently been shown to harbor large intragenic deletions in *CTNNB1*. Interestingly, desmoid fibromatosis of the breast appears to be enriched in *APC* mutations compared to all other sites, even in sporadic cases (approximately 10.7% vs. 2.6%). These results underscore the significant pathogenetic contribution of *APC* alterations specifically to the development of fibromatosis of the breast. Accordingly, molecular testing for both *CTNNB1* and *APC* mutations/alterations might be necessary to confirm the diagnosis in difficult cases.

## Differential Diagnosis

As alluded to above, fibromatosis shows some resemblance to low-grade fibromatosis-like metaplastic carcinoma, a low-grade triple-negative metaplastic carcinoma with relatively bland-appearing spindle cell morphology imparting a myofibroblastic appearance. However, the cells of low-grade fibromatosis-like metaplastic carcinoma are not myofibroblasts and are therefore strongly immunoreactive to various cytokeratins, especially high molecular weight cytokeratins. Fibromatosis is negative for cytokeratins, underscoring their usefulness in this differential diagnosis. As discussed above, beta-catenin immunostain should be used with extreme caution in this context as the nuclear expression can also be observed in the stromal component of phyllodes tumors and in metaplastic carcinomas; metaplastic carcinomas can also show *APC* or *CTNNB1* mutations albeit in different codons (33, 37, 42) compared to desmoid fibromatosis (codons 41 and 45).

Another differential diagnostic consideration is the lipomatous variant of mammary myofibroblastoma, which can produce the impression of an infiltrative growth pattern and mimic fibromatosis. Since fibromatosis is almost always negative for CD34 and myofibroblastoma is nearly always strongly positive, CD34 is a useful marker for the distinction of these two entities. Of course, loss of Rb supports a diagnosis of myofibroblastoma, whereas the presence of exon 3 mutations in *CTNNB1* or alterations of the *APC* gene confirm a diagnosis of fibromatosis. The importance of separating these two entities is based on the known recurrent potential of fibromatosis as compared to myofibroblastoma, which practically never recurs, even after simple excision.

Finally, fibromatosis should be distinguished from a scar which, perhaps, is the most common pure spindle cell proliferation encountered in the breast. This distinction can be extremely difficult as certain phases of scar formation are decidedly similar in appearance to desmoid fibromatosis. The diagnosis depends upon investigating the patient's chart for a history of previous trauma or surgical procedures to the site of the biopsy, although these factors are, unfortunately, associated with the development of breast fibromatosis as well. The presence of fat necrosis, hemosiderin deposits, scattered mixed chronic inflammation, giant cell reaction and histiocytes would favor a scar. In difficult cases, molecular genetic testing for confirmatory features of fibromatosis (i.e., exon 3 mutations in *CTNNB1* or alterations of the *APC* gene) can be pursued.

## Prognosis and Treatment

Breast fibromatosis was traditionally treated with surgery, but those cases often showed positive margins (32–75%) and up to 40% of cases recurred locally. Most importantly, just like at other sites, the margin clearance in desmoid fibromatosis is a poor predictor of recurrence, and therefore aiming for an R0 resection may produce a potentially disfiguring result with little long-term benefit. Recent studies showed no difference in event-free survival and long-term disease control between patients undergoing surgery and those managed conservatively. Furthermore, it appears that patients with desmoid fibromatosis at high-risk sites (chest wall, head, and neck) paradoxically fare worse if managed by initial surgery than if managed non-surgically. Thus, the current consensus approach to the initial management of fibromatosis in most patients is active surveillance, with CT/MRI at 3–6-month intervals over 1–2 years. Many such patients will experience stabilization or regression of their disease requiring no further surgical intervention, whereas patients who show a persistent progression or significant morbidity can be selected for active treatment (surgery, radiation, or medical management). The watchful waiting strategy is highly applicable to breast fibromatosis: studies to date showed that 80–90% of patients with breast fibromatosis had stabilization of their disease without active intervention. This approach prevents overtreatment of desmoid fibromatosis and excessive morbidity from surgical intervention.

# Pseudoangiomatous Stromal Hyperplasia

## Clinical Features

Pseudoangiomatous stromal hyperplasia (PASH) is a benign proliferation of stromal myofibroblasts in the breast. PASH presents in one of three forms: a mass-forming lesion, a mammographic abnormality (see below), or an incidental histologic finding in the background of other breast lesions, including fibrocystic changes, fibroepithelial lesions, and gynecomastia. Rarely, it may accompany invasive carcinoma. Mass forming PASH is far more common in women than in men, especially in the premenopausal age group or in patients receiving hormone replacement therapy, consistent with the notion that PASH is a hormonally driven proliferation. Mass-forming PASH presents as a palpable, usually painless mass, up to 12 cm in size, and may grow rapidly prompting clinical concern. PASH can occur as a solitary finding but can be multifocal or bilateral.

## Imaging

Mass forming PASH presents as a well-circumscribed, oval lobulated non-calcified mass with mammographic and sonographic characteristics that overlap with those of fibroadenomas. PASH that is incidentally discovered by screening mammography often appears as an asymmetry (i.e., an area of breast tissue that is asymmetrically dense as compared to the background breast tissue) and is biopsied in order to rule out a small invasive ductal or lobular carcinoma. PASH may also be entirely occult radiologically.

## Pathologic Features

### Gross Features

Well-circumscribed, lobulated tan-white rubbery mass; PASH presenting as part of another lesion or incidentally has no distinctive gross findings.

### Microscopic Features

The classic appearance of PASH is that of slight expansion of the interlobular stroma by a mildly fibrotic process interrupted by evenly distributed, slit-like spaces that seem to have focal lining cells, but which lack red blood cells (Figs. 5.16 and 5.17). These "lining cells" are actually the constituent myofibroblasts of PASH and the spaces are artifactual spaces caused by stromal retraction. The "pseudoangiomatous" appearance of these non-vascular, artifactual spaces give PASH its name. Stromal fibrosis or hyalinization is invariably present. Noteworthy variant morphology includes the fascicular variant, which is morphologically in a continuum with mammary myofibroblastoma and can also mimic mammary fibromatosis. In this variant of PASH, the lesional myofibroblasts are arranged into cellular fascicles and the characteristic pseudovascular spaces of conventional PASH are conspicuously absent (Figs. 5.18 and 5.19). Finally, similar to mammary myofibroblastomas, PASH can show focal atypical stromal cells that represent degenerative changes, but which can appear somewhat alarming.

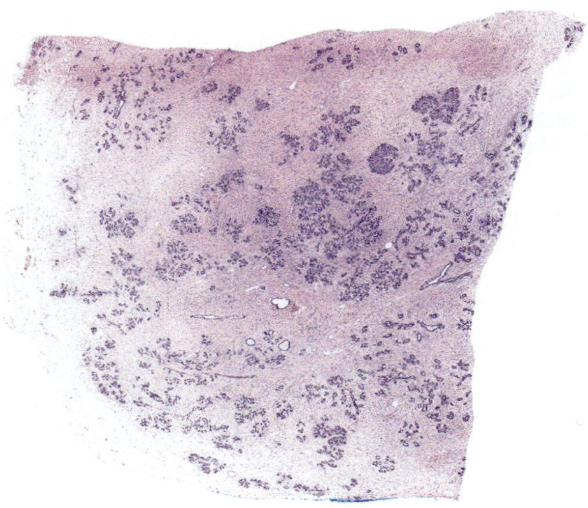

**Fig. 5.16** Pseudoangiomatous hyperplasia (PASH) showing a well-circumscribed, mass-like fibrous expansion of the interlobular breast stroma

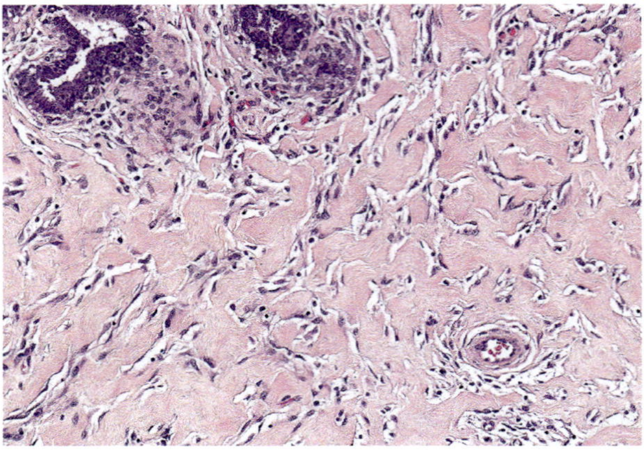

**Fig. 5.17** The constituent fibroblasts in PASH form evenly distributed, slit-like spaces imparting the "pseudoangiomatous" appearance; the spaces are artifactual due to stromal retraction

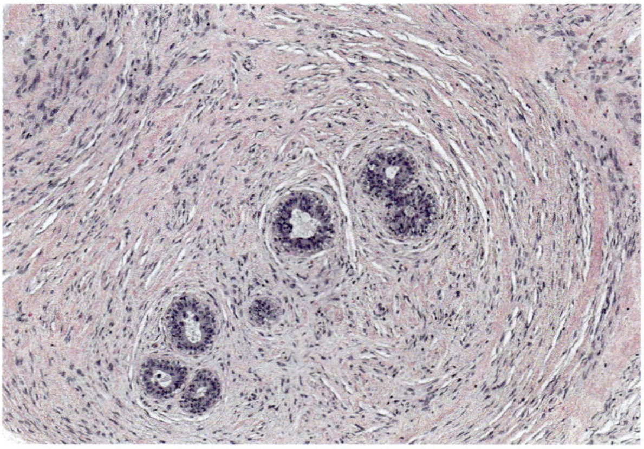

**Fig. 5.18** Fascicular PASH with bundles of stromal myofibroblasts arranged in a concentric fashion around breast lobules

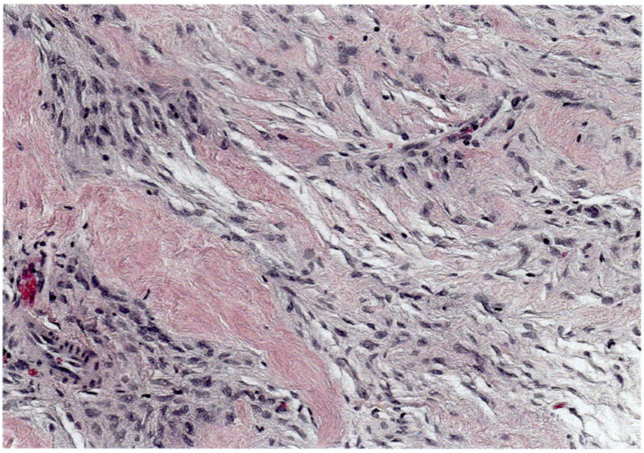

**Fig. 5.19** Some areas in fascicular PASH are devoid of breast glands and resemble mammary myofibroblastoma

## Immunohistochemistry

In that PASH is a proliferation of mammary myofibroblasts, it is not surprising that it stains for estrogen receptor, CD34, SMA, and desmin.

## Molecular

It is unclear whether PASH has the same 13q14 deletions and corresponding loss of Rb expression seen in mammary myofibroblastoma.

## Differential Diagnosis

An important differential diagnostic consideration for conventional PASH is low-grade primary angiosarcoma of the breast. The latter can be alarmingly low-grade in appearance, especially when only partially represented on small biopsy specimens. Key histological features that would favor PASH over angiosarcoma are a lack of red blood cells in the lesional spaces and the presence of lesion-associated fibrosis. The latter point is of great diagnostic utility since angiosarcomas are not typically associated with fibrosis and will involve both breast parenchyma and adipose tissue without eliciting a fibrotic response. This is in stark contrast to PASH which, almost by definition, produces a fibrotic stroma wherever it exists. Additionally, ERG and other vascular markers such as CD31 may also be used, as these would be negative in PASH, but positive in angiosarcoma; however, one must be careful with CD34, which would be positive in both lesions.

Fascicular PASH exists on a histologic continuum with myofibroblastoma and may closely resemble myofibroblastoma in core biopsies. Both lesions are positive for the same IHC markers (i.e., CD34, SMA, desmin, ER, and PR). While, to the best of our knowledge, Rb loss by IHC has not been systematically evaluated in PASH, loss of Rb staining in a cellular and fascicular myofibroblastic lesion of the breast would favor myofibroblastoma. In excision specimens, fascicular PASH can be readily separated from myofibroblastoma as it still maintains the close association of the cellular stromal component with mammary glands, feature not seen in myofibroblastoma. Slit-like spaces seen in conventional PASH are also not characteristic of myofibroblastoma.

The fascicular variant of PASH may mimic mammary fibromatosis due to its infiltrative appearance and fascicular growth pattern. Distinguishing these two entities may be aided by the positive staining for CD34 in PASH (which is nearly always negative in fibromatosis) and aberrant beta-catenin immunoreactivity in fibromatosis. However, as noted earlier, interpretation of beta-catenin staining in fibromatosis can be difficult. Accordingly, in difficult cases, molecular genetic testing for confirmatory features of fibromatosis (i.e., exon 3 mutations in *CTNNB1* or alterations of the *APC* gene) can be pursued.

## Prognosis and Treatment

PASH that is identified as an incidental finding on core needle biopsy with concordant imaging findings is not excised; however, surgical excision may be considered for patients with mass-forming PASH.

# Nodular Fasciitis

## Clinical Features

Nodular fasciitis is a benign, self-limited myofibroblastic neoplasm that has a predilection for the upper extremities, trunk and head and neck, but may occur at any site in the body, including the breast parenchyma. The most common presentation in the breast is as a palpable, rapidly growing mass of short duration.

## Imaging

Radiologically, nodular fasciitis most often forms an irregular or spiculated mass that can mimic invasive carcinoma; a less common presentation is that of a more circumscribed solid mass with internal vascularity.

## Pathological Features

### Gross Features

Partly circumscribed, fibrous to gelatinous mass with cystic areas.

### Microscopic Features

Microscopically, nodular fasciitis usually exhibits a predominantly well-circumscribed profile, with a mildly infiltrative periphery that can entrap mammary glands. The lesional cells are cytologically bland myofibroblasts arranged in short, haphazard fascicles that splay out at their ends, within a loose myxoid matrix with microcystic degeneration or a more fibrous stroma (Figs. 5.20, 5.21, 5.22, and 5.23). Extravasation of red blood cells, keloidal-like collagen, and scattered lymphocytes are common. Mitotic figures are often present and can be abundant, but atypical mitotic figures should not be seen. Some examples of nodular fasciitis show focal necrosis. Osteoclast-type giant cells, focal aneurysmal bone-cyst like changes, and occasionally, new bone formation can also occur (Fig. 5.24), in keeping with the recent observations that nodular fasciitis, aneurysmal bone cyst, and myositis ossificans are genetically related and represent different points on a histologic spectrum of a single disease process unified by *USP6* gene rearrangements.

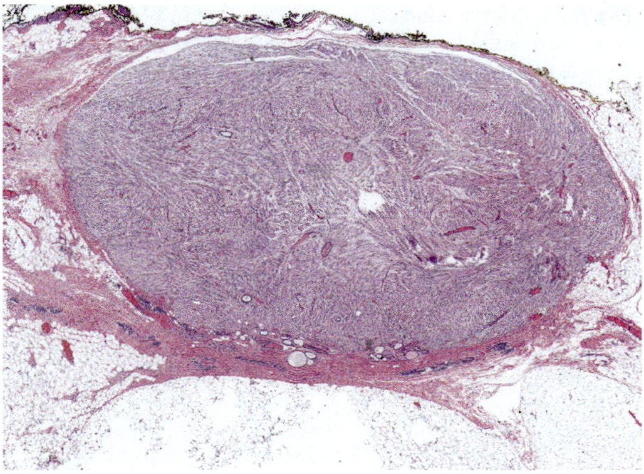

**Fig. 5.20** Nodular fasciitis of the breast showing a circumscribed myxoid nodule with focal entrapment of the mammary glands

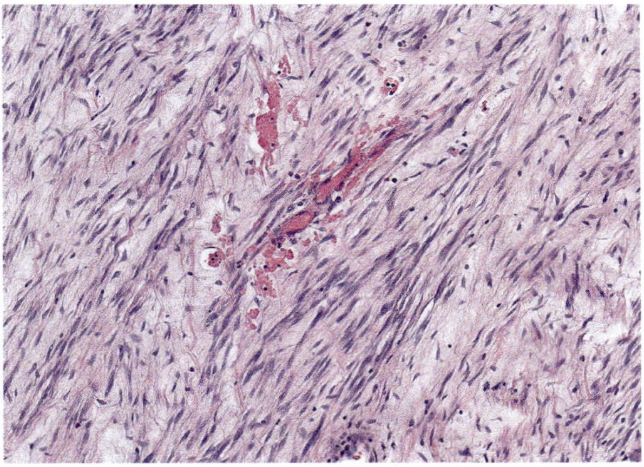

**Fig. 5.21** Nodular fasciitis showing a proliferation of cytologically bland myofibroblasts with tapered nuclei arranged in short, haphazard fascicles within a loose myxoid stroma; extravasated red blood cells and scattered inflammatory cells are present

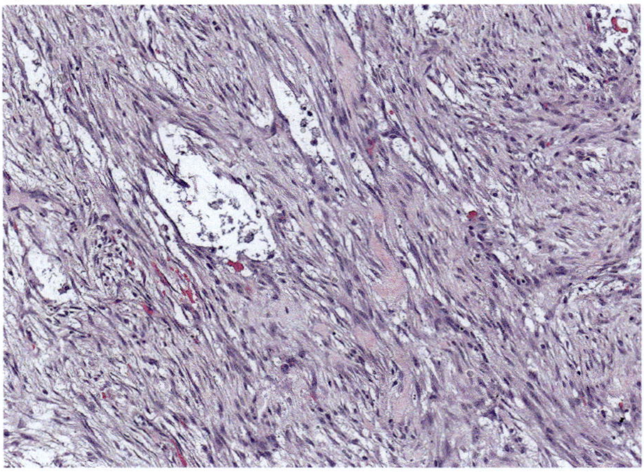

**Fig. 5.22** Another example of nodular fasciitis showing diffusely myxoid stroma, microcystic degeneration and keloidal-like collagen

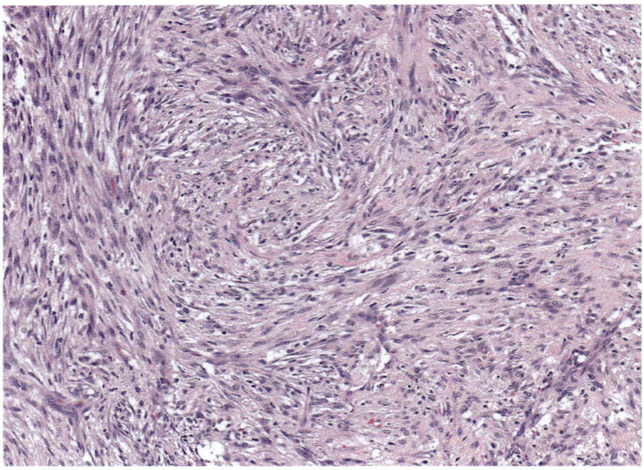

**Fig. 5.23** More cellular zones in nodular fasciitis; there is no significant nuclear atypia

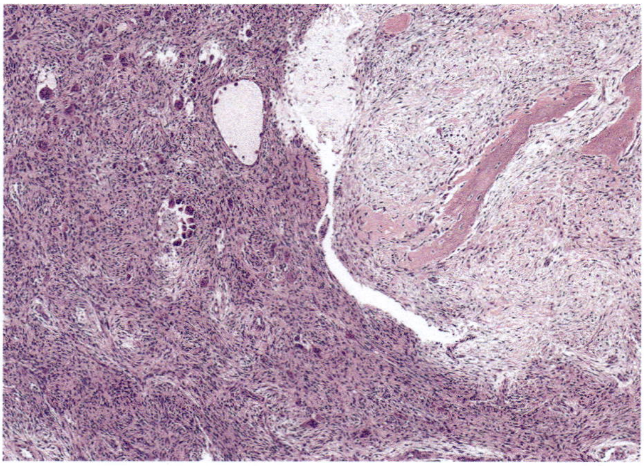

**Fig. 5.24** Osteoclast-type giant cells, aneurysmal bone-cyst like changes and new bone formation in a case with overlapping features of nodular fasciitis, aneurysmal bone cyst and myositis ossificans; these are genetically related lesions containing *USP6* gene rearrangements

## Immunohistochemistry

The constituent cells of nodular fasciitis are immunoreactive for muscle markers such as SMA and desmin with a characteristic myofibroblastic "tram-track"-like membranous staining pattern. CD34 is usually negative and cytokeratins are predominantly negative, though focal staining for both markers can occur.

## Molecular

Nodular fasciitis harbors an *MYH9-USP6* fusion, which can be useful in difficult cases (see below).

## Differential Diagnosis

In the breast, the most important differential diagnostic consideration for nodular fasciitis is low-grade fibromatosis-like metaplastic carcinoma (LGFMC), which can look very similar in appearance. Fortunately, LGFMC is diffusely positive for cytokeratins (especially high-molecular-weight cytokeratins) and p63 and has not been shown to harbor *MYH9-USP6* fusions. Nodular fasciitis can also look similar in appearance to benign cellular fibrous histiocytomas (FH). However, cellular FH shows at least focal peripheral collagen trapping, which is not a feature seen in association with nodular fasciitis, and typically lacks myxoid stroma. Cellular fibrous histiocytomas are discussed elsewhere in this chapter. Desmoid fibromatosis of the breast, also a myofibroblastic proliferation, can show some similarity to nodular fasciitis; however, the fascicles of fibromatosis are long and sweeping in appearance, as opposed to the short, haphazard fascicles of nodular fasciitis. Fasciitis-like areas with keloidal collagen may occur in fibromatosis but widespread myxoid stroma and microcystic changes are uncharacteristic; furthermore, fibromatosis shows markedly infiltrative borders, compared with the overall circumscription seen in nodular fasciitis. In difficult cases, FISH studies for the *MYH9-USP6* fusion or molecular studies to identify confirmatory features of fibromatosis (exon 3 mutations in *CTNNB1* or alterations of the *APC* gene) can be performed. Fibromatosis is also discussed elsewhere in this chapter.

Nodular fasciitis can also look very similar to inflammatory myofibroblastic tumor (IMT). IMT typically has a more brisk lymphoplasmacytic inflammatory infiltrate and, in most cases, a sharply defined edge. ALK IHC is almost always positive. Finally, owing to its loosely fascicular architecture and misleading immunophenotype, nodular fasciitis can look astonishingly similar to low-grade myofibroblastic sarcoma and spindle cell/sclerosing rhabdomyosarcoma, which can arise in the breast parenchyma or in the chest wall. All of these lesions are uncommon, requiring a high index of suspicion. In both scenarios, the degree of tissue infiltration and nuclear atypia is invariably greater than that of nodular fasciitis. Helpful ancillary tools include immunostaining for the skeletal muscle nuclear transcription factors myogenin and myoD1 (positive in rhabdomyosarcoma) or identification of *USP* gene alteration by FISH or RT-PCR.

## Prognosis and Treatment

While excision is traditionally performed in order to exclude its malignant mimickers, nodular fasciitis is an entirely benign, self-limited process that resolves spontaneously and is not expected to recur. Arguably, histologically classic or genetically confirmed cases in the breast can be managed expectantly.

## Inflammatory Myofibroblastic Tumor

### Clinical Findings

Inflammatory myofibroblastic tumor (IMT) is a low-grade translocation-associated neoplasm that most commonly harbors rearrangements involving the *ALK* gene, with corresponding positive staining for ALK by IHC. In children, a subset of ALK-negative IMTs may involve other kinase-encoding genes, including *NTRK*, *ROS1,* and *RET*. As a primary breast tumor, IMT is extremely rare and the English literature on this subject is limited to a handful of case reports and small series. However, even this small number is drastically reduced in number if ALK-negative cases or cases reported prior to the widespread use of ALK IHC or FISH testing (so-called inflammatory pseudotumors) are excluded. In the few remaining well-documented cases of mammary IMT, patients' ages ranged from 23 to 56 years old (mean age: 41 years old). Patients in these case reports all presented with a solitary palpable mass that ranged in size from 1.1 to 4.5 cm in size (mean size: 2.9 cm). Cutaneous, chest wall, and axillary IMTs can also occur and show clinical features similar to those reported at other sites.

### Imaging

Solitary, hypoechoic lesion with irregular borders on sonography; limited reported mammographic findings were classified as BI-RADS 4 (suspicious), prompting a biopsy.

### Pathologic Findings

#### Gross Features

Well-circumscribed, yellow-tan mass with or without central necrosis.

#### Microscopic Features

IMT is typically very well-delineated at scanning magnification and is composed of fascicles of fibroblastic/myofibroblastic cells, admixed with a conspicuous inflammatory infiltrate containing lymphocytes, plasma cells and less often, neutrophils, or eosinophils. The background stroma can be minimal, resulting in a densely fascicular growth pattern resembling low-grade myofibroblastic sarcoma or other low-grade spindle cell sarcomas with a fascicular pattern. Other cases show a prominent loose myxoid background with numerous blood vessels resembling nodular fasciitis (Figs. 5.25, 5.26, and 5.27). Some IMTs exhibit a densely collagenized stroma with diminished inflammatory cells, similar in appearance to a scar. The constituent cells of IMT are myofibroblasts that show characteristic morphologic features in keeping with this cell lineage, including ovoid nuclei, even chromatin, small discreet nucleoli, and slightly basophilic or pale eosinophilic cytoplasm (Fig. 5.28). Mitotic figures may be present but are usually not conspicuous.

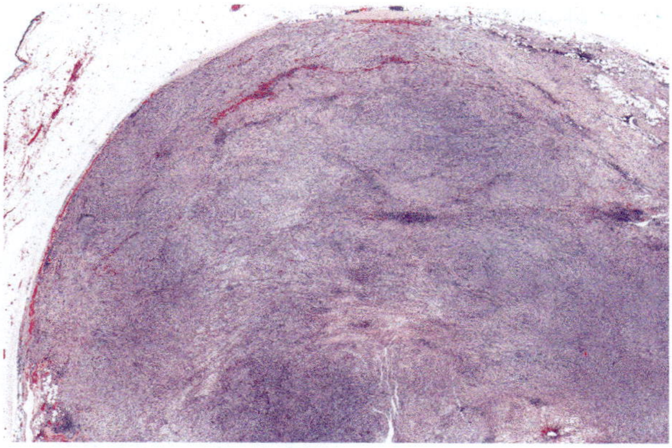

**Fig. 5.25** Inflammatory myofibroblastic tumor showing a modestly cellular fibromyxoid mass sharply demarcated from the surrounding tissue; focal fat entrapment can be seen

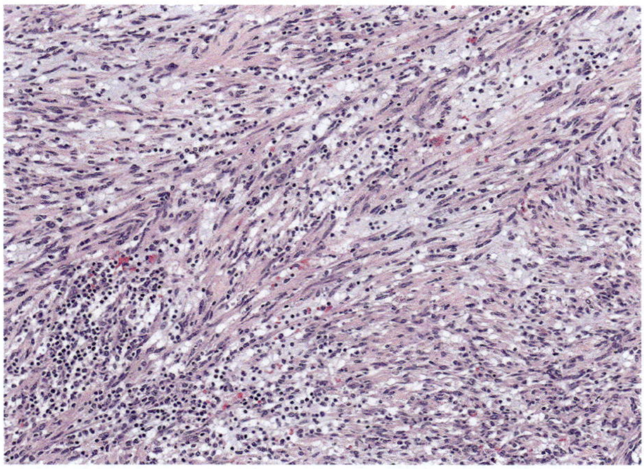

**Fig. 5.26** Inflammatory myofibroblastic tumor showing loose fascicles in a myxoid background with numerous blood vessels resembling nodular fasciitis; conspicuous inflammatory infiltrate is present

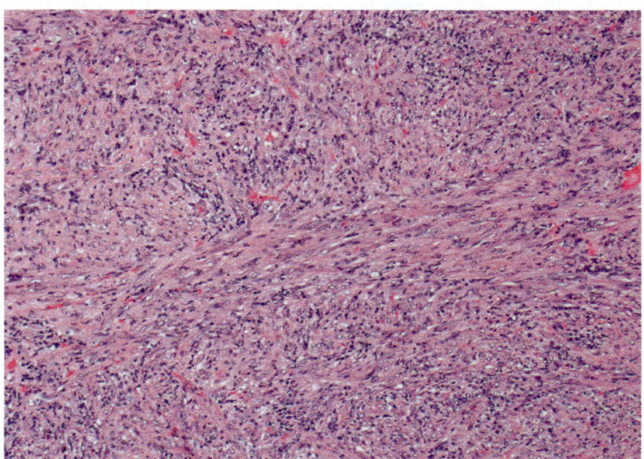

**Fig. 5.27** Inflammatory myofibroblastic tumor with more dense fascicular growth pattern resembling other low-grade spindle cell sarcomas

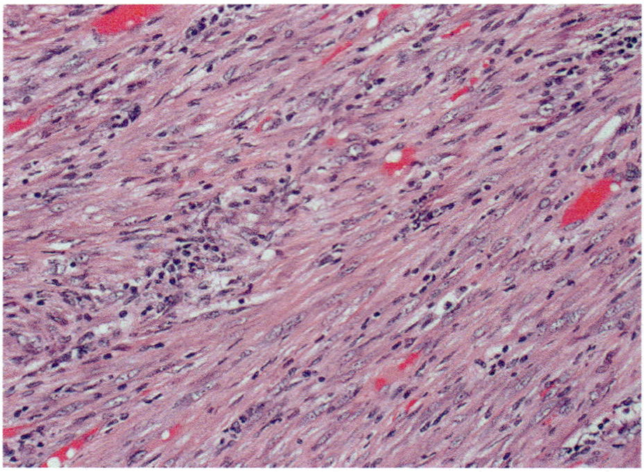

**Fig. 5.28** Inflammatory myofibroblastic tumor showing ovoid nuclei, open chromatin, small discreet nucleoli, and slightly basophilic or pale eosinophilic cytoplasm, features consistent with myofibroblastic lineage

## Immunohistochemistry

IMT is positive for muscle markers, such as SMA and desmin, negative for CD34 and may show cytokeratin positivity in about 30% of cases. ALK expression is seen in approximately 60% of cases and is very supportive of the diagnosis in this setting. A small subset of IMTs expresses ROS-1, in keeping the corresponding gene rearrangement.

## Molecular

As noted above, the majority of IMTs including those in breast harbor rearrangements in *ALK* that may be confirmed using break-apart FISH or next-generation sequencing platforms. A small subset of IMTs (5–10%), especially those in the pediatric population, harbor *ROS1*, *RET*, *NTRK*, and *PDGFR* rearrangements. That being said, many reported cases of breast IMT are insufficiently characterized at the immunohistochemical or genetic level; thus, the true frequency of *ALK* and other rearrangements in mammary IMTs is unknown. To the best of our knowledge, the more aggressive epithelioid variant of IMT (harboring an *ALK-RANBP2* fusion) has not yet been reported in the breast.

## Differential Diagnosis

Especially due to the proclivity of IMT to express cytokeratins, a major differential diagnostic consideration in the breast is low-grade fibromatosis-like metaplastic breast carcinoma. Differential diagnosis depends upon ALK testing (by IHC, next generation sequencing or FISH), although the pattern of cytokeratin expression in this instance is also helpful as IMTs typically do not show the robust, diffuse expression of high molecular weight cytokeratin or p63 as observed with many fibromatosis-like metaplastic breast carcinomas. Another differential diagnostic consideration is the lesion discussed elsewhere in this book known as cellular and spindled histiocytic pseudotumor complicating mammary fat necrosis (CSHP). True to its name, spindled histiocytic pseudotumor complicating mammary fat necrosis is a histiocytic lesion and should be negative for muscle markers, cytokeratins, and ALK, while showing diffuse immunoreactivity for histiocytic markers such as CD68 and CD163.

IMTs presenting with a loosely myxoid stroma can show a striking similarity to nodular fasciitis, especially in core biopsies. Nodular fasciitis is negative for ALK and also harbors its own gene rearrangements involving *USP6*; nodular fasciitis is discussed elsewhere in this chapter. Other low-grade fascicular spindle cell sarcomas that can mimic IMT (such as low-grade myofibroblastic sarcoma, fibrosarcomatous DSFP, or fibrosarcoma) typically lack the brisk inflammatory infiltrate of IMT or ALK expression.

## Prognosis and Treatment

Among the reported immunohistochemically confirmed breast IMT cases, 3 of 4 showed no recurrence but one patient experienced both local recurrence and distant metastasis (to the groin area) all within one year of diagnosis. While the data in the breast are still quite sparse, these variable outcomes are in keeping with those of IMT arising at other anatomic locations and underscore the observation that, despite its low-grade appearance and frequent indolent behavior, IMT may occasionally recur and/or metastasize.

## Dermatofibrosarcoma Protuberans

Dermatofibrosarcoma protuberans (DFSP) is a relatively common dermal or neoplasm of intermediate malignancy that has a predilection for the trunk and proximal extremities. As such, cases arising in the skin and subcutis overlying the breast or in the axillary region are not uncommon and may be seen by breast pathologists. Young to middle-aged patients are the most frequently affected (with a slight male predominance), though some cases can occur in very young children. DFSP presents as a nodular cutaneous mass with slow, but persistent growth; rapid growth usually heralds transformation to fibrosarcomatous DFSP. Cases reported specifically in the breast range from 1–2 cm in size and are centered on the subcutaneous tissue with occasional infiltration between breast lobules.

### Imaging

Typical DFSP cases are usually not imaged.

## Pathological Features

### Gross Features

Grossly, most cases of DFSP appear as an ill-defined indurated dermal/subcutaneous nodule or nodules in a background of a depressed plaque or scar. Cases with fibrosarcomatous transformation have a circumscribed, solid appearance, and a pushing border; in these situations, the background conventional DFSP in the surrounding adipose tissue is often underappreciated during surgical procedures or gross examination and may lead to an incomplete resection or inaccurate assessment of margin status.

### Microscopic Features

Microscopically, DFSP is characterized by an epicenter in the dermis and subcutaneous tissue with markedly infiltrative growth into the adipose tissue of the latter, in the form of both infiltrative tumor septa as well as entrapment of individual adipocytes, forming the characteristic "honeycombed" appearance (Figs. 5.29 and 5.30). The tumor cells are monotonous, bland-appearing fibroblastic spindle cells arranged in a storiform to the whorled pattern (Fig. 5.31). Myoid nodules, composed of pink bundles or whorls of spindled cells are an occasionally encountered, and nuclear palisading reminiscent of that seen in a schwannoma can be seen (Fig. 5.32). Myxoid stroma rich in small vessels is not uncommon and can be misleading as it resembles the stromal component of phyllodes tumor or pseudoangiomatous stromal hyperplasia (Figs. 5.33 and 5.34). A variable amount of melanin-containing dendritic cells can be present imparting a pigmented appearance (Bednar tumor, Fig. 5.35). Mitotic activity is inconspicuous and cytological atypia is minimal at best. By contrast, fibrosarcomatous DFSP shows a far more densely fascicular to herringbone monotonous growth pattern with moderate nuclear atypia and an elevated mitotic index (Figs. 5.36 and 5.37). Fibrosarcomatous DFSP can

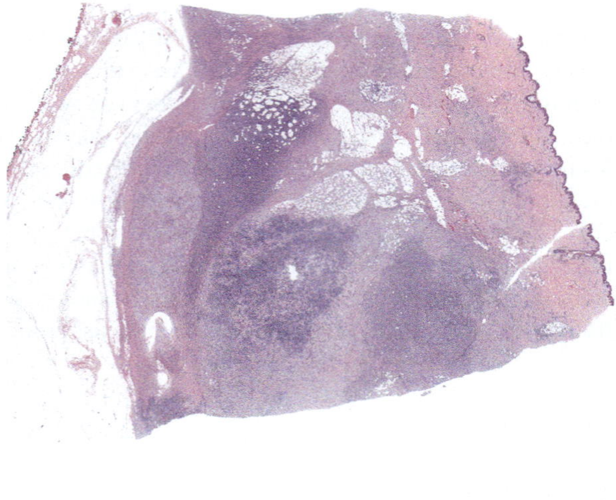

**Fig. 5.29** Dermatofibrosarcoma protuberans (DFSP) at scanning magnification showing an ill-defined nodule in the dermis and subcutaneous tissue

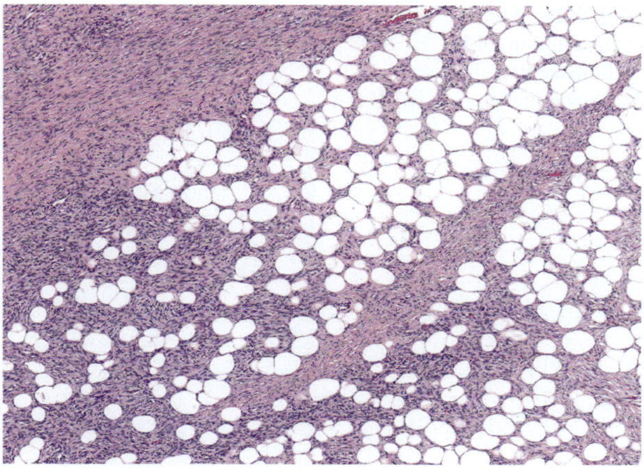

**Fig. 5.30** DFSP with markedly infiltrative growth into the adipose tissue in the form of both infiltrative tumor septa as well as entrapment of individual adipocytes, forming the characteristic "honeycombed" appearance

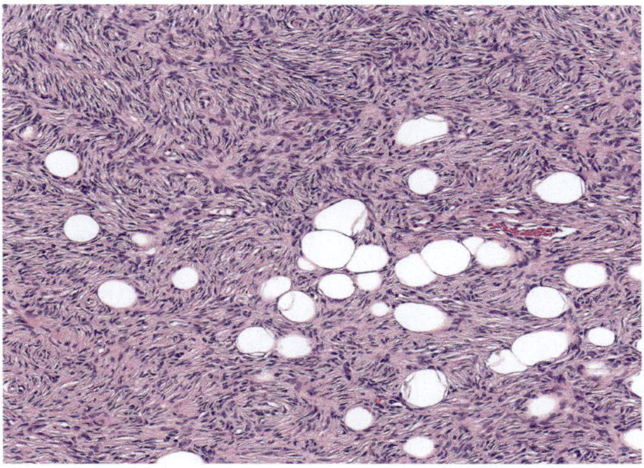

**Fig. 5.31** DFSP is composed of monotonous, bland-appearing fibroblastic spindle cells arranged in a storiform to whorled pattern

paradoxically show more of a pushing tumor border with the exclusion of adipocytes within the interior of the tumor and corresponding loss of the "honeycombed" appearance seen in conventional DFSP (Fig. 5.38).

## Immunohistochemistry

By immunohistochemistry, DFSP is diffusely and strongly positive for CD34 and is negative for SMA, desmin, S100, SOX10, STAT6, and cytokeratins, all of which are important in excluding its key mimickers (especially in relation to the fibrosarcomatous variant). CD34 expression is often diminished in areas with fibrosarcomatous transformation.

**Fig. 5.32** Areas of nuclear palisading in DFSP reminiscent of that seen in schwannoma

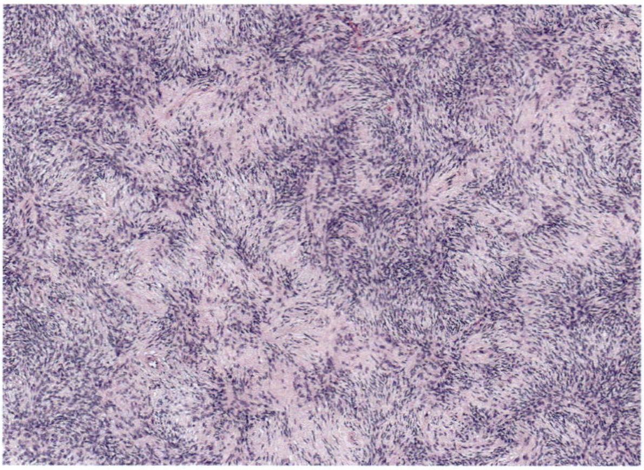

**Fig. 5.33** Myxoid DFSP with tumor cells arranged loosely in a diffusely myxoid stroma

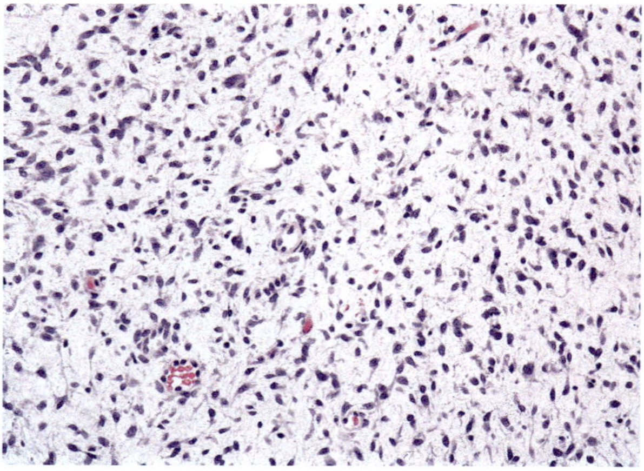

**Fig. 5.34** Another example of myxoid DFSP resembling pseudoangiomatous stromal hyperplasia

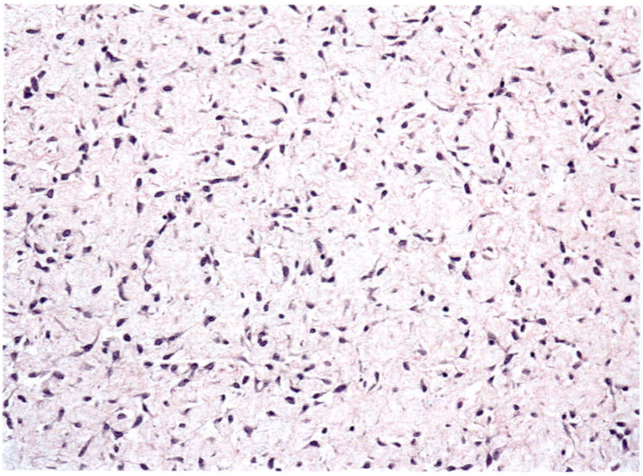

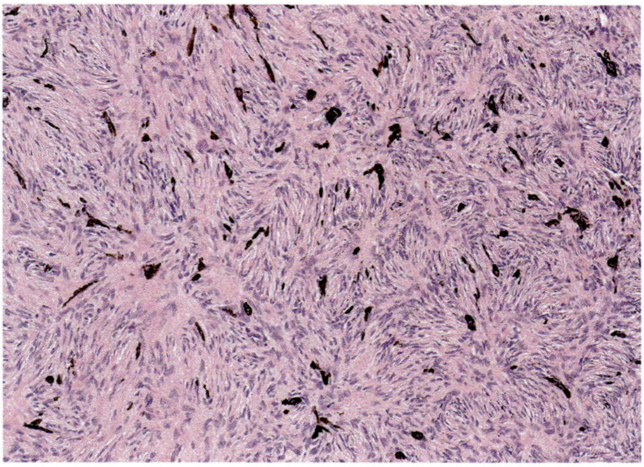

**Fig. 5.35** Pigmented DFSP (Bednar tumor) showing an admixture of melanin-containing dendritic cells

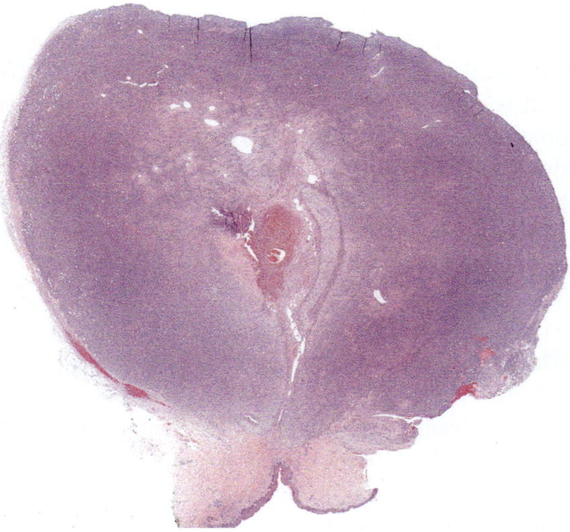

**Fig. 5.36** Fibrosarcomatous DFSP is a densely cellular tumor, which at scanning magnification can produce an impression of a well-circumscribed neoplasm with a pushing border

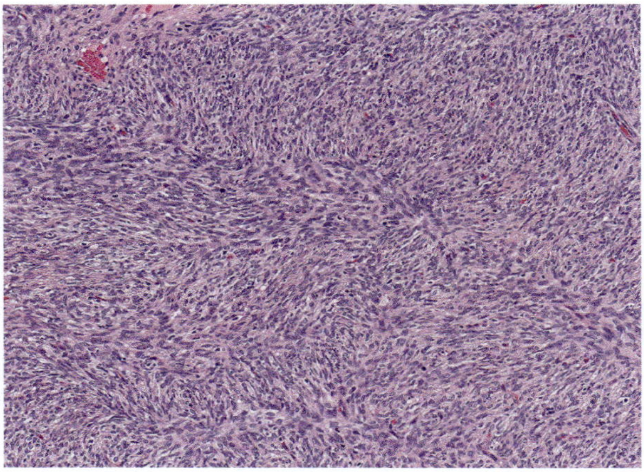

**Fig. 5.37** Fibrosarcomatous DFSP composed of densely cellular, monotonous intersecting fascicles with moderate nuclear atypia and an increase in mitotic activity; the honeycombing growth pattern of the conventional DFSP is no longer seen

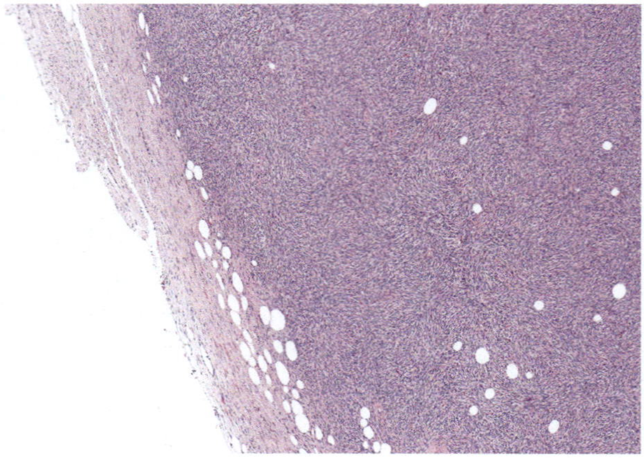

**Fig. 5.38** The conventional DFSP component at the periphery of fibrosarcomatous DFSP often gets compressed and may be mistaken for the surrounding non-neoplastic adipose tissue; in such cases, the margin can be misinterpreted as negative for tumor

## Molecular

DFSP at all sites is characterized by the canonical *COL1A1-PDGFRB* gene fusion, which is retained in the fibrosarcomatous component and can be very helpful in problematic cases. Interestingly, specifically in the female breast, DFSPs often show a novel variant *COL6A3-PDGFD* fusion, which still results in downstream expression of PDGFRB, driving DFSP tumorigenesis; all cases with this variant fusion described to date have shown conventional DFSP morphology without fibrosarcomatous transformation.

## Differential Diagnosis

In our experience, the biggest diagnostic pitfalls when evaluating a conventional DFSP in the breast region are low-grade fibromatosis-like metaplastic breast carcinoma, lipomatous mammary myofibroblastoma and, just as at extramammary sites, cellular fibrous histiocytoma. Unlike low-grade fibromatosis-like metaplastic breast carcinoma, DFSP is negative for cytokeratins and diffusely expresses CD34. The presence of ductal carcinoma in situ (DCIS) or foci of conventional invasive ductal carcinoma would favor low-grade fibromatosis-like metaplastic breast carcinoma. DFSP overlaps with cellular fibrous histiocytoma owing to the monotonous, vaguely fascicular, and somewhat infiltrative appearance and variable CD34 immunoreactivity of the latter; this differential diagnosis is discussed in detail in the next section. The most helpful histologic clue distinguishing lipomatous mammary myofibroblastoma from DFSP is the assessment at scanning magnification: while the close intermingling of lesional spindle cells and adipocytes in myofibroblastoma can give the impression of infiltrative growth, the outer border of myofibroblastoma is always circumscribed and entrapment of breast glands is very uncommon. This is in stark contrast to DFSP which has a truly infiltrative, ill-defined border producing the classic "honeycombing" appearance. Both DFSP and myofibroblastoma are diffusely positive for CD34; however, expression of myofibroblastic markers (desmin, SMA) and hormone receptors in DFSP is highly uncharacteristic.

Fibrosarcomatous DFSP invokes a different set of differential diagnostic considerations due to its higher-grade morphology. The first would be a high-grade spindle cell metaplastic carcinoma of the breast. Fibrosarcomatous DFSP, like its conventional counterpart, is negative for cytokeratins and would lack a component of DCIS or conventional ductal carcinoma of the breast, all of which would favor a metaplastic carcinoma, which is also typically negative for CD34. Another differential diagnostic consideration is a malignant phyllodes tumor, which often exhibits monotonous spindle cells in a fascicular or storiform pattern. In small biopsy material, the distinction between phyllodes tumor with sarcomatous overgrowth and fibrosarcomatous DFSP may be impossible on histological grounds alone and testing for the *COL1A1-PDGFRB* or the above variant gene fusion may be the only means to arrive at a definitive diagnosis in this setting.

Perhaps the most difficult differential diagnosis for a pure fibrosarcomatous DFSP at any site is an adult fibrosarcoma, from which fibrosarcomatous DFSP derives its name. Both tumors can look histologically identical, being composed of long and monotonous cellular fascicles, and both are variably positive for CD34. There is increasing evidence that most adult fibrosarcomas are also driven by tyrosine kinase gene fusions, most often involving *NTRK* or *RET*, as opposed to the *PDGFRB* gene fusions seen in fibrosarcomatous DFSP. In an excisional specimen, the presence of an often compressed, conventional DFSP component at the periphery of the fibrosarcomatous component would make this distinction easy; however, in small biopsy material, molecular testing for these rearrangements may be the only means for separating these pathogenetically related entities. As fusion-specific targeted therapies are available for both adult fibrosarcomas and fibrosarcomatous DFSP, this distinction has therapeutic implications in advanced or unresectable disease.

Fibrosarcomatous DFSP has a number of other mimickers that are rare in the breast, including malignant SFT, high-grade spindle cell malignant peripheral nerve sheath tumor (MPNST), synovial sarcoma, and atypical dermal smooth muscle tumor/leiomyosarcoma. These are covered in detail elsewhere in this text. Given that fibrosarcomatous DFSP is negative for STAT6, S100, SOX10, and cytokeratins, and virtually never expresses muscle markers to a significant extent (except, perhaps, occasional immunoreactivity in myoid nodules) this helps to exclude all of the above mimickers.

In all of the diagnostic dilemmas described above, especially with limited sampling, molecular or FISH testing for the pathognomonic *PDGFRB* gene fusion can be used to confirm the diagnosis of DFSP, although it is worth noting that FISH is likely to miss the variant *COL6A3-PDGFD* fusion, which thus far appears to be more prevalent in mammary cases of DFSP.

### Prognosis and Treatment

Conventional DFSP has a high rate of local recurrence (20–50%) and treatment accordingly involves an excision with wide margins. Conventional DFSP has essentially no metastatic potential. Conversely, high-grade progression to fibrosarcomatous DFSP is associated with acquisition of metastatic potential (10–15%). Targeted therapies are also available for patients with DFSP, making a distinction from its mimickers clinically relevant.

## Cellular Dermatofibroma (Cellular Benign Fibrous Histiocytoma)

### Clinical Features

A comprehensive review of fibrohistiocytic tumors is beyond the scope of this chapter, but we include cutaneous cellular dermatofibroma (DF) variant due to its frequent subcutaneous extension, myofibroblastic phenotype, and a somewhat infiltrative fascicular arrangement mimicking other fibroblastic and myofibroblastic lesions described herein. While most common in the head and neck region, cellular DF can occur at any location in the body, including skin of the breast, chest, and axillary region.

### Imaging

Most of these lesions are based in the dermis and subcutis and are not imaged.

### Pathological Features

#### Gross Features

A dermal or subcutaneous fibrous lesion with a somewhat irregular border.

#### Microscopic Features

Cellular dermatofibroma (cellular benign fibrous histiocytoma) is characterized by an increased cellularity relative to its conventional counterparts, and a predominantly fascicular growth pattern. At scanning magnification, the lesion acquires a somewhat stellate configuration, with focal infiltration of the subcutaneous tissue (Figs. 5.39 and 5.40). While all variants of DF by definition have a somewhat feathery edge with characteristic collagen trapping, in which thin strands of tumor cells at the periphery of the lesion insinuate themselves around dermal collagen fibers, this feature is only focally present in cellular DF (Fig. 5.41). The constituent cells in cellular DF appear a lot more monotonous and myofibroblastic in quality than their conventional counterparts, with ovoid nuclei, small nucleoli, and pale eosinophilic or basophilic cytoplasm (Figs. 5.42 and 5.43); the presence of mitotic activity

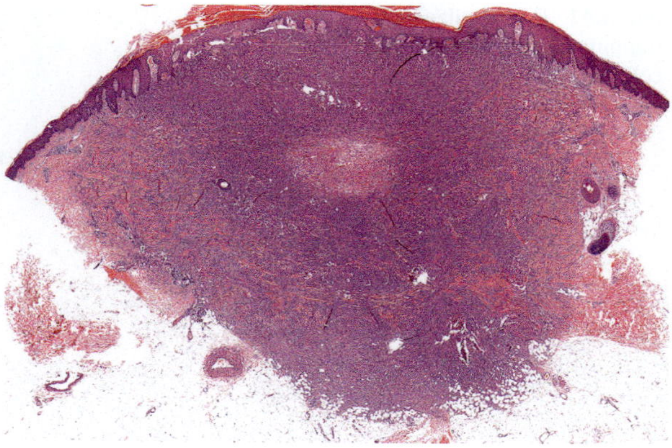

**Fig. 5.39** Cellular dermatofibroma (Cellular benign fibrous histiocytoma: at scanning magnification, the tumor is more cellular than its conventional counterpart, and shows a stellate configuration with focal infiltration of the subcutaneous tissue

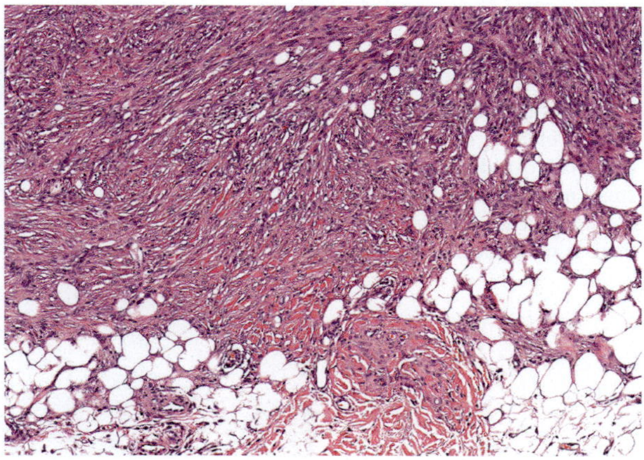

**Fig. 5.40** The infiltration of subcutaneous tissue in cellular dermatofibroma is focal and finger-like and never as diffuse as seen in DFSP

(5–10/10 HPF) and even occasional necrosis contribute further to an appearance that is reminiscent of more aggressive tumors (see differential diagnosis section below). Of note, various secondary elements that are typically present in conventional benign DF (inflammatory cells, foamy histiocytes, giant cells, and hemosiderin deposits) are not usually seen in cellular DF. However, cellular DF may coexist with other DF variants including the atypical variant, characterized by bizarre cells with considerable nuclear atypia and aneurysmal DF, characterized by copious amounts of extravasated red blood cells (Figs. 5.44 and 5.45). In these instances, the diagnosis of a variant of fibrous histiocytoma is more straightforward.

## Immunohistochemistry

For most variants of DF immunohistochemistry (IHC) is not necessary, as the characteristic cytomorphological features of the constituent tumor cells together with the collagen trapping at the tumor periphery and the overlying epidermal

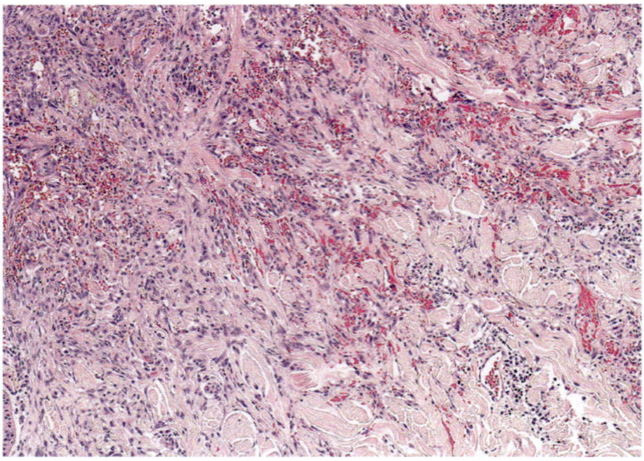

**Fig. 5.41** Focal collagen trapping at the periphery of cellular fibrous histiocytoma is an important diagnostic clue

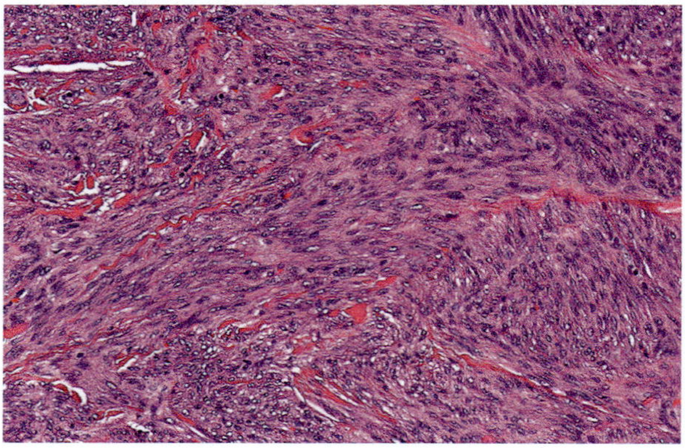

**Fig. 5.42** Cellular dermatofibroma composed of monotonous fascicles of myofibroblastic spindle cells with ovoid nuclei, small nucleoli, and pale eosinophilic cytoplasm; there is mild nuclear atypia

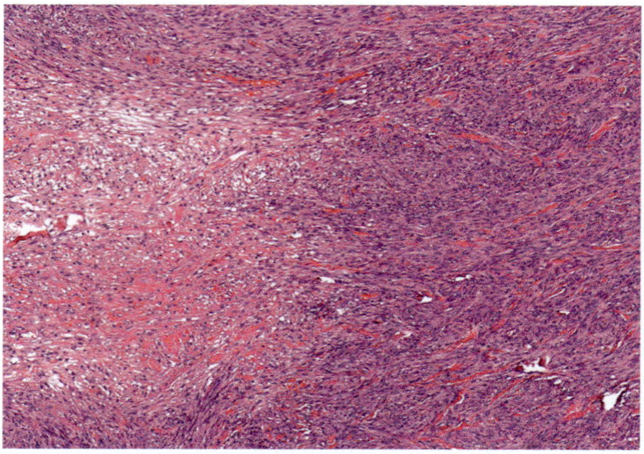

**Fig. 5.43** Occasional necrosis can be seen in cellular dermatofibroma; while it may be alarming, this feature does not imply malignancy

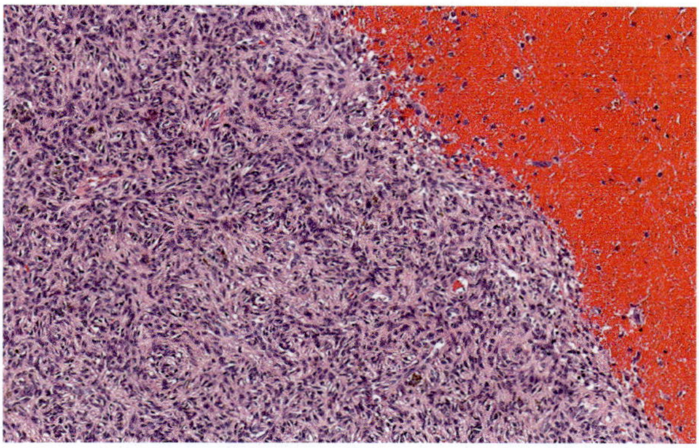

**Fig. 5.44** Aneurysmal fibrous histiocytoma showing a large cystic space filled with extravasated red blood cells; of note, the tumor cells are polymorphous and admixed with various secondary elements including inflammatory cells, foamy histiocytes, giant cells, and hemosiderin deposits; these features are usually not seen in pure cellular fibrous histiocytoma

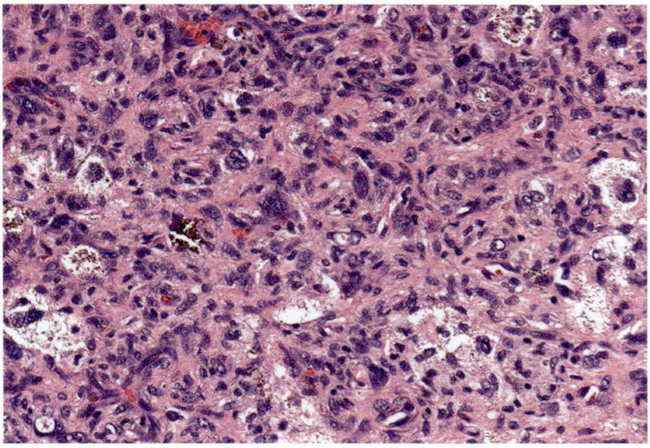

**Fig. 5.45** Atypical variant of fibrous histiocytoma characterized by bizarre cells with considerable nuclear atypia; when features of aneurysmal or atypical variant are present along with the spindle cells, the diagnosis of a variant of fibrous histiocytoma is straightforward

hyperplasia are sufficient for diagnosis. However, the cellular variant of DF is almost always positive for SMA in a myofibroblastic pattern, can show desmin expression and can show more CD34 expression than most pathologists are comfortable with, more often at the lesional periphery where the lesional cells intermingle with dermal collagen. This immunophenotype may overlap with that of nodular fasciitis, myofibroblastoma, and DFSP; however, cellular DF does not show strong, diffuse CD34 positivity expected in DFSP or myofibroblastoma, and estrogen and progesterone receptor expression is either focal or absent.

## Molecular

Like other variants of DF, a subset of cellular DF harbors rearrangements involving the *PKC* gene.

## Differential Diagnosis

As already alluded to, cellular DF can appear quite alarming and potential overdiagnosis as malignancy is more than a theoretical possibility. In particular, cellular DF can closely resemble both atypical dermal smooth muscle tumors and leiomyosarcomas. The positivity of cellular DF for both desmin and SMA can further confound this differential diagnosis since these are both positive in smooth muscle tumors. However, like its conventional counterpart, cellular DF consistently shows collagen trapping and in more superficial cases, also epidermal hyperplasia, features that are not seen in its smooth muscle mimics. Cellular DF can also resemble conventional and fibrosarcomatous DFSP; given that cellular DF can also show a considerable degree of CD34 expression, this can confound the situation even further. As noted above, cellular DF is also positive for desmin and SMA, markers that are consistently negative in all variants of DFSP. In difficult situations, testing for the *COL1A1-PDGFRB* rearrangement may be performed, which is pathognomonic for DFSP in this setting. DFSP is discussed elsewhere in this chapter.

Spindle cell metaplastic carcinoma and malignant phyllodes tumor may also enter the differential diagnosis with cellular DF occurring in the breast. The key pathognomonic histological features mentioned above (i.e., collagen trapping, epidermal hyperplasia) are not expected to be seen in either of these lesions. Application of a basic cytokeratin stain will easily distinguish cellular DF from low-grade fibromatosis-like metaplastic carcinoma.

On the benign end of the spectrum, both nodular fasciitis and myofibroblastoma can enter the differential diagnosis. We find that more cellular examples of nodular fasciitis might be especially difficult to separate from cellular DF as both lesions will show fascicular myofibroblastic architecture and a mildly infiltrative edge. FISH testing for *USP6* gene rearrangement can be employed but from a pragmatic standpoint, this distinction has relevance only in situations in which expectant management is considered, as cellular DF will tend to progress with time if not excised, whereas nodular fasciitis will likely regress. Myofibroblastoma can be separated from cellular DF by identifying (in the former) a sharply demarcated edge without collagen trapping, more uniformly diffuse CD34 immunoreactivity, and diffuse expression of ER, PR, and androgen receptor.

## Prognosis and Treatment

Cellular, atypical, and aneurysmal variants of fibrous histiocytoma are benign but have a reasonably significant rate of non-destructive local recurrence (up to 20% in some series), which can be multiple. The cellular variant of DF is responsible for most recurrences. Very rare metastases and death from the disease have been reported with these variants but these are truly exceptional events. Most cases of cellular DF will cause no problems outside of non-destructive local recurrence; therefore, in patients with these variants, conservative re-excision may be considered if cosmetically feasible.

## Myxoma and Superficial Angiomyxoma

### Clinical Features

Outside of the well-established intramuscular myxoma with *GNAS* mutation, the descriptive term "myxoma" is used for a number of benign lesions with overlapping features, all of which are superficial and poorly demarcated with very low cellularity, bland fibroblastic cells, and diffusely myxoid stroma. These lesions occur over a wide age range with a slight male predominance, and at numerous anatomical sites, including the skin and subcutaneous tissue of the breast and chest wall as well as the breast parenchyma and the nipple. When the vascular component is conspicuous and accompanied by scattered neutrophils, such lesions are often referred to as superficial angiomyxomas. Breast and cutaneous myxomas and superficial angiomyxomas may occur either sporadically or in association with Carney complex, in which case these lesions are often multiple.

### Imaging

Not applicable.

### Pathological Features

#### Gross Features

Poorly circumscribed, often multilobulated gelatinous lesions.

#### Microscopic Features

Microscopically, myxomas and superficial angiomyxoma show a poorly defined, infiltrative to multinodular profile involving the dermis, subcutis, or breast parenchyma. The tumor stroma is paucicellular and diffusely myxoid (Fig. 5.46). The tumor cells show fibroblastic morphology with a small amount of eosinophilic cytoplasm and nuclei with vesicular chromatin and inconspicuous nucleoli (Fig. 5.47). Atypia, if present at all, is often focal and mild and mitotic figures are scant to absent. As mentioned above, myxomas have a sparse, non-descript vasculature, while superficial angiomyxoma is notably more vascular, with scattered curvilinear blood vessels and a sprinkle of perivascular mixed inflammatory

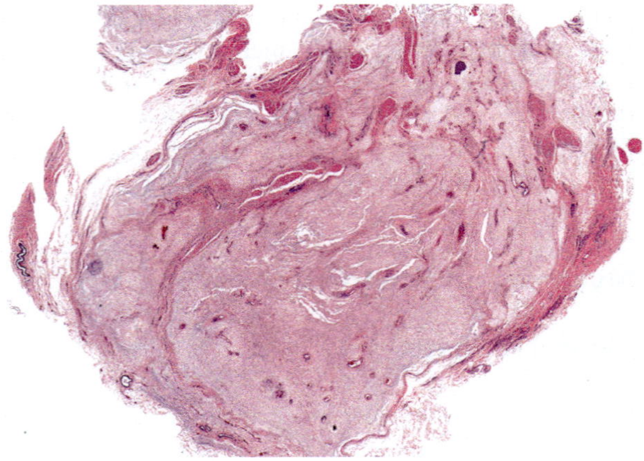

**Fig. 5.46** Superficial angiomyxoma of the nipple forming a poorly defined, multinodular mass with diffusely myxoid stroma

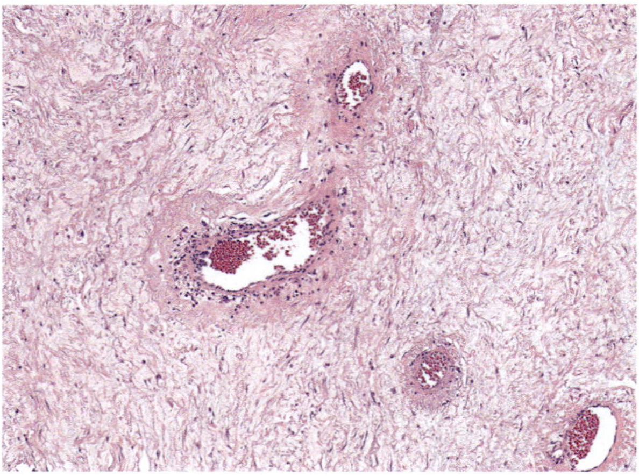

**Fig. 5.47** Superficial angiomyxoma showing a markedly paucicellular myxoid stroma with scattered benign fibroblastic cells with vesicular chromatin, inconspicuous nucleoli, and a small amount of pale eosinophilic cytoplasm

infiltrate; the most characteristic inflammatory cells are neutrophils that are present despite the lack of overlying epidermal ulceration (Fig. 5.48). Occasionally, the more superficially located superficial angiomyxomas may entrap and distort pre-existing epithelial adnexal structures (Fig. 5.49), producing an appearance that, to the breast pathologist, can resemble a myxoid fibroadenoma; however, careful scrutiny may demonstrate a connection of these epithelial structures to the overlying epidermis.

## Immunohistochemistry

By immunohistochemistry, the neoplastic cells of myxomas and superficial angiomyxoma are variably positive for SMA and consistently negative for CD34, desmin, cytokeratins, S100, and SOX10.

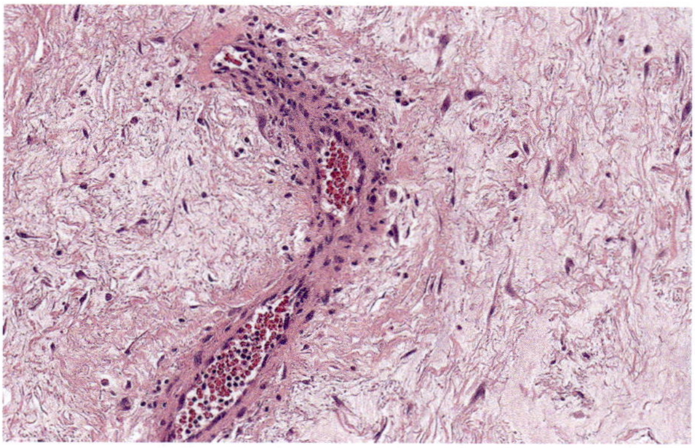

**Fig. 5.48** A distinctive feature in superficial angiomyxoma is the presence of curvilinear blood vessels with a sprinkle of inflammatory cells, most characteristically neutrophils

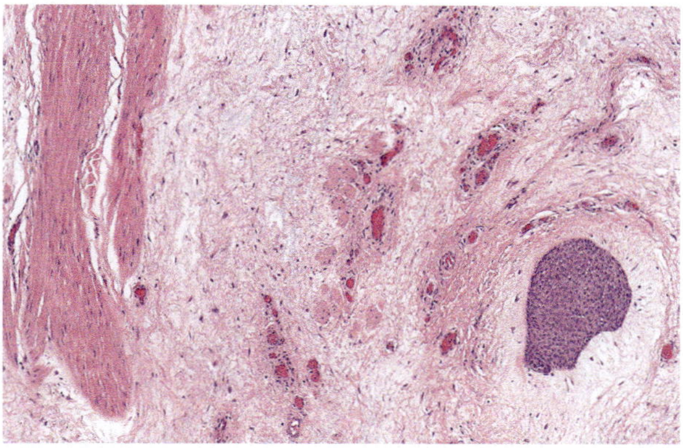

**Fig. 5.49** Superficial angiomyxoma showing an entrapment of a preexisting squamous adnexal structure

## Molecular

Myxomas associated with Carney complex harbor *PRKAR1A* gene mutations. Nodular mucinosis of the breast is a paucicellular, diffusely myxoid lesion with overlapping morphology that has classically been described in the areola and nipple of young female patients without Carney complex. The genetic signature of nodular mucinosis remains to be defined but it probably falls into two categories: CD34 and SMA-positive lesions likely representing myxoid variants of mammary myofibroblastoma, and those more similar to myxomas and angiomyxomas of the nipple region.

## Differential Diagnosis

For the breast pathologist, the most likely lesion to be confused with both breast myxoma and superficial angiomyxoma is a myxoid fibroadenoma. This can be difficult in cases of superficial angiomyxoma with epithelial entrapment/distortion, as

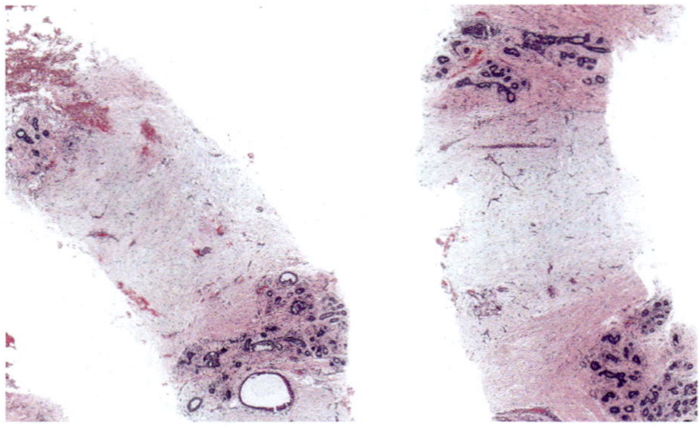

**Fig. 5.50** Diffusely myxoid lesion involving breast parenchyma without any additional defining characteristics

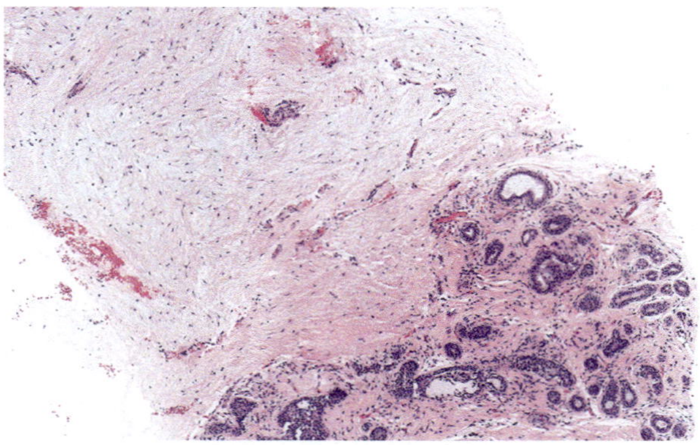

**Fig. 5.51** Diffusely myxoid lesion abuts histologically normal breast glands and shows no proliferative epithelial component or distinctive perivascular neutrophils. Separating myxoid fibroadenoma, breast myxoma or superficial angiomyxoma may not be possible in this small biopsy. All of these lesions are benign and may be associated with Carney complex, including myxoid fibroadenoma

described above; a careful search for evidence of adnexal structures and/or connection of the epithelial structures to the epidermal surface may help in this distinction as only superficial angiomyxoma would be expected to show this arrangement. In small core biopsies (Figs. 5.50 and 5.51), separating these three lesions may not be possible and may not be necessary, since all of them are benign and may be associated with Carney complex, including myxoid fibroadenoma. Recognizing the possible syndromic association for all of these lesions represents perhaps the most clinically important point here, since cardiac imaging may be recommended in order to identify an occult cardiac myxoma.

Myxoid myofibroblastoma is another myxoid primary breast lesion that may resemble both myxoma and superficial angiomyxoma. Myxoid myofibroblastoma lacks the curvilinear vascular pattern and neutrophilic infiltrate that typify superficial angiomyxoma and, in keeping with its origin from mammary stromal fibroblasts, myofibroblastoma is typically diffusely positive for CD34. In difficult cases, Rb IHC or FISH for 13q14 (using probes directed against *FOXO1*) could be performed in order to rule out myxoid myofibroblastoma; however, as both of these lesions are benign, this is unlikely to be necessary. Cutaneous lesions such as nerve sheath myxomas also enter the differential diagnosis with superficial angiomyxoma. Unlike nerve sheath myxomas, superficial angiomyxoma is negative for S100 and SOX10.

In our opinion, the only malignant lesion that has a real possibility of being mistaken for myxoma or superficial angiomyxoma is a low-grade myxofibrosarcoma given its characteristically subcutaneous location, relatively paucicellular stroma, curvilinear vasculature, and sparse chronic inflammation. An important pitfall is that the infiltrative, multinodular growth pattern is very similar in both superficial angiomyxoma and low-grade myxofibrosarcoma. But even in low-grade myxofibrosarcoma, the degree of nuclear atypia usually exceeds that of superficial angiomyxoma. While low-grade myxofibrosarcomas rarely metastasize, they invariably progress if incompletely excised and have a significant potential for local recurrence; therefore, in contrast to myxomas and superficial angiomyxoma, myxofibrosarcomas require a wide re-excision. Myxofibrosarcoma is discussed below.

### Prognosis and Treatment

Myxomas and superficial angiomyxoma are benign but due to their ill-defined multinodular nature, they can locally recur.

## Primary Breast Sarcomas with Fibroblastic/Myofibroblastic Differentiation

In general, sarcomas of the breast are exceedingly rare (< 0.1% of all breast malignancies based on more rigorous studies, and < 5% of all sarcomas). Sarcomas in the setting of prior radiation for breast carcinoma are more common than primary breast sarcomas, the most frequent being angiosarcoma and undifferentiated pleomorphic sarcoma. But even these are very rare, occurring in less than 0.2% of patients with breast cancer. Thus, if a sarcomatoid malignant neoplasm is encountered by a breast pathologist, it is statistically far more likely to represent a metaplastic breast carcinoma, malignant phyllodes tumor, fibrosarcomatous DFSP, or a spindle cell/pleomorphic sarcoma of the skin or underlying chest wall. Primary and radiation-associated sarcomas of the breast have the same morphologic features, immunophenotype, grading, and management approach as their soft tissue counterparts. Here, we discuss a few select sarcomas with fibroblastic/myofibroblastic differentiation that can occur in the breast region and revisit the diagnosis of adult fibrosarcoma in light of recent molecular genetic findings that have therapeutic implications.

## Adult Fibrosarcoma and Kinase-Rearranged Spindle Cell Sarcomas

### Clinical Features

In series that predate the current sarcoma classification, fibrosarcomas were the third most common sarcoma in the breast after angiosarcoma and undifferentiated pleomorphic sarcoma. However, true adult fibrosarcomas at all sites have long been considered to be extremely rare, as most of them can be classified by modern immunohistochemical and genetic/molecular techniques as another sarcoma type with a fibrosarcoma-like pattern (such as synovial sarcoma, MPNST, malignant solitary fibrous tumor, leiomyosarcoma, or fibrosarcomatous DFSP). By contrast, infantile fibrosarcomas represent well-established molecularly defined entities, characterized by an *NTRK3-ETV6* gene fusion. More recently, targeted RNA sequencing technology has been uncovering *NTRK3* and related *NTRK1, BRAF,* and *RET* tyrosine kinase fusions in infantile fibrosarcoma-like tumors in the pediatric population and in similar tumors in bone, soft tissue, and viscera of adults, revitalizing the concept of "adult fibrosarcoma" and suggesting that some of the strictly defined adult fibrosarcoma cases fall into this category. As these kinase fusion-based fibrosarcomas are being increasingly recognized at various sites, including the trunk and chest wall, they could conceivably involve the breast tissue. Recognition of these tumors is important because of the availability of targeted therapeutic options.

Clinically, most adult fibrosarcomas present as a firm, well-defined mass, which may grow rapidly.

### Imaging

The imaging appearance of most spindle cell sarcomas of the breast is non-specific; most often, they present as a solid mass without spiculation or calcification on mammograms and as an irregular mass with indistinct edges on ultrasound.

### Pathologic Features

#### Gross Features

Usually a single, well-defined solid fibrous or fleshy mass.

#### Microscopic Features

Adult fibrosarcomas show a circumscribed to the infiltrative border with the surrounding tissue and exhibit a fascicular, herringbone to storiform growth pattern (Figs. 5.52, 5.53, and 5.54). The stroma ranges from collagenous to somewhat myxoid. Mitotic activity is variable and may be not conspicuous. In many kinase-rearranged spindle cell sarcomas, a frequent and helpful finding is perivascular hyalinized collagen deposition (Figs. 5.55 and 5.56). There is variability in the

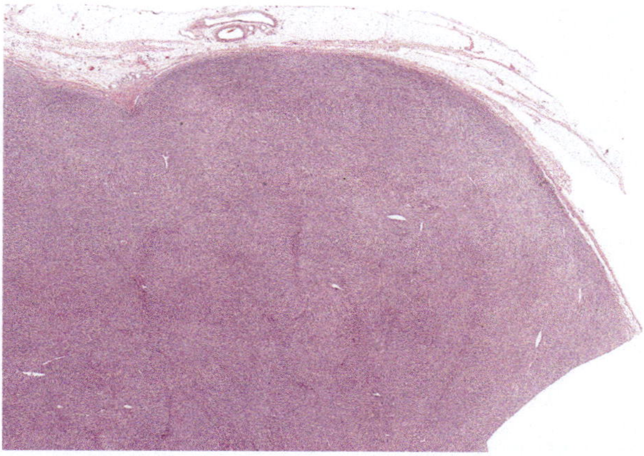

**Fig. 5.52** Adult fibrosarcoma showing a circumscribed, densely cellular mass

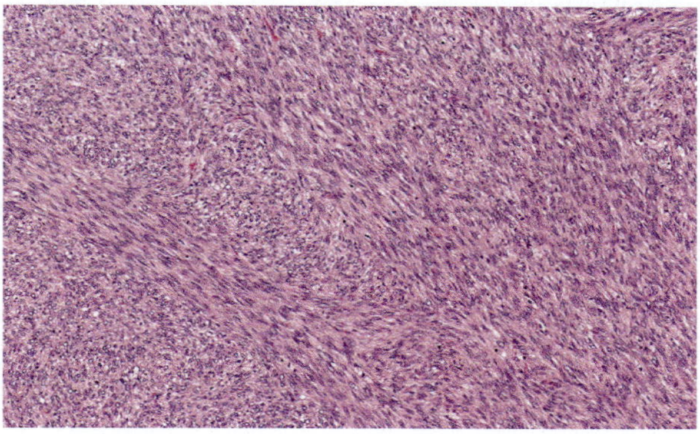

**Fig. 5.53** Adult fibrosarcoma composed of dense, monotonous fascicles arranged in a herringbone growth pattern

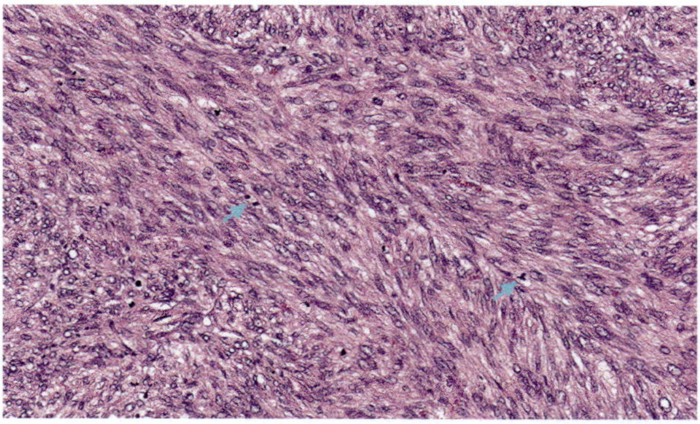

**Fig. 5.54** Adult fibrosarcoma showing overt nuclear atypia and mitotic activity

degree of nuclear atypia, ranging from rather bland-appearing spindle cells to more epithelioid cells with moderate to focally severe nuclear atypia. However, most adult fibrosarcomas histologically fall under the monomorphic fascicular spindle cell pattern rather than a "pleomorphic sarcoma" pattern; the latter should be

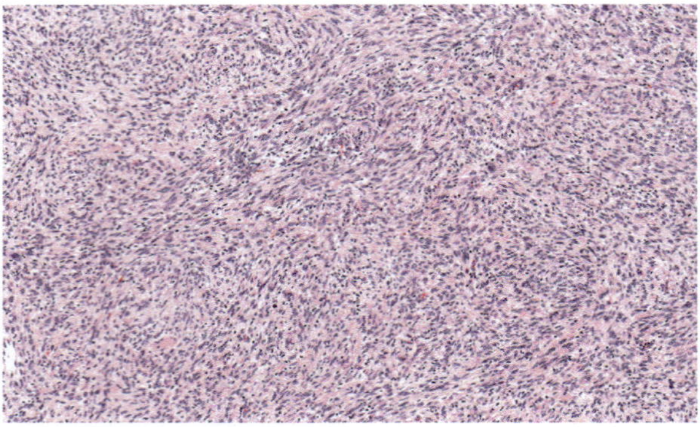

**Fig. 5.55** An example of fibrosarcoma with *RET* gene rearrangement showing a fascicular growth pattern and a collagenous background

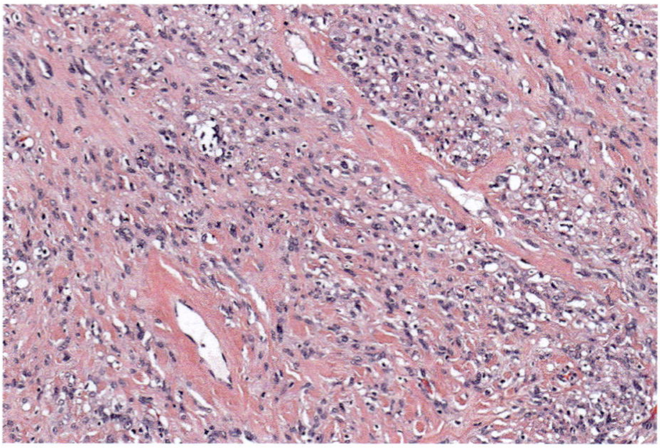

**Fig. 5.56** Perivascular hyalinized collagen deposition is a frequent and helpful finding in kinase-rearranged spindle cell sarcomas (showing here in a *RET*-rearranged fibrosarcoma). Kinase-rearranged sarcomas also show greater variability in the degree of nuclear atypia

diagnosed as undifferentiated pleomorphic sarcoma provided that other lineages were rigorously excluded.

## Immunohistochemistry

Most kinase fusion-based fibrosarcomas do not have a clear-cut lineage-specific immunoprofile. Rather, they often (albeit somewhat inconsistently) show a partial neural immunophenotype, with co-expression of S100 and CD34 without SOX10 expression.

## Molecular

The above unusual immunoprofile, when present, can trigger molecular testing for rearrangements in kinase-encoding genes such as *NTRK1, NTRK3, BRAF, ALK,* and *RET*, a feature that has both diagnostic and therapeutic value. Adult fibrosarcomas that are negative for these fusions show an essentially null immunohistochemical profile with the exception of an occasional expression of SMA in keeping with a fibroblastic phenotype.

## Differential Diagnosis

The principal differential diagnosis for adult fibrosarcoma in the breast includes spindle cell metaplastic carcinoma and malignant phyllodes tumor with sarcomatous overgrowth. Cases with a lesser degree of nuclear atypia need to be distinguished from low-grade fibromatosis-like metaplastic carcinoma. Fortunately, all subtypes of metaplastic carcinoma are usually positive for at least one cytokeratin, especially high molecular weight cytokeratin, and p63 while adult fibrosarcoma is negative for these markers and instead often expresses CD34. In biopsy material, the distinction between phyllodes tumor with sarcomatous overgrowth and adult fibrosarcoma might not be possible on histological grounds alone as CD34 can stain positive in phyllodes tumors as well, particularly in the stroma of benign and borderline variants. That said, molecular testing for *NTRK* or related fusions may be necessary for a definitive diagnosis of adult fibrosarcoma. Of note, we (Xu et al) have recently observed a dedifferentiated secretory carcinoma of the breast harboring an *ETV6-NTRK3* fusion in which the dedifferentiated component (also *ETV6-NTRK3* positive) acquired a fibrosarcoma-like morphology and focal CD34 immunoreactivity that, for practical purposes, was indistinguishable from a primary fibrosarcoma driven by an *NTRK* fusion (Figs. 5.57 and 5.58). Secretory carcinomas, in addition to the canonical *ETV6-NTRK3* gene fusion, may also harbor other kinase-encoding gene fusions such as *RET, MET,* or *ALK*, all of which have also been reported in pediatric and adult kinase-rearranged fibrosarcomas. Accordingly, if the conventional secretory carcinoma component is overgrown, it might not be possible to distinguish a secretory carcinoma of the breast with fibrosarcomatous dedifferentiation from a primary kinase-rearranged adult fibrosarcoma.

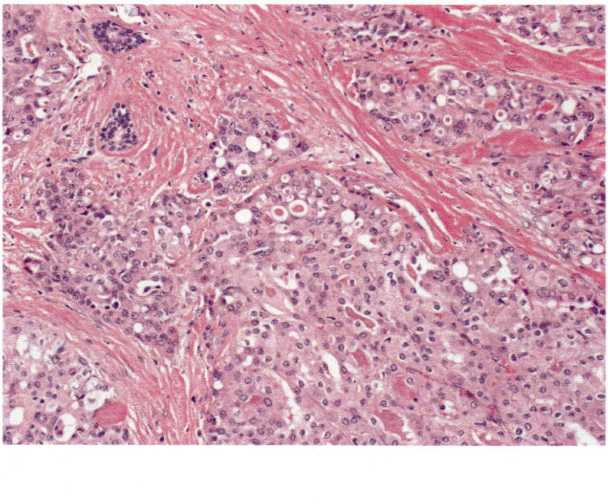

**Fig. 5.57** Conventional secretory carcinoma with *ETV6-NTRK3* gene fusion

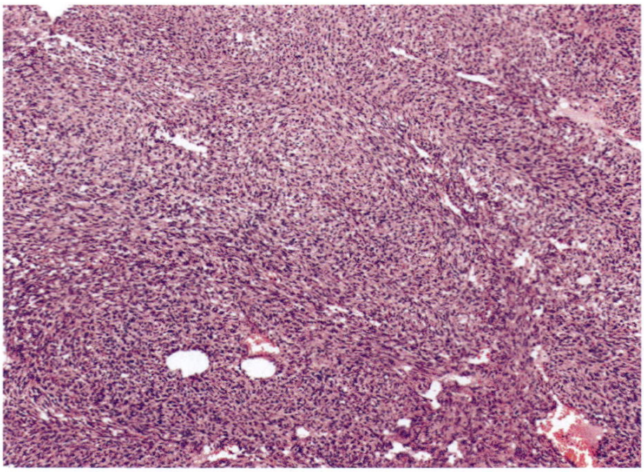

**Fig. 5.58** Dedifferentiated component with fibrosarcoma-like pattern in secretory carcinoma with *ETV6-NTRK3* gene fusion. The dedifferentiated component is also positive for the same fusion, and would be indistinguishable histologically or by ancillary testing from a primary kinase-rearranged adult fibrosarcoma unless a conventional secretory carcinoma component is identified

As mentioned above, other sarcomas with a fascicular growth pattern can resemble adult fibrosarcoma. Malignant solitary fibrous tumor, which often acquires a fascicular growth pattern and is CD34 positive, can be distinguished by STAT6 expression, which is virtually pathognomonic for solitary fibrous tumor in this setting. Malignant peripheral nerve sheath tumor (MPNST) can also mimic adult fibrosarcoma. While both tumors may be positive for S100, staining is far more diffuse in adult fibrosarcoma; furthermore, SOX10 is uniformly negative in adult fibrosarcoma, but is frequently expressed in MPNST. H3K27me2 or H3K27me3 staining by IHC, which is often lost in sporadic cases of MPNST, would be expected to be retained in adult fibrosarcoma whereas rearrangements in the above-mentioned kinase-encoding genes (*NTRK1, NTRK3, BRAF,* or *RET*) would strongly favor kinase fusion-based fibrosarcoma. Synovial sarcoma can be distinguished by focal expression of cytokeratins or EMA and a characteristic lack of CD34 expression since at least the kinase fusion-based adult fibrosarcomas show the opposite result for both IHC markers. However, testing for the *SS18-SSX* fusion (synovial sarcoma), its corresponding fusion-specific IHC antibody, or for adult fibrosarcoma-specific rearrangements is recommended to objectively confirm the diagnosis and to guide treatment. The differential diagnosis with fibrosarcomatous DFSP is discussed separately in this chapter.

Low-grade fibromyxoid sarcoma (Evans tumor) can also resemble adult fibrosarcoma, especially in small biopsies. MUC4 IHC would be the most useful stain for differentiating adult fibrosarcoma from Evans tumor, since it would be negative in the former and positive in the latter. Evans tumor is discussed further below.

### Prognosis and Treatment

When diagnosed on histological grounds alone by the rigorous exclusion of other lineages, adult fibrosarcomas are associated with a poor prognosis, with high rates of local recurrence and systemic metastasis. However, the prognosis of kinase fusion-based fibrosarcomas is guarded as the few reports in the literature include only a small series with variable outcomes ranging from no recurrence to deaths from tumor recurrence or metastasis. Breast sarcomas are best managed by a multidisciplinary team with a combination of surgery and radiation as an initial approach to resectable disease. As targeted therapies are now available for *NTRK-, RET-*, and *ALK*-rearranged solid tumors, the accurate diagnosis of adult fibrosarcomas and their substratification into fusion-defined subtypes is becoming increasingly important for optimal management.

## Myxofibrosarcoma

### Clinical Features

Myxofibrosarcoma is one of the most common sarcomas in older adults, with a peak in the sixth to eighth decades of life. The vast majority of these tumors arise in the extremities with only rare examples in the trunk and at other anatomic sites. Myxofibrosarcoma arising as a primary breast sarcoma is very uncommon but the latter may involve subcutaneous tissue of the breast region, or chest wall. Myxofibrosarcoma most commonly presents as a slowly enlarging painless mass and has a marked predilection for superficial locations (i.e., superficial to the deep fascia), where it shows a multinodular growth pattern with substantial infiltration along the underlying fascial planes. MFS can present at a range of histological grades, from low-grade to high-grade tumors.

### Imaging

Myxofibrosarcomas present as infiltrative, non-calcified single or multinodular superficial masses with irregular borders, suspicious for malignancy.

### Pathological Features

#### Gross Features

Multiple, variably firm to purely myxoid nodules with an invariably infiltrative margin and a variable degree of necrosis.

## Microscopic Features

Similar to its clinically infiltrative growth pattern, myxofibrosarcoma shows extensive infiltration microscopically, often evident as a multinodular growth pattern (Fig. 5.59). The tumor cells grow within an overtly myxoid stroma, punctuated by curvilinear vessels around which the tumor cells often loosely aggregate (Figs. 5.60 and 5.61). The tumor cells show a variable degree of nuclear hyperchromasia and pleomorphism, which can range from mild to severe but is invariably present. Cytoplasmic vacuolization imparting a "pseudolipoblastic" appearance is often present. Some of the higher-grade tumors have a more epithelioid appearance, resembling carcinoma or malignant melanoma (Fig. 5.62). Sparse chronic inflammatory

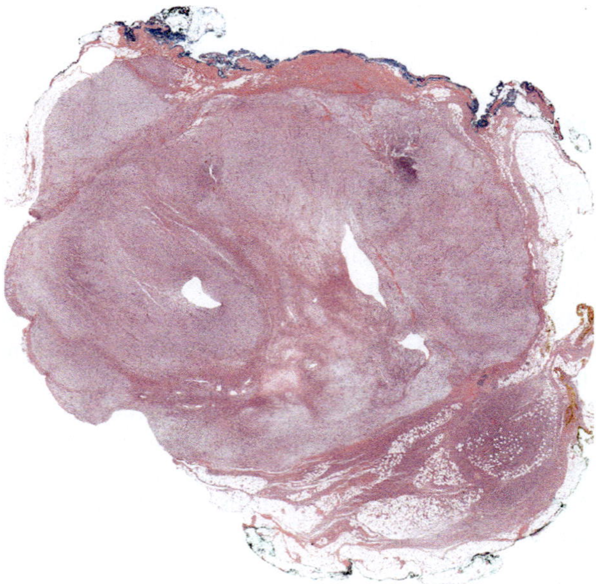

**Fig. 5.59** Myxofibrosarcoma showing a markedly infiltrative multinodular growth pattern in the subcutaneous tissue

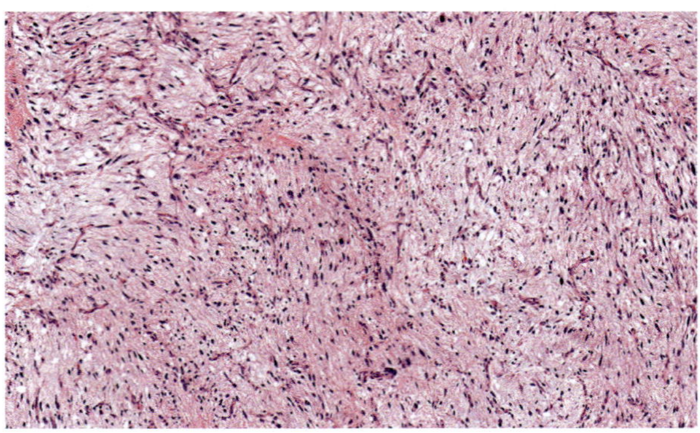

**Fig. 5.60** The tumor cells are loosely distributed within an overtly myxoid stroma containing prominent curvilinear vessels around which the tumor cells often congregate; there is mild nuclear atypia with occasional pleomorphic cells that can be picked up at low power

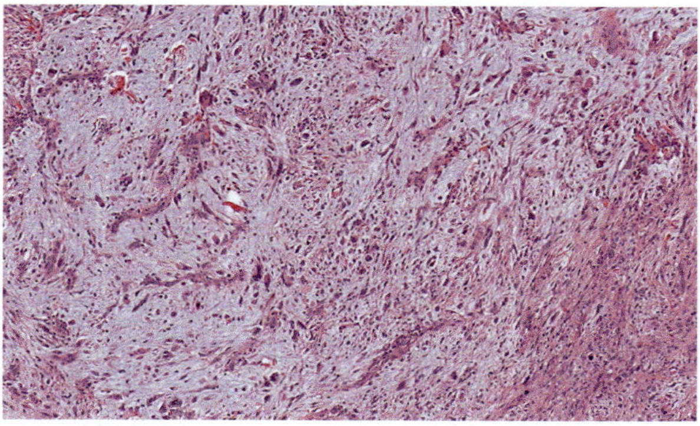

**Fig. 5.61** Another example of myxofibrosarcoma with prominent curvilinear vasculature; there is marked nuclear atypia and pleomorphism in this example

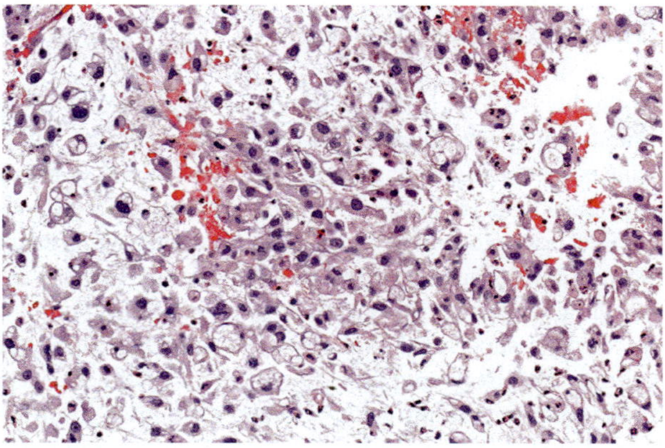

**Fig. 5.62** Epithelioid myxofibrosarcoma showing ovoid to polygonal cells with open chromatin and nucleoli reminiscent of carcinoma or malignant melanoma; multivacuolated cells with cytoplasmic vacuoles containing mucin are often present and can be mistaken for lipoblasts (so-called "pseudolipoblasts")

component is often seen. The degree of cellularity, pleomorphism, mitotic activity, and the presence or absence of necrosis depend upon (and, in fact, define) the tumor grade, which should be done based on the FNCLCC grading system. The infiltrative growth pattern of myxofibrosarcoma can make margin interpretation very problematic, especially when a low- to intermediate-grade example of MFS is encountered as it can be extremely difficult to distinguish a tumor of this grade from a reactive myofibroblastic reaction with myxoid stroma (Fig. 5.63).

## Immunohistochemistry

Immunohistochemistry in myxofibrosarcoma is non-specific and of limited value.

## Molecular

Currently, there are no disease-defining molecular characteristics for this tumor type.

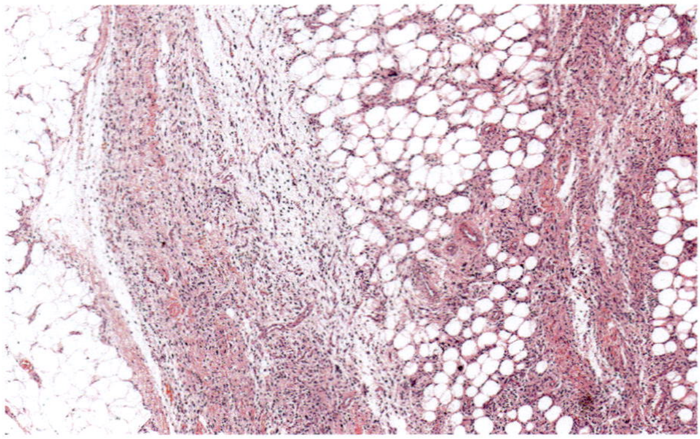

**Fig. 5.63** Low-grade myxofibrosarcoma permeating along the subcutaneous fibrous septa; a tumor of this grade might be difficult to distinguish from the reactive myofibroblasts at the periphery of the tumor and require a close scrutiny for nuclear hyperchromasia and pleomorphism

## Differential Diagnosis

In the breast, the primary differential diagnostic considerations are metaplastic carcinoma (especially the matrix-producing subtype) and malignant phyllodes tumor. Matrix-producing metaplastic breast carcinoma is positive for cytokeratin and often expresses SOX10; both of these markers are expected to be negative (or focal and weak at best) in myxofibrosarcoma. Differentiating malignant phyllodes tumor from myxofibrosarcoma could be more problematic; particularly if the pathognomonic leaf-like phyllodes architecture is absent. Low-grade myxofibrosarcoma can be mistaken for myxoma or superficial angiomyxoma as both tumors occur in the subcutis, have paucicellular, diffusely myxoid stroma and curvilinear vasculature with sparse chronic inflammation and, most importantly, display an infiltrative, multinodular growth pattern. The distinction can be challenging but even in low-grade myxofibrosarcoma, the degree of nuclear atypia usually exceeds that of myxoma or superficial angiomyxoma.

## Prognosis and Treatment

Low-grade tumors show very little metastatic potential, but have a high rate of local recurrence, while higher-grade tumors acquire a significant metastatic potential (approximately 30%). Recurrences may be associated with higher nuclear grade. Regardless of tumor grade, excision with wide margins is essential in order to minimize the risk of local recurrence.

# Low-Grade Fibromyxoid Sarcoma (Evans Tumor) and Sclerosing Epithelioid Fibrosarcoma

## Clinical Features

Low-grade fibromyxoid sarcoma (LGFMS), also known as Evans tumor, and the closely related sclerosing epithelioid fibrosarcoma are fibroblastic sarcomas that share the same genetic rearrangements. Low-grade fibromyxoid sarcoma occurs predominantly in young adults and may occur at a number of anatomic sites with a predilection for deep, subfascial locations, although up to 20% of cases may occur superficially. Sclerosing epithelioid fibrosarcoma occurs in an older population than LGFMS, predominantly affecting middle aged to elderly adults, and is also a deep-seated neoplasm. Both present as painless slow-growing masses with significant variation in tumor size; most LGFMS and sclerosing epithelioid fibrosarcomas are <10 cm but very large tumors exceeding 20 cm are not uncommon. Exceptionally rare cases of low-grade fibromyxoid sarcoma within the breast parenchyma have been reported. However, given that superficial/subcutaneous examples of LGFMS are well-established and both low-grade fibromyxoid sarcoma and sclerosing epithelioid fibrosarcoma can involve the trunk, chest wall, or axilla, breast pathologists should be aware of these entities. Therefore, both tumors are covered here given their deceptively low-grade morphology and their propensity to mimic several primary breast lesions.

## Imaging

The data on the appearance in the breast are limited to a single case report, showing a well-circumscribed, heterogenous low echogenicity mass by ultrasound.

## Pathologic Features

### Gross Features

Low-grade fibromyxoid sarcoma and sclerosing epithelioid fibrosarcoma are a sharply outlined, firm, white-tan fibrous or less often, focally mucoid masses. Microcalcifications may be present.

### Microscopic Features

Low-grade fibromyxoid sarcoma is characterized by the presence of both hypocellular densely collagenous areas juxtaposed to areas with a myxoid extracellular matrix and increased cellularity; these latter areas often have a nodular configuration (Fig. 5.64). The spindle cells of LGFMS are short and rather non-descript fibroblasts with characteristically bland nuclear features that may be arranged in a fascicular to the whorled pattern. Mitotic figures are usually inconspicuous (Figs. 5.65 and 5.66). Two additional classical histological features of LGFMS can greatly aid in its recognition. The first is the presence of curvilinear vessels which are most pronounced in the areas with myxoid stroma (Fig. 5.67). The second is the occasional presence of collagenous rosettes composed of a core of densely hyalinized stroma surrounded by a rim of palisading spindle to epithelioid tumor cells (Fig. 5.68). This variant morphology is often referred to as hyalinizing spindle cell tumor with giant rosettes.

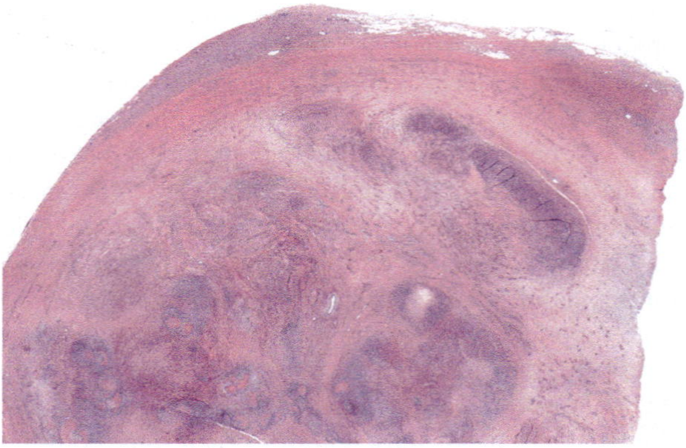

**Fig. 5.64** Low-grade fibromyxoid sarcoma (LGFMS): a circumscribed tumor with focal infiltration. At scanning magnification, one can appreciate a somewhat nodular configuration with alternating hypocellular collagenous areas and areas with increased cellularity and a myxoid stroma

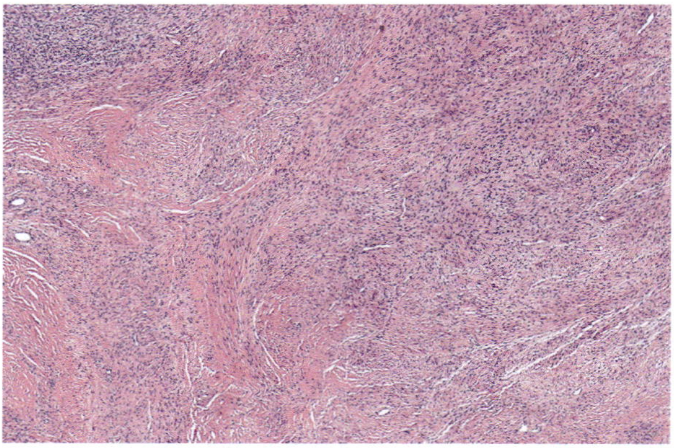

**Fig. 5.65** LGFMS showing a variation in cellularity and a combination of a fascicular and a whorled growth pattern

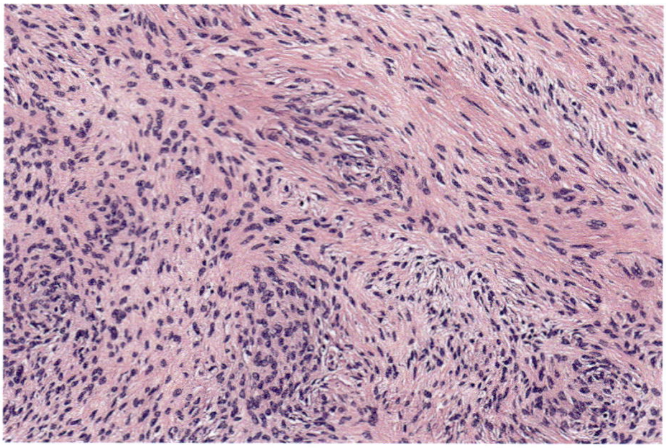

**Fig. 5.66** Cytologically, LGMFS is composed of short non-descript fibroblasts with characteristically bland nuclear features and inconspicuous mitotic figures

Sclerosing epithelioid fibrosarcoma often shows a more infiltrative growth pattern than that of low-grade fibromyxoid sarcoma, often with extension into the surrounding skeletal muscle and fascia. The tumor is composed of bland-appearing epithelioid cells with irregular vesicular nuclei and small nucleoli that grow singly

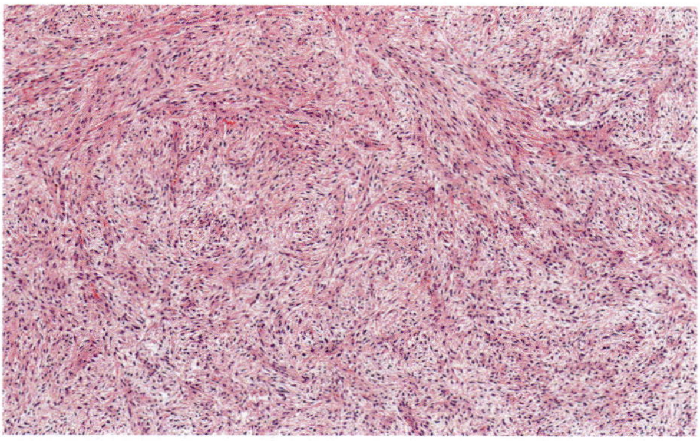

**Fig. 5.67** LGFMS showing arcades of curvilinear vessels which are most pronounced in the areas with myxoid stroma

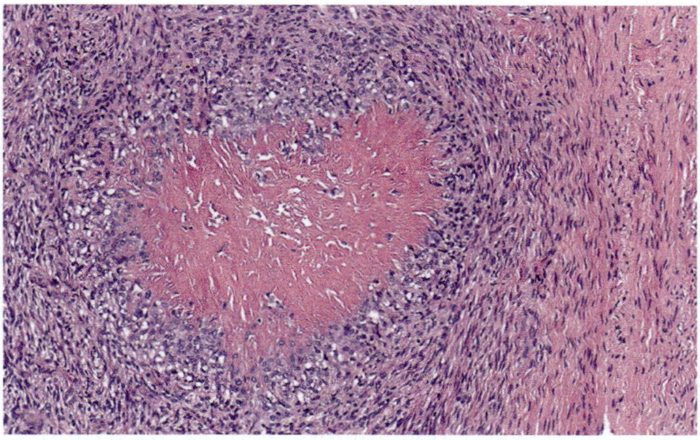

**Fig. 5.68** Collagenous rosettes in LGFMS composed of a core of densely hyalinized stroma surrounded by a rim of palisading spindle to epithelioid tumor cells. This variant morphology may be referred to as hyalinizing spindle cell tumor with giant rosettes

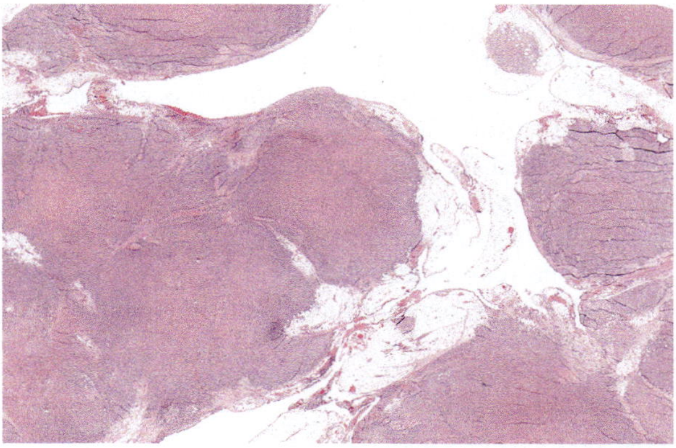

**Fig. 5.69** Sclerosing epithelioid fibrosarcoma showing an overtly infiltrative multinodular growth pattern at scanning magnification, and a more uniformly collagenous stroma

or arranged into cords and trabeculae within a densely collagenous stroma—an appearance that has been classically compared to infiltrating lobular carcinoma of the breast (Figs. 5.69 and 5.70). Mitotic figures are typically inconspicuous. However, rarely, areas with more severe nuclear atypia, increased mitotic rate, and necrosis may be seen.

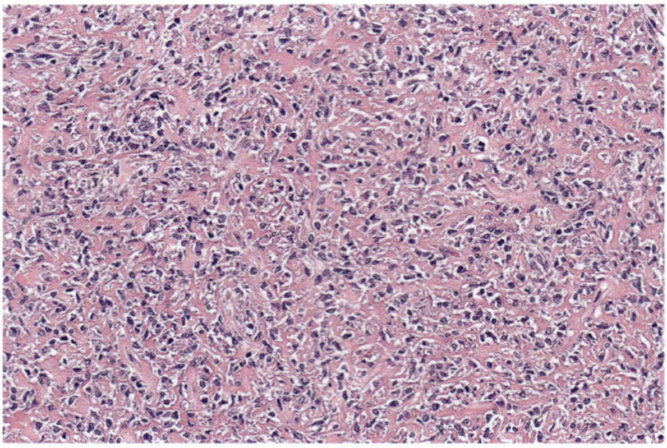

**Fig. 5.70** Sclerosing epithelioid fibrosarcoma showing bland epithelioid cells with irregular vesicular nuclei and small nucleoli arranged singly or into cords within a densely collagenous stroma—an appearance that can mimic lobular carcinoma of the breast

## Immunohistochemistry

Both low-grade fibromyxoid sarcoma and sclerosing epithelioid fibrosarcoma express MUC4, which is highly sensitive and specific in this setting, being present in nearly 100% of LGFMS and at least 80% of sclerosing epithelioid fibrosarcoma. There may be a variable expression of EMA, SMA, or S100 in these tumors. Of note, cytokeratins and CD34 are reliably negative in these tumors.

## Molecular

On a genetic level, both tumors share *FUS-CREB3L1* and *FUS-CREB3L2* fusions, although these are far more common in LGFMS and in hybrid tumors with features of both LGFMS and sclerosing epithelioid fibrosarcoma. Pure sclerosing epithelioid fibrosarcoma is more commonly associated with *EWSR1-CREB3L1* and *EWSR1-CREB3L2* fusions, though occasional cases of LGFMS may also harbor these fusions. Recently, the spectrum of sclerosing epithelioid fibrosarcoma was expanded by the identification of *YAP1* and *KMT2A* gene rearrangements, and these tumors are MUC4-negative. Because different fusion combinations are possible in these closely related tumors, molecular testing for *FUS*, *EWSR1,* and *YAP1* gene rearrangements (the latter is present as part of some commercially available next-generation sarcoma fusion panels) may be necessary to confirm the diagnosis.

## Differential Diagnosis

The most important mimicker of low-grade fibromyxoid sarcoma in the breast is low-grade fibromatosis-like metaplastic carcinoma. Low-grade fibromatosis-like metaplastic carcinoma is positive for cytokeratins, especially high molecular weight cytokeratins, while LGFMS is negative for cytokeratins. MUC4 may be very useful in this setting, as it would be expected to be negative in low-grade fibromatosis-like metaplastic carcinoma. Because low-grade fibromyxoid sarcoma is notoriously bland-looking, other clinically significant fibroblastic tumors can closely mimic LGFMS including myofibroblastoma, desmoid fibromatosis, dermatofibrosarcoma protuberans, and solitary fibrous tumor (SFT). All of the above mimics are expected to be negative for MUC4. CD34 can also serve as a quick screening tool as it is diffusely positive in myofibroblastoma, SFT, and DFSP but generally negative in LGFMS. Positive staining for STAT6 by IHC is virtually diagnostic for SFT in this setting; conversely, MUC4 is negative in SFT. In difficult cases, confirmatory testing for rearrangements involving *FUS*, *EWSR1,* or *YAP1* is required in establishing the diagnosis of low-grade fibromyxoid sarcoma and represents the definitive test for distinguishing LGFMS from all of its mimickers in the breast or elsewhere.

In the breast, the tumors with the greatest propensity for mimicking sclerosing epithelioid fibrosarcoma are invasive lobular carcinoma and the epithelioid variant of myofibroblastoma. Invasive lobular carcinoma is diffusely and strongly positive for cytokeratins and, while EMA may be focally expressed in sclerosing epithelioid fibrosarcoma, cytokeratin stains are negative. Epithelioid myofibroblastoma is positive for CD34, SMA, and desmin, while these markers are negative in sclerosing epithelioid fibrosarcoma. While MUC4 can be very useful in differentiating epithelioid myofibroblastoma from sclerosing epithelioid fibrosarcoma, it is not advised for differentiating sclerosing epithelioid fibrosarcoma from invasive lobular carcinoma, as adenocarcinomas from numerous anatomical sites may express MUC4. In all cases in which sclerosing epithelioid fibrosarcoma is strongly suspected, confirmatory testing for rearrangements involving *FUS* or *EWSR1* will provide accurate classification.

### Prognosis and Treatment

Despite its highly misleading name, low-grade fibromyxoid sarcoma is well-known for developing late recurrences and metastases in up to 40% of cases, sometimes decades after the initial diagnosis. Sclerosing epithelioid fibrosarcoma behaves more aggressively, with frequent recurrences and metastases to lung, bone, soft tissue, and liver in 50% of cases. Both tumors, irrespective of location, should be managed by a multidisciplinary team.

## Low-Grade Myofibroblastic Sarcoma

### Clinical Features

Low-grade myofibroblastic sarcoma is an uncommon myofibroblastic neoplasm with a fascicular architecture resembling fibromatosis or nodular fasciitis, significant potential for local recurrence, but very low rates of metastasis. Low-grade myofibroblastic sarcoma occurs predominantly in adults, with a predilection for the head and neck region and oral cavity but has been described in the subcutaneous soft tissue and in the breast parenchyma. Low-grade myofibroblastic sarcoma in the breast presents as a slow growing, well-defined palpable mass, and can grow relatively large (2–22 cm based on reported cases).

## Imaging

On mammography, low-grade myofibroblastic sarcoma presents as a well-circumscribed high-density mass suggestive of fibroadenoma or phyllodes tumor.

## Pathological Features

### Gross Features

Firm, fibrous mass with ill-defined or circumscribed borders.

### Microscopic Features

Low-grade myofibroblastic sarcoma is characterized by a diffusely infiltrative growth pattern and can extend along connective tissue septa or infiltrate between muscle bundles, similar to the pattern seen in fibromatosis. Fewer cases are well-circumscribed, with a pushing margin, including some reported in the breast. The tumor cells, which are arranged in a fascicular to storiform pattern, show typical myofibroblastic morphology, with spindled fusiform nuclei, vesicular chromatin, small nucleoli, and pale eosinophilic to amphophilic cytoplasm. Some cases superficially resemble nodular fasciitis, with a loose arrangement of lesional cells in a myxoid stroma containing extravasated red blood cells and scattered inflammatory cells. The vasculature is usually inconspicuous (Figs. 5.71, 5.72, and 5.73). By definition, low-grade myofibroblastic sarcoma does not have diffuse high-grade nuclear atypia and pleomorphism; however, some degree of nuclear atypia with hyperchromasia and increased mitotic activity is required to qualify for the diagnosis. Scattered enlarged pleomorphic cells may also be observed.

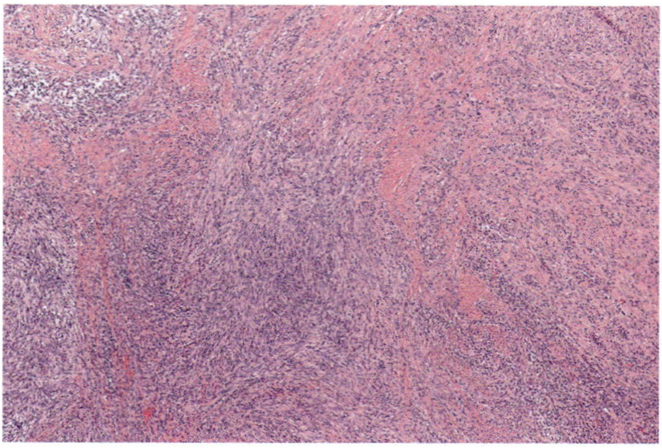

**Fig. 5.71** Low-grade myofibroblastic sarcoma composed of myofibroblastic cells arranged in a fascicular to storiform pattern, infiltrating between collagen bundles

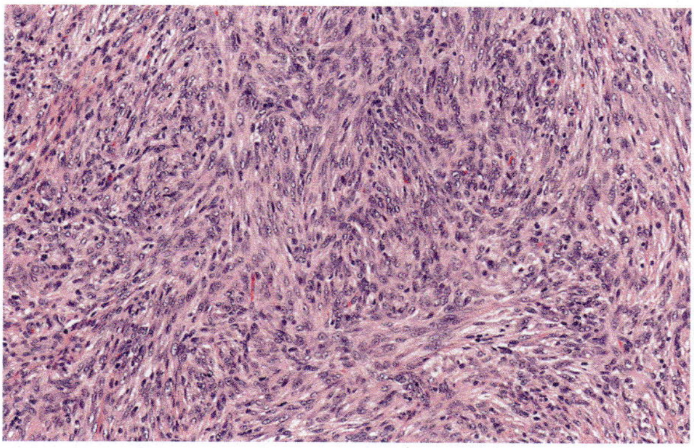

**Fig. 5.72** The spindle cells in LGMS show a typical myofibroblastic appearance with spindled fusiform nuclei, vesicular chromatin, small nucleoli, and pale eosinophilic to amphophilic cytoplasm. There is recognizable mild nuclear atypia but an overtly high-grade nuclear atypia and pleomorphism is not a feature in this tumor

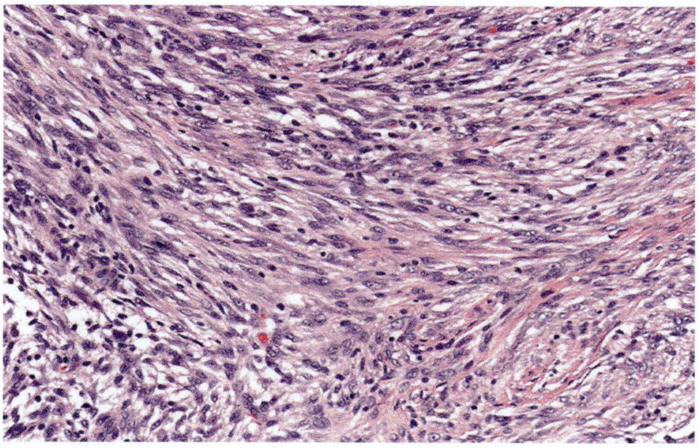

**Fig. 5.73** LGMS with a loose arrangement of the lesional cells resembling nodular fasciitis

## Immunohistochemistry

Low-grade myofibroblastic sarcoma shows the expected myofibroblastic immunophenotype, with variable staining for SMA, desmin, and calponin, usually in the characteristic membranous "tram-track" pattern typical of myofibroblasts. Epithelial markers, S100, h-caldesmon, and skeletal muscle markers are negative but nuclear expression of beta-catenin can occasionally be observed.

## Molecular

To date, no defining genetic aberrations have been identified for low-grade myofibroblastic sarcoma.

## Differential Diagnosis

The differential diagnosis for low-grade myofibroblastic sarcoma in the breast includes several lesions. Low-grade fibromatosis-like metaplastic carcinoma of the breast is the principal consideration. Unlike low-grade myofibroblastic sarcoma, low-grade fibromatosis-like metaplastic carcinoma is positive for cytokeratin stains, especially high molecular weight cytokeratins, and p63. Desmoid fibromatosis can also resemble low-grade myofibroblastic sarcoma in that both are composed of variable SMA and desmin-positive myofibroblastic fascicles with a markedly infiltrative pattern. However, low-grade myofibroblastic sarcoma is expected to have a much greater degree of nuclear atypia, including some nuclear hyperchromasia, and a higher mitotic index. Molecular testing for mutations in exon 3 of *CTNNB1* or alterations in *APC* can also be of great utility in this setting as a positive finding would be confirmatory for fibromatosis. Beta-catenin immunostaining should be interpreted with caution as nuclear immunoreactivity has been reported in low-grade myofibroblastic sarcoma.

Nodular fasciitis of the breast also often resembles low-grade myofibroblastic sarcoma architecturally and cytologically but just as was the case for fibromatosis, the degree of cytological atypia (especially hyperchromasia) is expected to be greater in low-grade myofibroblastic sarcoma than in nodular fasciitis. The mitotic activity in nodular fasciitis can approximate that of low-grade myofibroblastic sarcoma and is less helpful in this setting. As the immunoprofile of nodular fasciitis cannot distinguish it from low-grade myofibroblastic sarcoma, FISH or molecular testing for rearrangements involving *USP6* can be very helpful, as they are diagnostic of nodular fasciitis. Inflammatory myofibroblastic tumor can be distinguished based on a circumscribed growth pattern, a brisk chronic inflammatory infiltrate much in excess of what would be expected in nodular fasciitis or low-grade myofibroblastic sarcoma, and immunohistochemistry or FISH/molecular testing for *ALK* gene rearrangements. This distinction can be quite difficult on histological grounds alone, and confirmatory IHC and/or molecular testing is necessary to confidently separate inflammatory myofibroblastic tumor and low-grade myofibroblastic sarcoma.

Fibrosarcomatous DFSP can be easily separated based on the classical features of the precursor conventional component of the tumor. However, in limited material, testing for the *PDGFRB* or variant gene rearrangements may be very helpful, as it is pathognomonic for DFSP. Finally, the aforementioned adult fibrosarcoma and kinase fusion-based sarcomas can show a considerable degree of histological overlap with low-grade myofibroblastic sarcoma. However, given the fact that S100 and CD34 are frequently positive in kinase fusion-based fibrosarcomas and negative in low-grade myofibroblastic sarcoma, this distinction is less problematic than it may seem. In difficult cases, a sarcoma fusion panel including rearrangements involving the *NTRK* family of genes and *RET* can be of both diagnostic and theragnostic value, since rearrangements in these genes facilitate targeted therapy against their fusion products.

## Prognosis and Treatment

Due to its infiltrative nature, low-grade myofibroblastic sarcoma is prone to local recurrence, even after complete resection. Metastases are rare and usually associated with higher grade tumors. The tumor may progress to a high-grade myofibroblastic sarcoma, especially in recurrent cases.

# Soft Tissue Angiofibroma

## Clinical Features

Soft tissue angiofibroma is a low-grade fibroblastic tumor with a very low rate of local recurrence and no risk of metastasis. Soft tissue angiofibroma occurs over a large age range and shows a female predominance. Tumors present as painless deep-seated or superficial masses that may arise at a number of anatomical sites, most often upper and lower extremities. As examples of soft tissue angiofibroma arising in the breast and chest wall have already been reported, albeit in small numbers, we have included soft tissue angiofibroma in this chapter.

## Imaging

In the soft tissue, the imaging appearance of soft tissue angiofibroma is broad ranging from a well-circumscribed mass with benign characteristics to that with hypervascularity and ill-defined margins worrisome for malignancy.

## Pathologic Features

### Gross Features

A firm, rubbery to gelatinous mass, which can be well-circumscribed or multilobulated with infiltration of the surrounding tissues. The size ranges from 1 to 12 cm (median size, 5 cm).

### Microscopic Features

While soft tissue angiofibroma is often a circumscribed tumor, focal infiltration into the surrounding soft tissue may be seen (Fig. 5.74). The tumor is composed of bland, non-descript fibroblastic cells with ovoid nuclei, uniform chromatin, and pale eosinophilic cytoplasm, set within a loose myxoid to collagenous connective tissue matrix but thick collagenous bands as seen in some of its mimics like myofibroblastoma or solitary fibrous tumor, are uncharacteristic. The most striking feature of soft tissue angiofibroma is its vascularity, which is characterized by a rich network of evenly spaced curvilinear to branched small caliber vessels. Occasional additional

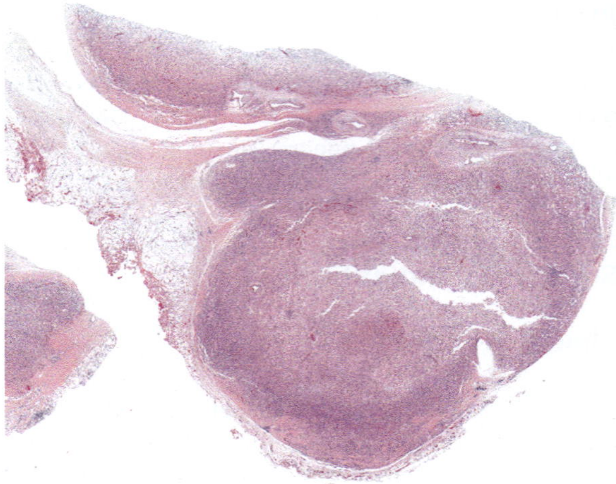

**Fig. 5.74** Soft tissue angiofibroma showing focal infiltration into the surrounding soft tissue at low magnification

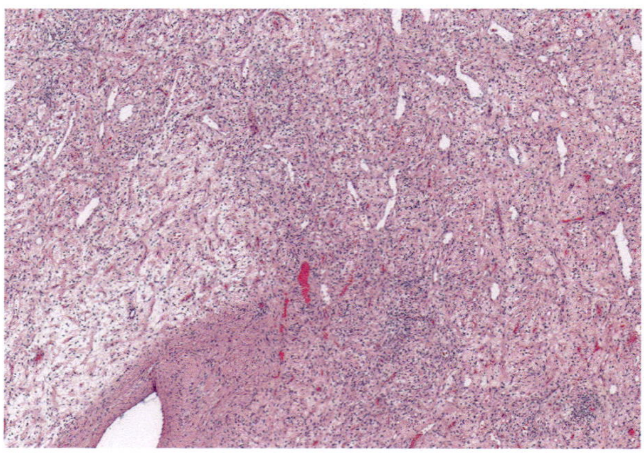

**Fig. 5.75** Soft tissue angiofibroma showing a very distinctive network of evenly spaced curvilinear to branched small caliber vessels admixed with staghorn vessels. Background stroma varies from myxoid to collagenous

vascular patterns may also be present, including medium to large-sized staghorn vessels, perivascular collagen deposition, and fibrinoid necrosis (Figs. 5.75 and 5.76). Nuclear atypia is typically absent, but degenerative atypia may be focally seen, typically accompanied by edema and other features of ischemic necrosis. Mitotic figures, if present at all, are not conspicuous (Fig. 5.77).

## Immunohistochemistry

As is often the case with translocation-driven neoplasms, soft tissue angiofibroma has a complex immunophenotype most frequently expressing estrogen receptor and CD163, EMA (approximately 50%) and, in about 10–20% of cases, SMA, desmin, and CD34 (often focally). Cytokeratins, S100 and SOX10, are consistently negative. Focal and weak STAT6 expression has been reported in 7% of cases and can be misleading.

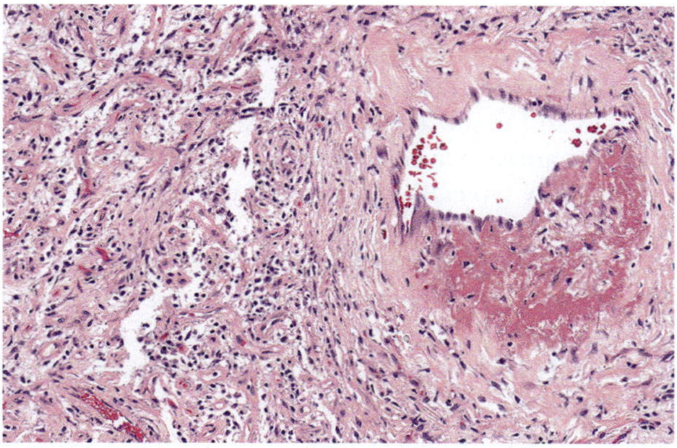

**Fig. 5.76** Soft tissue angiofibroma showing numerous small branching vessels and a large vessel with fibrinoid necrosis

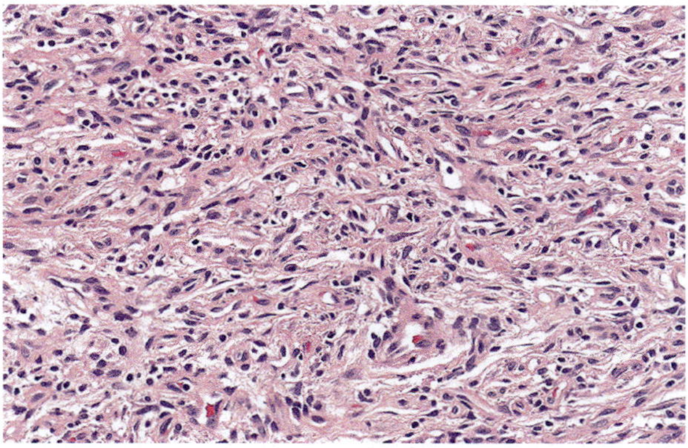

**Fig. 5.77** Soft tissue angiofibroma composed of bland, non-descript fibroblastic cells with ovoid nuclei, uniform chromatin, pale eosinophilic cytoplasm, and little mitotic activity

## Molecular

Molecularly, soft tissue angiofibroma harbors rearrangements involving *NCOA2* in more than half of the cases with *AHRR*, *GTF21,* and *ETV4* fusion partners; recently, a *GAB1-ABL1* fusion was also described. Of note, *NCOA2* IHC is a very sensitive marker of soft tissue angiofibroma but it lacks specificity.

## Differential Diagnosis

The most likely primary breast tumors to be confused with soft tissue angiofibroma are myofibroblastoma, especially the more myxoid examples, and solitary fibrous tumor (SFT). Myofibroblastoma has an overlapping immunoprofile (SMA, desmin, and estrogen receptor) and may occasionally show a prominent vascular pattern, though not typically to the extent seen in soft tissue angiofibroma. If necessary, Rb IHC (lost in myofibroblastoma) or molecular testing (for rearrangements in *NCOA2* for soft tissue angiofibroma and deletions in *RB1/FOXO1* for myofibroblastoma) can be performed. A staghorn vascular pattern in soft tissue angiofibroma can closely mimic an SFT. SFTs are usually more cellular and collagenous than soft tissue angiofibroma, and IHC for STAT6 can easily remedy this dilemma. STAT6 is usually strongly, diffusely positive in SFT but shows only focal staining in less than 10% of soft tissue angiofibroma cases. Of note, the prominent thick collagen bundles that are seen in both myofibroblastoma and SFT, and the extent of CD34 immunoreactivity typically encountered with both of these tumors, are not characteristic of soft tissue angiofibroma.

Soft tissue angiofibroma can mimic low-grade malignant tumors such as low-grade fibromatosis-like metaplastic carcinoma or low-grade fibromyxoid sarcomas. Low-grade fibromatosis-like metaplastic carcinoma is positive for cytokeratins (especially high molecular weight cytokeratins), which are expected to be negative in soft tissue angiofibroma. Low-grade fibromyxoid sarcomas are positive for MUC4 by IHC, which is highly sensitive and specific in this setting. FISH or molecular testing for rearrangements in *FUS* and *EWSR1* (LGFMS) or *NCOA2* (soft tissue angiofibroma) may help to distinguish these tumors.

## Prognosis and Treatment

Soft tissue angiofibromas are benign but local recurrence has been reported in a small subset of cases. Treatment is surgical excision.

## Selected References


1. Adem C, Reynolds C, Ingle JN, Nascimento AG. Primary breast sarcoma: clinicopathologic series from the Mayo Clinic and review of the literature. Br J Cancer. 2004;91(2):237–41.
2. Antonescu CR. Emerging soft tissue tumors with kinase fusions: an overview of the recent literature with an emphasis on diagnostic criteria. Genes Chromosomes Cancer. 2020;59(8):437–44.
3. Bahrami A, Folpe AL. Adult-type fibrosarcoma: a reevaluation of 163 putative cases diagnosed at a single institution over a 48-year period. Am J Surg Pathol. 2010;34(10):1504–13.
4. Billings SD, Giblen G, Fanburg-Smith JC. Superficial low-grade fibromyxoid sarcoma (Evans tumor): a clinicopathologic analysis of 19 cases with a unique observation in the pediatric population. Am J Surg Pathol. 2005;29(2):204–10.
5. Bosse K, Ott C, Biegner T, Fend F, Siegmann-Luz K, Wallwiener D, Hahn M. 23-year-old female with an inflammatory myofibroblastic tumour of the breast: a case report and a review of the literature. Geburtshilfe Frauenheilkd. 2014;74(2):167–70. PMID: 24741129
6. Bowman E, Oprea G, Okoli J, Gundry K, Rizzo M, Gabram-Mendola S, Manne U, Smith G, Pambuccian S, Bumpers HL. Pseudoangiomatous stromal hyperplasia (PASH) of the breast: a series of 24 patients. Breast J. 2012;18(3):242–7. PMID: 22583194.
7. Calonje E, Guerin D, McCormick D, Fletcher CD. Superficial angiomyxoma: clinicopathologic analysis of a series of distinctive but poorly recognized cutaneous tumors with tendency for recurrence. Am J Surg Pathol. 1999;23(8):910–7.
8. Calonje E, Mentzel T, Fletcher CD. Cellular benign fibrous histiocytoma. Clinicopathologic analysis of 74 cases of a distinctive variant of cutaneous fibrous histiocytoma with frequent recurrence. Am J Surg Pathol. 1994;18(7):668–76.
9. Cheah AL, Billings SD, Rowe JJ. Mesenchymal tumours of the breast and their mimics: a review with approach to diagnosis. Pathology. 2016;48(5):406–24. Epub 2016 Jun 16

10. Colombo C, Urbini M, Astolfi A, Collini P, Indio V, Belfiore A, Paielli N, Perrone F, Tarantino G, Palassini E, Fiore M, Pession A, Stacchiotti S, Pantaleo MA, Gronchi A. Novel intragenic large deletions of CTNNB1 gene identified in WT desmoid-type fibromatosis. Genes Chromosomes Cancer. 2018;57(10):495–503.
11. D'Alfonso TM, Subramaniyam S, Ginter PS, Mosquera JM, Croyle J, Liu YF, Rubin MA, Shin SJ. Characterization of CD34-deficient myofibroblastomas of the breast. Breast J. 2018;24(1):55–61. Epub 2017 May 30
12. D'Alfonso TM, Subramaniyam S, Ginter PS, Mosquera JM, MacDonald TY, Noorzad Z, Orta LY, Liu YF, Rubin MA, Shin SJ. Characterization of the leiomyomatous variant of myofibroblastoma: a rare subset distinct from other smooth muscle tumors of the breast. Hum Pathol. 2016;58:54–61.
13. Desmoid Tumor Working Group. The management of desmoid tumours: a joint global consensus-based guideline approach for adult and paediatric patients. Eur J Cancer. 2020;127:96–107.
14. Dickson BC, Hornick JL, Fletcher CDM, Demicco EG, Howarth DJ, Swanson D, Zhang L, Sung YS, Antonescu CR. Dermatofibrosarcoma protuberans with a novel COL6A3-PDGFD fusion gene and apparent predilection for breast. Genes Chromosomes Cancer. 2018;57(9):437–45.
15. Doyle LA, Möller E, Dal Cin P, Fletcher CD, Mertens F, Hornick JL. MUC4 is a highly sensitive and specific marker for low-grade fibromyxoid sarcoma. Am J Surg Pathol. 2011;35(5):733–41.
16. Drinka EK, Bargaje A, Erşahin ÇH, Patel P, Salhadar A, Sinacore J, Rajan P. Pseudoangiomatous stromal hyperplasia (PASH) of the breast: a clinicopathological study of 79 cases. Int J Surg Pathol. 2012;20(1):54–8.
17. East EG, Carter CS, Sciallis AP. Cellular spindled Histiocytic Pseudotumor: a benign mimic of spindle cell Neoplasia of the breast. Arch Pathol Lab Med. 2019;143(12):1497–503.
18. Erber R, Agaimy A. Misses and near misses in diagnosing nodular fasciitis and morphologically related reactive myofibroblastic proliferations: experience of a referral center with emphasis on frequency of USP6 gene rearrangements. Virchows Arch. 2018;473(3):351–60. PMID: 29623468.
19. Hartel PH, Bratthauer G, Hartel JV, Fanburg-Smith JC. Primary malignant fibrous histiocytoma (myxofibrosarcoma/pleomorphic sarcoma not otherwise specified) of the breast: clinicopathologic study of 19 cases. Ann Diagn Pathol. 2011;15(6):407–13.
20. Howitt BE, Fletcher CD. Mammary-type myofibroblastoma: clinicopathologic characterization in a series of 143 cases. Am J Surg Pathol. 2016;40(3):361–7.
21. Jones KN, Glazebrook KN, Reynolds C. Pseudoangiomatous stromal hyperplasia: imaging findings with pathologic and clinical correlation. AJR Am J Roentgenol. 2010;195(4):1036–42.
22. Lacroix-Triki M, Geyer FC, Lambros MB, Savage K, Ellis IO, Lee AH, Reis-Filho JS. β-Catenin/Wnt signalling pathway in fibromatosis, metaplastic carcinomas and phyllodes tumours of the breast. Mod Pathol. 2010;23(11):1438–48.
23. Magro G, Angelico G, Righi A, Benini S, Salvatorelli L, Palazzo J. Utility of STAT6 and 13q14 deletion in the classification of the benign spindle cell stromal tumors of the breast. Hum Pathol. 2018;81:55–64.
24. Magro G. Mammary myofibroblastoma: an update with emphasis on the most diagnostically challenging variants. Histol Histopathol. 2016;31(1):1–23.
25. Mariño-Enríquez A, Fletcher CD. Angiofibroma of soft tissue: clinicopathologic characterization of a distinctive benign fibrovascular neoplasm in a series of 37 cases. Am J Surg Pathol. 2012;36(4):500–8.
26. Mentzel T, Calonje E, Wadden C, Camplejohn RS, Beham A, Smith MA, Fletcher CD. Myxofibrosarcoma. Clinicopathologic analysis of 75 cases with emphasis on the low-grade variant. Am J Surg Pathol. 1996;20(4):391–405.
27. Michal M, Ludvíková M, Zámecník M. Nodular mucinosis of the breast: report of three cases. Pathol Int. 1998;48(7):542–4.
28. Mindiola-Romero AE, Maloney N, Bridge JA, Korkolopoulou P, Sakellariou S, Linos K. A concise review of angiofibroma of soft tissue: a rare newly described entity that can be encountered by dermatopathologists. J Cutan Pathol. 2020;47(2):179–85.

29. Montgomery E, Goldblum JR, Fisher C. Myofibrosarcoma: a clinicopathologic study. Am J Surg Pathol. 2001;25(2):219–28.
30. Myong NH, Min JW. Low-grade myofibroblastic sarcoma arising in fibroadenoma of the breast-a case report. Diagn Pathol. 2016;11:33. https://doi.org/10.1186/s13000-016-0480-8.
31. Norkowski E, Masliah-Planchon J, Le Guellec S, Trassard M, Courrèges JB, Charron-Barra C, Terrier P, Bonvalot S, Coindre JM, Laé M. Lower rate of CTNNB1 mutations and higher rate of APC mutations in desmoid fibromatosis of the breast: a series of 134 tumors. Am J Surg Pathol. 2020;44(9):1266–73.
32. Paliogiannis P, Cossu A, Palmieri G, Scognamillo F, Pala C, Nonnis R, Sotgiu G, Fois A, Palomba G, Attene F. Breast nodular fasciitis: a comprehensive review. Breast Care (Basel). 2016;11(4):270–4. PMID: 27721715.
33. Patel KU, Szabo SS, Hernandez VS, Prieto VG, Abruzzo LV, Lazar AJ, López-Terrada D. Dermatofibrosarcoma protuberans COL1A1-PDGFB fusion is identified in virtually all dermatofibrosarcoma protuberans cases when investigated by newly developed multiplex reverse transcription polymerase chain reaction and fluorescence in situ hybridization assays. Hum Pathol. 2008;39(2):184–93.
34. Sandberg AA, Anderson WD, Fredenberg C, Hashimoto H. Dermatofibrosarcoma protuberans of breast. Cancer Genet Cytogenet. 2003;142(1):56–9.
35. Schwartz CJ, Schandl CA, Morse J, Ralston J, Rapkiewicz A, Darvishian F. Benign Fibromyxoid lesion of the breast: a distinct entity from benign spindle cell tumors of the mammary Stroma? Int J Surg Pathol. 2018;26(6):488–93.
36. Sciallis AP, Chen B, Folpe AL. Cellular spindled histiocytic pseudotumor complicating mammary fat necrosis: a potential diagnostic pitfall. Am J Surg Pathol. 2012;36(10):1571–8.
37. Sfeir MM, Schuetz A, Van Besien K, Borczuk AC, Soave R, Jenkins SG, Walsh TJ, Small CB. Mycobacterial spindle cell pseudotumour: epidemiology and clinical outcomes. J Clin Pathol. 2018;71(7):626–30.
38. Strait AM, Linos K, Tafe LJ, Muller KE. A novel case of mammary-type myofibroblastoma with sarcomatous features. Int J Surg Pathol. 2020.
39. Suurmeijer AJH, Dickson BC, Swanson D, Zhang L, Sung YS, Cotzia P, Fletcher CDM, Antonescu CR. A novel group of spindle cell tumors defined by S100 and CD34 co-expression shows recurrent fusions involving RAF1, BRAF, and NTRK1/2 genes. Genes Chromosomes Cancer. 2018;57(12):611–21. PMID: 30276917.
40. Suurmeijer AJH, Kao YC, Antonescu CR. New advances in the molecular classification of pediatric mesenchymal tumors. Genes Chromosomes Cancer. 2019;58(2):100–10. PMID: 30187985.
41. Taccagni G, Rovere E, Masullo M, Christensen L, Eyden B. Myofibrosarcoma of the breast: review of the literature on myofibroblastic tumors and criteria for defining myofibroblastic differentiation. Am J Surg Pathol. 1997;21(4):489–96.
42. Tan PH, Harada O, Thike AA, Tse GM. Histiocytoid breast carcinoma: an enigmatic lobular entity. J Clin Pathol. 2011;64(8):654–9.
43. Virk RK, Khan A. Pseudoangiomatous stromal hyperplasia: an overview. Arch Pathol Lab Med. 2010;134(7):1070–4.
44. Volpicelli ER, Fletcher CD. Desmin and CD34 positivity in cellular fibrous histiocytoma: an immunohistochemical analysis of 100 cases. J Cutan Pathol. 2012;39(8):747–52.
45. Walther C, Hofvander J, Nilsson J, Magnusson L, Domanski HA, Gisselsson D, Tayebwa J, Doyle LA, Fletcher CD, Mertens F. Gene fusion detection in formalin-fixed paraffin-embedded benign fibrous histiocytomas using fluorescence in situ hybridization and RNA sequencing. Lab Investig. 2015;95(9):1071–6.
46. Warmke LM, Meis JM. Sclerosing epithelioid fibrosarcoma: a distinct sarcoma with aggressive features. Am J Surg Pathol. 2020.
47. Xu J, Weisman P. Dedifferentiated secretory breast carcinoma with fibrosarcomatous features harboring an ETV6-NTRK3 fusion in both components. Genes Chromosomes Cancer 2020; 20.

48. Zhang Y, Wan D, Gao F. Primary low-grade fibromyxoid sarcoma of the breast: a rare case report with immunohistochemical and fluorescence in situ hybridization detection. Hum Pathol. 2018;79:208–11.
49. Zhao HD, Wu T, Wang JQ, Zhang WD, He XL, Bao GQ, Li Y, Gong L, Wang Q. Primary inflammatory myofibroblastic tumor of the breast with rapid recurrence and metastasis: a case report. Oncol Lett. 2013;5(1):97–100. PMID: 23255901.
50. Zhou Y, Zhu J, Zhang Y, Jiang J, Jia M. An inflammatory myofibroblastic tumour of the breast with ALK overexpression. BMJ Case Rep. 2013;4:2013. PMID: 23386486.

# Adipocytic Tumors

# 6

Alison L. Cheah

## Contents



A. L. Cheah (✉)
Douglass Hanly Moir Pathology, Department of Histopathology,
Macquarie Park, NSW, Australia
e-mail: acheah@dhm.com.au



J. J. Rowe, E. Downs-Kelly (eds.), *Mesenchymal Tumors of the Breast and Their Mimics*, https://doi.org/10.1007/978-3-030-74474-8_6

## Reactive Processes with Prominent Fat

### Fat Necrosis

#### Clinical Features

Some patients have a history of prior trauma or surgery; however, most cases have no known history of antecedent injury or intervention.

## Imaging

Fat necrosis is often a mimic of a malignancy clinically and mammographically owing to its presentation as a firm mass that may be spiculated and associated with calcifications.

## Pathologic Features

**Gross Features** Early fat necrosis is typically an area of indurated fat with hemorrhage. More mature lesions are mass-like with a firm, heterogeneous yellow-gray cut surface and variable cystic change.

**Microscopic Features** The histologic appearances depend on the time course of the lesion. In early fat necrosis, zones filled with lipid, hemorrhage, and cystic spaces of various sizes are surrounded by a histiocytic and foreign body-type giant cell response (Fig. 6.1). Lipomembranous fat necrosis is a variant in which densely eosinophilic membranes outline the residua of necrotic adipocytes. Older lesions have a dense collagenous stroma or scar-like appearance, often with hemosiderin deposition and dystrophic calcification, and may be entirely cystic.

## Immunohistochemistry

By immunohistochemistry, the lipid-laden histiocytes are positive for CD68 and CD163. One caveat to bear in mind is that CD68 is not lineage-specific and will highlight cells that have abundant lysosomes.

## Differential Diagnosis

Granular cell tumor and some carcinomas with granular cytoplasm are among tumors in which CD68 is expressed. A cytokeratin stain should readily exclude the possibility of histiocytoid carcinoma.

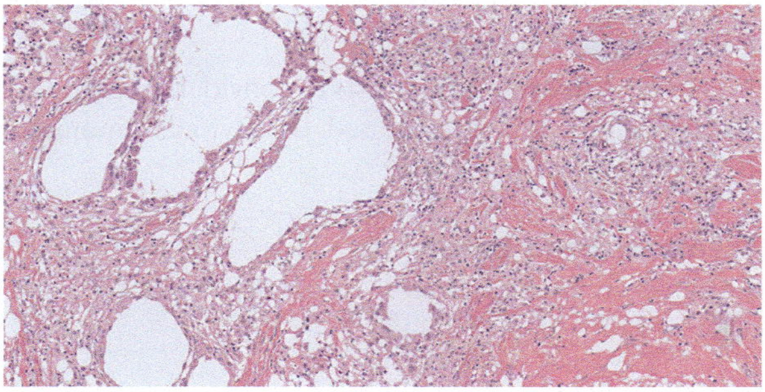

**Fig. 6.1** Fat necrosis. Cystic spaces and sheets of foamy histiocytes are characteristic early in the course of the lesion

#### Treatment and Prognosis

Fat necrosis is benign and no definitive treatment is necessary.

## Benign Adipocytic Tumors Occurring in Breast

### Lipoma

#### Clinical Features

Conventional lipoma is the most commonly encountered adipocytic tumor in the breast and is indistinguishable from lipomas in other sites. The usual presentation is a superficial palpable mass reflecting frequent origin in the subcutis.

#### Imaging

The typical appearance is that of a discrete, encapsulated homogeneous fatty mass.

#### Pathologic Features

**Gross Features** Lipomas are lobulated masses of homogeneous yellow adipose tissue surrounded by a thin capsule.

**Microscopic Features** Histologically, breast lipomas are characterized by mature fat surrounded by a delicate fibrous capsule in the absence of ducts and lobular units (Fig. 6.2). It may not be possible to make an unequivocal diagnosis of lipoma on core biopsy, particularly since biopsies of prominent fatty lobules in post-menopausal breasts can show a similar appearance.

#### Immunohistochemistry

Immunohistochemistry is generally not necessary in the diagnosis of lipoma.

#### Molecular Features

Lipomas lack amplification of MDM2.

#### Differential Diagnosis

The main differential diagnosis to consider in samples of mature lipomatous lesions, particularly when deep-seated, is atypical lipomatous tumor/well-differentiated liposarcoma (see below).

#### Treatment and Prognosis

Lipomas are benign. Simple excision is curative.

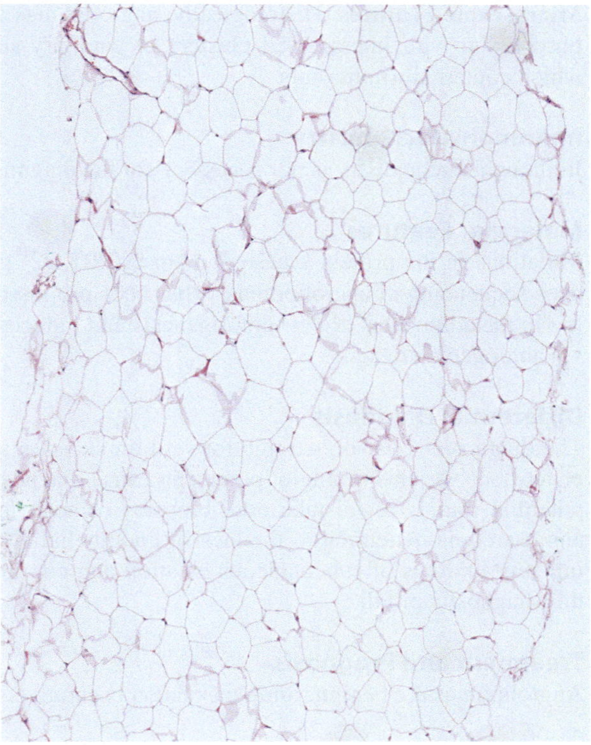

**Fig. 6.2** Lipoma. It may not be possible to make an unequivocal diagnosis of lipoma on core biopsy since prominent fat lobules in post-menopausal breast can show a similar appearance

## Angiolipoma

### Clinical Features

Angiolipomas are encountered not infrequently in the trunk wall, including subcutaneous tissue overlying the breast. They commonly occur as multiple lesions and may be tender.

### Imaging

There is no typical radiographic appearance. Angiolipomas may be indistinguishable from lipomas. Prominent vascularity may be detected.

### Pathologic Features

**Gross Features** Angiolipomas are encapsulated masses of yellow adipose tissue which may be grossly indistinguishable from lipomas. They may have a slightly reddish hue, depending on the proportion of vessels present.

**Microscopic Features** Histologically, angiolipomas are composed of mature adipose tissue with interspersed clusters of capillary-sized blood vessels, some of which contain fibrin thrombi.

### Immunohistochemistry

Immunohistochemistry is not necessary for the diagnosis of angiolipoma.

### Molecular Features

Mutations in the protein kinase domain 2 (PRKD2) gene have been identified by deep sequencing of angiolipomas. It has been proposed that altered PRKD2 signaling in the adipocytes drives tumorigenesis and induces secondary vessel formation via angiogenic effects.

### Differential Diagnosis

The diagnosis is usually straightforward on excision specimens; however, cellular or fat-poor variants of angiolipoma can cause diagnostic difficulty (Fig. 6.3). One potential trap is to mistake core biopsies of such lesions as well-differentiated angiosarcoma. Attention to the lack of endothelial atypia and correlation with the imaging findings of subcutaneous location and circumscription should help avoid this diagnostic pitfall.

### Treatment and Prognosis

Angiolipomas are benign. Simple excision is curative.

## Hibernoma

### Clinical Features

Mammary hibernoma is extremely rare, accounting for less than 2% of all hibernomas. They typically present as slow-growing painless masses.

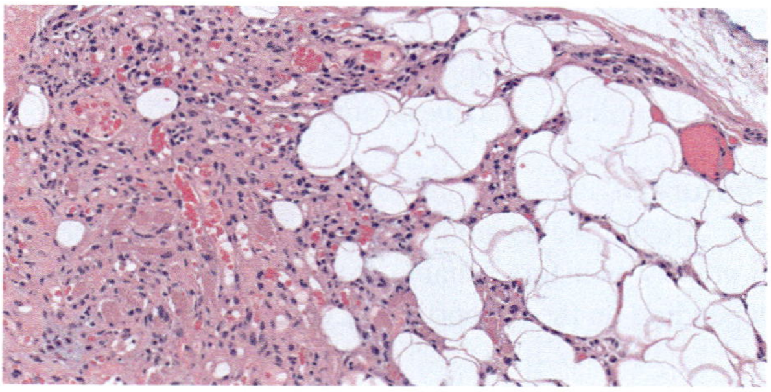

**Fig. 6.3** Angiolipoma in subcutaneous tissue overlying breast. Core biopsies of cellular angiolipomas can be confused with angiosarcoma if the subcutaneous location and circumscription is not recognized. Note the presence of numerous fibrin thrombi

## Imaging

On mammography, hibernomas are radiodense relative to the surrounding fatty breast tissue and on ultrasound appear as well-circumscribed hyperechoic lesions with increased vascularity. Hibernomas show signal intensity intermediate between skeletal muscle and subcutaneous fat on MRI studies and contrast enhancement due to their rich vascularity. Unlike conventional lipomas, lipomas are fluorodeoxyglucose (FDG)-avid on positron emission tomography (PET) scan due to their abundant mitochondria.

## Pathologic Features

**Gross Features** On gross examination, hibernomas are tan to brown in color.

**Microscopic Features** Histologically, they are circumscribed proliferations of adipocytes with finely vacuolated eosinophilic cytoplasm and central round nuclei, consistent with brown fat (Fig. 6.4). The proportion of brown fat is variable and may account for part or most of the tumor. A subset of hibernomas contain predominantly mature fat and only a minor component of brown fat (so-called "lipoma-like" variants).

## Immunohistochemistry

Hibernomas are positive for S100 protein.

## Molecular Features

Hibernomas show simultaneous loss of the tumor suppressor genes *MEN1* and *AIP* as a result of translocations involving chromosome 11q13. Loss of *AIP* in particular is thought to drive the brown fat phenotype.

## Differential Diagnosis

Attention to the morphologic features on hematoxylin and eosin-stained slides should lead to the correct diagnosis. Hibernomas are positive for S100 and this may

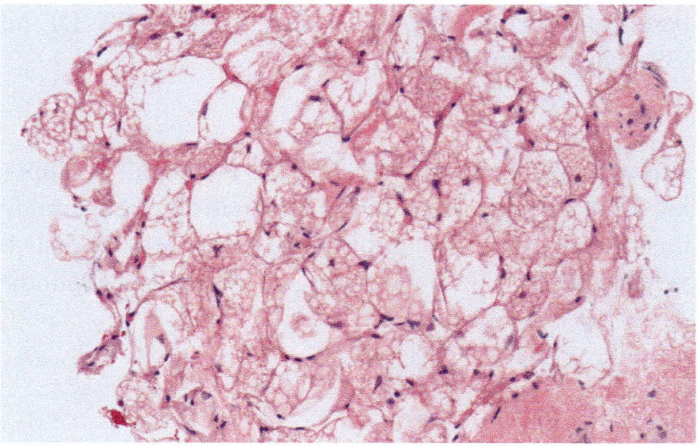

**Fig. 6.4** Hibernoma of breast consisting of finely vacuolated eosinophilic cells

cause confusion with granular cell tumor. Granular cell tumors are generally less well-circumscribed and have coarsely granular cytoplasm as opposed to the microvesicular cytoplasm present in hibernomas.

### Treatment and Prognosis

Hibernomas are benign. Simple excision is curative.

## Liposarcomas Occurring in Breast

True liposarcomas arising de novo within breast parenchyma are distinctly rare. The diagnosis of primary liposarcoma of the breast should only be made after thorough sampling to exclude a fibroepithelial lesion as liposarcomatous tumours encountered in breast most often represent heterologous differentiation in a malignant phyllodes tumor. Depending on the context, application of molecular diagnostic techniques such as FISH for *MDM2* amplification or *DDIT3* rearrangement is also helpful (see below).

### Atypical Lipomatous Tumor/Well-Differentiated Liposarcoma (ALT/WDL)

#### Clinical Features

ALT/WDL can rarely occur in the mammary parenchyma, or it may arise as an intramuscular mass within the pectoralis muscle, mimicking a primary breast tumor.

#### Imaging

MRI features that raise suspicion for ALT/WDL include thickened or nodular septa, prominent foci of high T2-weighted signal, non-fatty areas, and prominent areas of contrast enhancement.

#### Pathologic Features

**Gross Features** ALT/WDL is often a large, multinodular fatty tumor with fibrous bands and variable myxoid zones. Some ALT/WDL may be macroscopically indistinguishable from lipoma.

**Microscopic Features** ALT/WDL is typically composed of mature fat with irregular fibrous septa and scattered hyperchromatic pleomorphic cells within a loose collagenous matrix. The atypical cells are variably distributed; they may be focal and very difficult to find, consisting of rare cells surrounding blood vessels (Fig. 6.5).

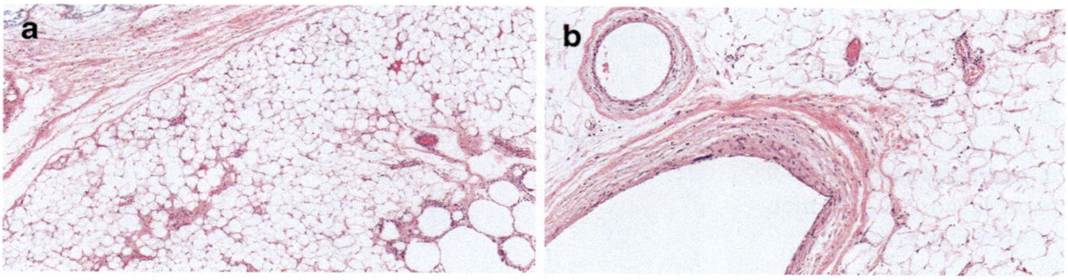


**Fig. 6.5** Atypical lipomatous tumor in breast/chest wall, positive for MDM2 amplification by FISH. (**a**) The tumor is composed of mature adipose tissue with fat necrosis and fibrous septae containing mildly atypical spindle cells. (**b**) Atypical cells focally within blood vessel walls

### Immunohistochemistry

Immunohistochemistry for MDM2 and CDK4 may be used as a surrogate for molecular testing; however, in our experience, immunohistochemistry for these markers has been difficult to optimize and interpret in lipomatous lesions.

### Molecular Features

The cytogenetic alterations that are characteristic of ALT/WDL are supernumerary ring or giant chromosomes derived from the long arm of chromosome 12. This abnormality results in amplification of chromosomal region 12q13-15, which includes the *MDM2* gene locus. A positive FISH study for *MDM2* amplification supports a diagnosis of ALT/WDL because *MDM2* amplification is not seen in lipoma or the liposarcomatous differentiation in phyllodes tumor. FISH analysis for *MDM2* amplification should be considered for any large deep-seated lipomatous tumor in the breast or chest wall, especially in tumors lacking convincing atypia and in which breast epithelial elements are absent.

### Differential Diagnosis

At the most well-differentiated end of the spectrum, tumors with minimal or no atypia may resemble a lipoma. Thorough sampling is prudent to ensure that the atypical areas are submitted for microscopic examination. Dedifferentiation is characterized by non-lipogenic zones typically accompanied by increased cellularity and mitotic activity (Fig. 6.6).

### Treatment and Prognosis

ALT/WDL shows a high rate of local recurrence, in part, due to the difficulty in distinguishing neoplastic fat from normal adipose tissue of the breast. The usual treatment is local excision and clinical follow-up. Unless there is evidence of dedifferentiation, there is no risk of metastasis.

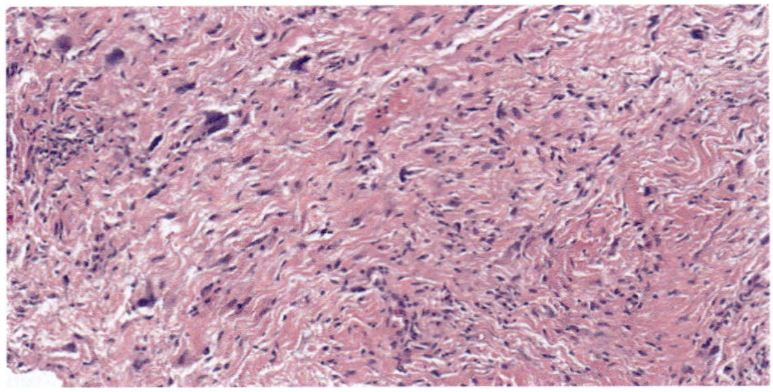

**Fig. 6.6** Dedifferentiated liposarcoma in axillary tail. The tumor is non-lipogenic and consists of pleomorphic spindled cells in a collagenous background. Amplification of MDM2 was detected by FISH

## Myxoid Liposarcoma

### Clinical Features

The presentation of myxoid liposarcoma as a primary breast tumor is highly unusual and should prompt consideration of a metastasis or component of a malignant phyllodes tumor. The concern for a metastasis to the breast is based on the known proclivity of myxoid liposarcoma to metastasize to other soft tissue sites. On occasion, the breast tumor may represent a solitary metastasis of myxoid liposarcoma of the extremity.

### Imaging

Myxoid liposarcomas are uniformly T1 isointense and T2 hyperintense lesions. T2 heterogeneity may be present. There may be thick internal septations. They mostly show intense contrast enhancement. A small amount of visible fat may be present. Imaging of the extremities to exclude an extramammary primary is most helpful.

### Pathologic Features

**Gross Features** The cut surface of myxoid liposarcoma is nodular and gelatinous. Tumors with high-grade areas may show a solid, fleshy component.

**Microscopic Features** Histologically, myxoid liposarcoma is composed of small hyperchromatic spindle cells in an abundant myxoid stroma containing a delicate plexiform capillary vasculature. A variable number of lipoblasts are present, usually univacuolar in type, typically at the edge of tumor nodules. High-grade transformation may take the form of round cell change with increased cellularity, overlapping tumor nuclei, greater nuclear atypia, and mitotic activity. Spindle cell and pleomorphic features may occasionally be present. A hypercellular/round cell component that comprises more than 5% of the tumor is considered an adverse prognostic factor. In our practice, we include an estimate of the percentage of the high-grade component in the diagnostic line for myxoid liposarcoma.

### Immunohistochemistry

Immunohistochemistry does not play a major role in the diagnosis of myxoid liposarcoma. The lesional cells are positive for S100 protein.

### Molecular Features

The characteristic cytogenetic alteration in myxoid liposarcoma is a t(12;16) translocation resulting in *FUS-DDIT3* fusion gene. In a small subset of cases, *EWSR1-DDIT3* fusions have been demonstrated. FISH for *DDIT3* gene rearrangement can be performed in ambiguous cases to confirm the diagnosis of myxoid liposarcoma, particularly in core biopsy specimens.

### Differential Diagnosis

If the breast is the primary site, liposarcomatous differentiation in a phyllodes tumor is a major consideration, and thorough sampling to identify epithelial elements would be desirable. A subset of dedifferentiated liposarcomas can also show areas resembling myxoid liposarcoma (particularly if DDIT3 is co-amplified, as it lies within the 12q13-15 amplicon that includes MDM2 and CDK4). Dedifferentiated liposarcoma typically shows greater morphologic heterogeneity than myxoid liposarcoma, and scrutiny of the background fat may show features of ALT/WDL. In difficult cases, FISH analysis for MDM2 amplification and DDIT3 rearrangement should allow distinction.

### Treatment and Prognosis

Myxoid liposarcoma metastasizes to lung, bone, and distant soft tissue locations including abdominal cavity. The amount of high-grade/round cell component correlates with metastasis and adverse outcome. Wide excision is the treatment of choice. Adjuvant therapy may be considered for high-grade, unresectable, or metastatic tumors. Options include radiotherapy and/or chemotherapy including anthracycline-based regimens and newer agents such as trabectedin and eribulin.

## Pleomorphic Liposarcoma

### Clinical Features

Pleomorphic liposarcoma is a less commonly encountered liposarcoma subtype in the breast. Rare cases have arisen as radiation-induced sarcomas. Areas resembling pleomorphic liposarcoma can also be encountered as a component of malignant phyllodes tumor.

### Imaging

There are no specific imaging characteristics. Pleomorphic liposarcoma tends to be heterogeneously T2 hyperintense with intense contrast enhancement. There is commonly peritumoral edema, intratumoral hemorrhage, and necrosis.

### Pathologic Features

**Gross Features** Pleomorphic liposarcoma resembles other high-grade sarcomas grossly. The cut surface is fleshy and variably myxoid. Necrosis and hemorrhage may be present. Fat is often not evident.

**Microscopic Features** A variety of histologic appearances may be present, including spindled, pleomorphic, or epithelioid; however, the defining histological feature is the presence of often bizarre-appearing pleomorphic lipoblasts. These unusual cells may be focal, reinforcing the need for adequate sampling and thorough examination of an apparently undifferentiated tumor for a line of differentiation.

### Immunohistochemistry

Immunohistochemical studies are generally not helpful. One pitfall is the presence of cytokeratin immunoreactivity in the epithelioid variant of pleomorphic liposarcoma potentially causing confusion with a poorly differentiated or metaplastic carcinoma.

### Molecular Features

Pleomorphic liposarcoma shows a complex karyotype and is not known to harbor recurrent chromosomal translocations that would aid in diagnosis.

### Differential Diagnosis

Exclusion of dedifferentiated liposarcoma with homologous lipoblastic (pleomorphic liposarcoma-like) dedifferentiation could be considered in ambiguous cases with the aid of FISH for *MDM2* amplification.

### Treatment and Prognosis

The clinical behavior of pleomorphic liposarcoma is usually that of a high-grade sarcoma, with a 5-year mortality rate of 60%. The mainstay of therapy is wide resection or mastectomy. Involvement of axillary lymph nodes has not been reported and axillary lymph node sampling is not recommended.

## Mammary Tumors with Adipocytic Components

Myofibroblastoma (Fig. 6.7), phyllodes tumors (Fig. 6.8), and periductal stromal tumors (Fig. 6.9) are all mammary tumors containing varying proportions of adipocytes. All of these neoplasms are discussed individually within their respective chapters.

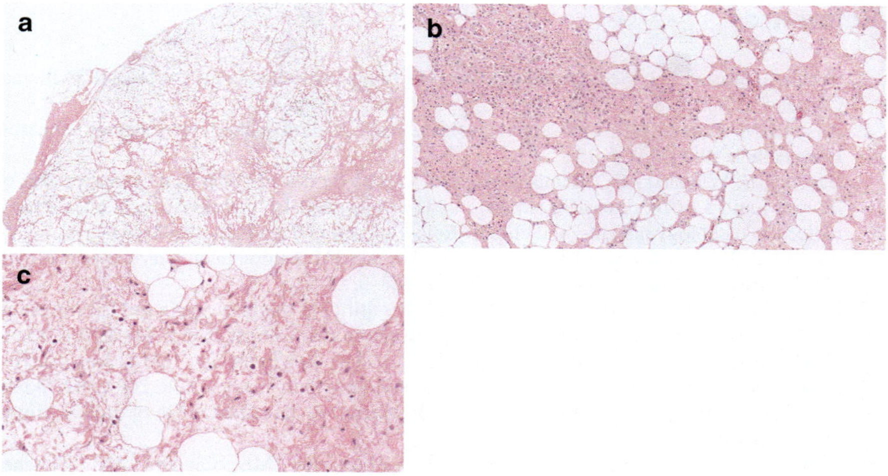


**Fig. 6.7** Lipomatous epithelioid myofibroblastoma. (**a**) The adipose tissue component in myofibroblastoma can be so prominent that it resembles a lipomatous neoplasm. (**b**) The tumor cells are epithelioid in a lightly collagenous background. (**c**) Focal areas show myxoid zones with ropey collagen fibers and mast cells, reminiscent of spindle cell lipoma

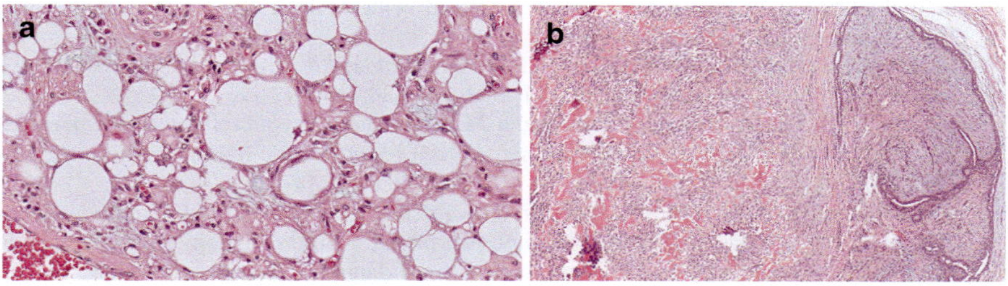


**Fig. 6.8** Malignant phyllodes tumor with liposarcomatous differentiation. (**a**) The liposarcomatous component consists of pleomorphic liposarcoma-like areas. (**b**) Zones of osteosarcomatous differentiation are also present

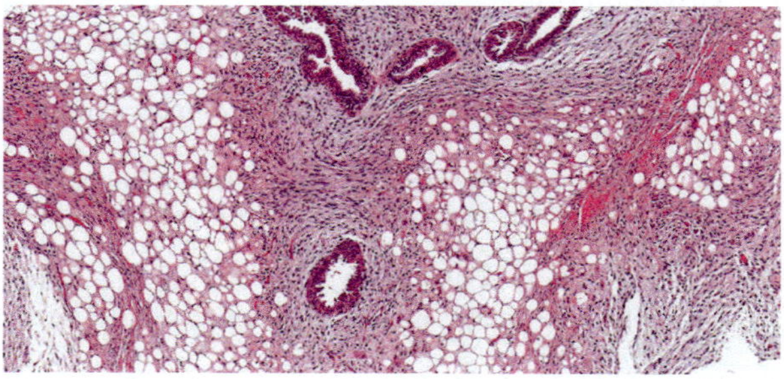

**Fig. 6.9** Periductal stromal sarcoma. Periductal cuffs of atypical stromal cells and associated fat, most likely representing entrapped adipose tissue

## References


1. Arbabi L, Warhol MJ. Pleomorphic liposarcoma following radiotherapy for breast carcinoma. Cancer. 1982;49:878–80.
2. Austin RM, Dupree WB. Liposarcoma of the breast: a clinicopathologic study of 20 cases. Hum Pathol. 1986;17:906–13.
3. Bacchi CE, Wludarski SC, Lamovec J, et al. Lipophyllodes of the breast. A reappraisal of fat-rich tumors of the breast based on 22 cases integrated by immunohistochemical study, molecular pathology insights, and clinical follow-up. Ann Diagn Pathol. 2016;21:1–6.
4. Baxendine-Jones J, Baldwin LJ, Bateman AC, Theaker JM. Predominant fatty variant of myofibroblastoma of breast. J Clin Pathol. 2001;54:568–9.
5. Downs-Kelly E, Goldblum JR, Patel RM, et al. The utility of fluorescence in situ hybridization (FISH) in the diagnosis of myxoid soft tissue neoplasms. Am J Surg Pathol. 2008;32:8–13.
6. Gaskin CM, Helms CA. Lipomas, lipoma variants, and well-differentiated liposarcomas (atypical lipomas): results of MRI evaluations of 126 consecutive fatty masses. AJR. 2004;182:733–9.
7. Hofvander J, Arbajian E, Stenkula KG, et al. Frequent low-level mutations of protein kinase D2 in angiolipoma. J Pathol. 2017;241:578–82.
8. Hornick JL, Bosenberg MW, Mentzel T, McMenamin ME, Oliveira AM, Fletcher CDM. Pleomorphic liposarcoma: clinicopathologic analysis of 57 cases. Am J Surg Pathol. 2004;28:1257–67.
9. Inyang A, Thomas DG, Jorns J. Heterologous liposarcomatous differentiation in malignant phyllodes tumor is histologically similar but immunohistochemically and molecularly distinct from well-differentiated liposarcoma of soft tissue. Breast J. 2016;22:282–6.
10. Lyle PL, Bridge JA, Simpson JF, Cates JM, Sanders ME. Liposarcomatous differentiation in malignant phyllodes tumours is unassociated with MDM2 or CDK4 amplification. Histopathology. 2016;68:1040–5.
11. Magnusson L, Hansen N, Saba KH, et al. Loss of the tumour suppressor gene AIP mediates the browning of human brown fat tumours. J Pathol. 2017;243:160–4.
12. Magro G, Michal M, Vasquez E, Bisceglia M. Lipomatous myofibroblastoma: a potential diagnostic pitfall in the spectrum of the spindle cell lesions of the breast. Virchows Archiv. 2000;437:540–4.
13. Marino-Enriquez A, Fletcher CD, Dal Cin P, Hornick JL. Dedifferentiated liposarcoma with "homologous" lipoblastic (pleomorphic liposarcoma-like) differentiation: clinicopathologic and molecular analysis of a series suggesting revised diagnostic criteria. Am J Surg Pathol. 2010;34:1122–31.
14. Martini N, Londero V, Machin P, et al. An unusual breast lesion: the ultrasonographic, mammographic, MRI and nuclear medicine findings of mammary hibernoma. Br J Radiol. 2010;83:e1–4.
15. Pilotti S, Della Torre G, Lavarino C, et al. Molecular abnormalities in liposarcoma: role of MDM2 and CDK4-containing amplicons at 12q13-22. J Pathol. 1998;185:188–90.
16. Powell CM, Rosen PP. Adipose differentiation in cystosarcoma phyllodes: a study of 14 cases. Am J Surg Pathol. 1994;18:720–7.
17. Riley MP, Karamchandani DM. Mammary hibernoma: a rare entity. Arch Pathol Lab Med. 2015;139:1565–7.
18. Salemis NS. Intramuscular atypical lipomatous tumor/well-differentiated liposarcoma of the pectoralis major masquerading as a breast tumor: management and review of the literature. Int Surg. 2015;100:194–8.
19. Weaver J, Rao P, Goldblum JR, et al. Can MDM2 analytical tests performed on core needle biopsy be relied upon to diagnose well-differentiated liposarcoma? Mod Pathol. 2010;23:1301–6.
20. Yokouchi M, Nagano S, Kijima Y, et al. Solitary breast metastasis from myxoid liposarcoma. BMC Cancer. 2014;14:482.

# Inflammatory Lesions and Inflammatory-Like Lesions

# 7

J. Jordi Rowe, Darya Buehler, Paul Weisman, and Erinn Downs-Kelly

## Contents



J. J. Rowe · E. Downs-Kelly (✉)
Cleveland Clinic, Department of Pathology, Robert J. Tomsich Pathology and Laboratory Medicine Institute, Cleveland, OH, USA
e-mail: downske@ccf.org

D. Buehler · P. Weisman
Department of Pathology and Laboratory Medicine, School of Medicine and Public Health, University of Wisconsin-Madison, Madison, WI, USA



J. J. Rowe, E. Downs-Kelly (eds.), *Mesenchymal Tumors of the Breast and Their Mimics*, https://doi.org/10.1007/978-3-030-74474-8_7

## Overview

Several inflammatory or inflammatory-like lesions that involve the breast have an overall spindle cell appearance or may develop focal areas with spindled or histiocytoid morphology. Such lesions can present diagnostic challenges given the broad differential that arises from their often overlapping histologies, especially on the limited sampling of a core needle biopsy. Some of these lesions are specific to the breast, while others are more ubiquitous and are known to involve multiple anatomic sites. As such, remembering that they may occur in the breast is key in their diagnosis and subsequent appropriate management which is especially relevant as the biologic behavior of this group ranges from benign to malignant.

## Invasive Histiocytoid Carcinoma

### Introduction

There has been debate in the literature about the histogenesis of invasive histiocytoid carcinoma and if this lesion represents a variant of ductal, lobular, or apocrine carcinoma. The 5th edition of the WHO Classification of Breast Tumors has given a brief mention of histiocytoid morphology as a pattern of invasive lobular carcinoma. As the name implies, this primary breast carcinoma is composed of cells morphologically resembling spindled or epithelioid histiocytes. This lesion deserves recognition given how cytologically bland it can appear and hence has the potential for misdiagnosis as simply fat necrosis or other benign lesions with prominent histiocytes.

### Clinical Features

Invasive histiocytoid carcinoma is a rare morphologic pattern of invasive mammary carcinoma, representing a very small percentage (<1%) of invasive breast cancers. As mentioned above, its histogenesis remains controversial; however, a subset of these tumors described in the literature have lacked E-cadherin expression and have had associated lobular neoplasia. In light of this, there are certain features of invasive lobular carcinoma that apply to this lesion including multifocality, multicentricity, and higher rates of bilaterality than invasive ductal carcinoma, NOS. Age at diagnosis has ranged from 35 to 87 years (mean 61 years), and tumor size has been noted to be widely variable ranging from 1 cm up to 10 cm with involvement of all four quadrants of the breast. Clinical presentation may include a palpable mass or mammographic abnormality.

### Imaging

The imaging characteristics are widely variable and likely related to the size of the lesion. A subset of lesions have been described as subtle on imaging and similar to invasive lobular carcinoma, with the findings described as vague areas of thickening or an increased density. Conversely, patients can present with mammographic abnormalities or palpable masses as is seen with invasive ductal carcinoma, NOS. Often, ruptured cysts and fat necrosis are within the imaging differential for invasive histiocytoid carcinoma.

## Pathologic Features

### Gross Features

Similar to invasive ductal carcinoma, NOS, invasive histiocytoid carcinoma may form a well-defined tan stellate mass. Other examples take on the appearance and feel of ill-defined areas of dense fibrosis.

### Microscopic

Histiocytoid invasive tumors appear to have no consistent architecture, save infiltrative, and are subtle and difficult to identify on low magnification as the scattered and dispersed pattern of cell infiltration can be complicated by adjacent background fibrocystic breast tissue and reactive changes including prior biopsy site (Fig. 7.1). The tumor cells of invasive histiocytoid carcinoma have a low nuclear to cytoplasmic ratio and contain abundant finely vacuolated to granular cytoplasm that ranges from clear to eosinophilic (Fig. 7.2). The nuclei can display slight pleomorphism with focal nucleoli, but do not have the classic reniform nuclei of histiocytes. The nuclei are grade 1 or grade 2 and mitotic activity is typically scarce. Invasive histiocytoid carcinoma typically infiltrates the breast stroma as single cells, sheets, clusters, and cords (Fig. 7.3). It also has been shown to mimic the single file linear stranding of classic invasive lobular carcinoma, with invasive cells circling normal ductal structures.

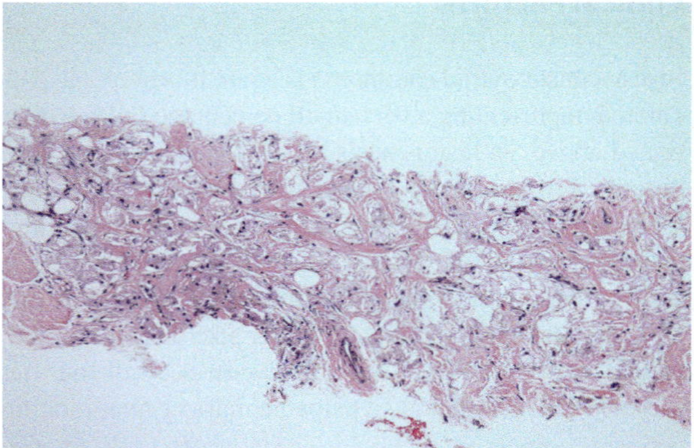

**Fig. 7.1** In this low-power image, the histiocytoid cells of this invasive histiocytoid carcinoma could be easily overlooked as fat necrosis

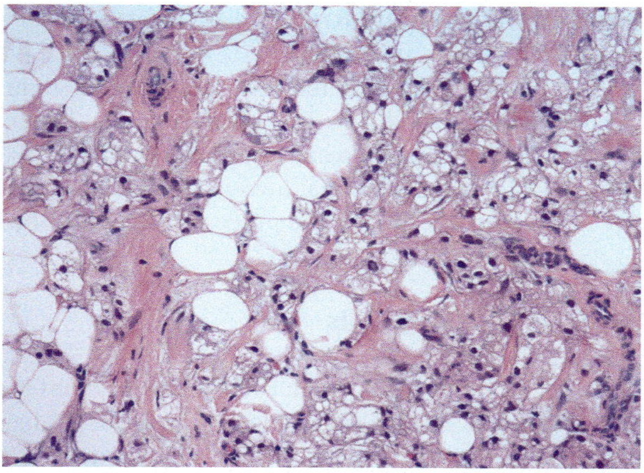

**Fig. 7.2** Note the paucity of inflammatory cell types, a clue that could help differentiate fat necrosis which typically has a mixed population of inflammatory cells from invasive histiocytoid carcinoma. The lack of nuclear pleomorphism, abundant frothy clear to eosinophilic cytoplasm, and the dispersed pattern throughout the stroma are key features of invasive histiocytoid carcinoma

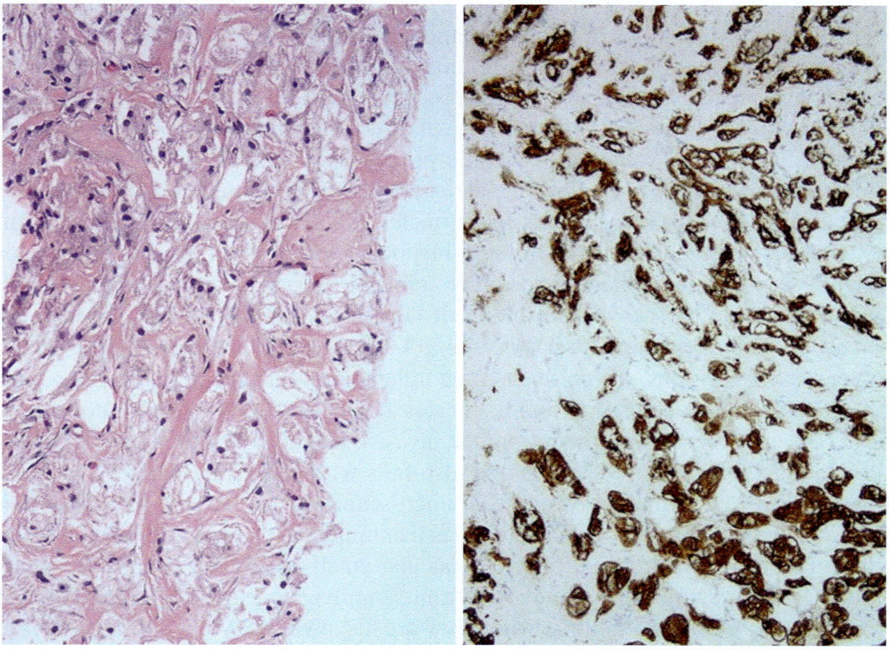

**Fig. 7.3** The panel on the left highlights the small, hyperchromatic nuclei and abundant cytoplasm of this invasive histiocytoid carcinoma. Mitotic activity is absent. The panel on the right is the corresponding cytokeratin AE1/3 confirming the epithelial nature of this process

## Immunohistochemistry

Invasive histiocytoid carcinoma stains with cytokeratin markers (AE1/3, cytokeratin 7, among others) and is negative for traditional histiocytic markers like CD68 and CD163. E-cadherin is typically negative, furthering the idea that these lesions are a variant of lobular carcinoma. Invasive histiocytoid carcinomas are variably positive for expression of estrogen and progesterone receptors. HER2 status is also variable.

## Differential Diagnosis

The bland cytomorphology and subtle pattern of infiltration of invasive histiocytoid carcinoma can lead to under-recognition and misdiagnosis. The judicious use of cytokeratins (pancytokeratin, AE1/3, and/or cytokeratin 7) can confirm the presence of an infiltrating epithelial process. The mimics of invasive histiocytoid carcinoma range from benign reactive histiocytic rich processes to neoplasms. Reactive histiocytic rich processes are common in the breast and are seen in response to injured ducts or in the setting of mammary duct ectasia where histiocytes fill the lumen and involve the surrounding soft tissue. Organizing fat necrosis is a similarly histiocyte-rich process that may develop post-trauma, after biopsy, or even spontaneously. In addition to histiocytes, these reactive processes have an additional inflammatory cell component including lymphocytes, plasma cells, and at times, foreign body giant cells. Cellular spindled histiocytic pseudotumor (CSHP, described in detail below) is a distinctive mass-forming histiocytic lesion composed of cells with ample granular to clear cytoplasm and small nuclei. CSHP is negative for cytokeratin expression while uniformly expressing histiocyte-specific markers like CD163 or CD68. As with any pathology specimen, clinical history is key as histiocyte-rich populations can be seen in the setting of neoadjuvant chemotherapy for invasive breast carcinoma when there has been a good response to treatment. In all of the above reactive lesions, the presence of an inflammatory cell component along with immunohistochemical stains for histiocytes (CD68 or CD163) and cytokeratins (AE1/3) can help separate them from the invasive histiocytoid carcinoma. Granular cell tumor (discussed in detail below) also falls within the differential of invasive histiocytoid carcinoma by virtue of its microscopically infiltrative growth pattern and its clinical and imaging characteristics that mimic carcinoma. Morphologically, the cells of granular cell tumor have vesicular small nuclei and abundant eosinophilic granular cytoplasm. Granular cell tumors uniformly express S100 protein and may express CD68 and inhibin, while they are negative for cytokeratin expression. Extranodal Rosai-Dorfman disease (RDD, discussed in detail below) also enters the differential diagnosis in this context, especially in limited core needle biopsies. RDD is composed of sheets of histiocytes with emperipolesis (engulfed intact inflammatory cells within the cytoplasm of histiocytes) and usually has a striking intervening lymphoplasmacytic infiltrate that includes lymphoid aggregates with well-defined germinal centers and prominent plasma cells. However, on a given core, the whole picture may not be clear and only variable components may be sampled. The histiocytes of RDD show staining for S100 protein and OCT-2 and are negative for cytokeratin expression. Clinical history is also important in the setting of metastatic disease to the breast as some metastases, most notably malignant melanoma, may have a histiocytoid appearance.

### Molecular

Specific molecular studies of invasive histiocytoid variant are currently lacking; however, extrapolating from other studies on lobular carcinoma and its variants (including those with apocrine differentiation and those with pleomorphic features), the genetic changes common to lobular lesions include mutations that result in loss of E-cadherin expression, as well as gains on chromosome 1q and losses on chromosome 16q.

### Treatment and Prognosis

If thought of as a variant of invasive lobular carcinoma, invasive histiocytoid carcinoma would then adopt the aforementioned increased risk of bilaterality and multifocality. The treatment remains the same as for conventional invasive mammary carcinoma, guided largely by size, grade, hormone receptor status, and HER2 status.

### Practical Tips

Many of the lesions that fall within the differential of invasive histiocytoid carcinoma have an admixed inflammatory cell component (plasma cells and lymphocytes), while this second inflammatory cell population is not typically seen in invasive histiocytoid carcinoma. Use of cytokeratins when faced with a histiocytoid population can help identify them as either epithelial in origin when positive and can help identify the pattern of infiltration. Clinical and pathologic history are important and may help guide the workup, especially in the setting of potential metastases.

## Cystic Neutrophilic Granulomatous Mastitis

### Introduction

Cystic neutrophilic granulomatous mastitis (CNGM) is a more recently recognized form of granulomatous mastitis that has similarities clinically, radiologically, and histologically with idiopathic granulomatous mastitis. One notable difference is that CNGM has been shown by histology with special stains, culture, and DNA analysis to harbor *Corynebacterium* species. That said, it is possible that with more stringent diagnostic criteria and awareness of CNGM along with tissue culture, these lesions will become better defined allowing for appropriate treatment.

## Clinical Features

Like many inflammatory mastitides, CNGM occurs in women of childbearing age and is often seen in the setting of pregnancy and/or lactation but has also been identified years following the cessation of lactation. Initial symptoms may include a painful breast mass, with or without erythema, nipple discharge and inversion, as well as sinus formation. Due to delays in diagnosis of this under-recognized lesion, women tend to be identified months after initial presentation.

## Imaging

CNGM can present as a mass-forming lesion seen on ultrasound and asymmetry identified on mammographic imaging with a size range of 7 mm to 96 mm, as noted in one recent study by Gautham et al. A large proportion of patients have highly worrisome imaging including BIRADS category 4 (suspicious of malignancy) or category 5 (highly suspicious of malignancy).

## Pathologic Features

### Gross

Gross findings in the literature have been limited; however, the one series to date with macroscopic descriptions had gross findings including solid mass lesions or masses with abscess cavities.

### Microscopic

CNGM is a lobulocentric based inflammatory lesion composed of mononuclear inflammatory cells, arranged in sheets that overtake and obliterate the normal terminal duct lobular unit architecture. The sheets of inflammation are pockmarked with occasional cystic spaces (Fig. 7.4). These empty small cystic spaces that are typically 200–800 μm are ringed by neutrophils which are then surrounded by epithelioid and spindled histiocytes. This configuration of microcysts surrounded by neutrophils and then histiocytes is a key histologic finding (Fig. 7.5). The number of microcysts within a given case is highly variable. A subtle but helpful feature is that the geographic areas of tissue necrosis with peripheral palisading such as those seen in fungal and mycobacterial infections are not typical of CNGM. Tissue Gram stain may highlight small numbers of intracystic Gram-positive bacilli (Fig. 7.6).

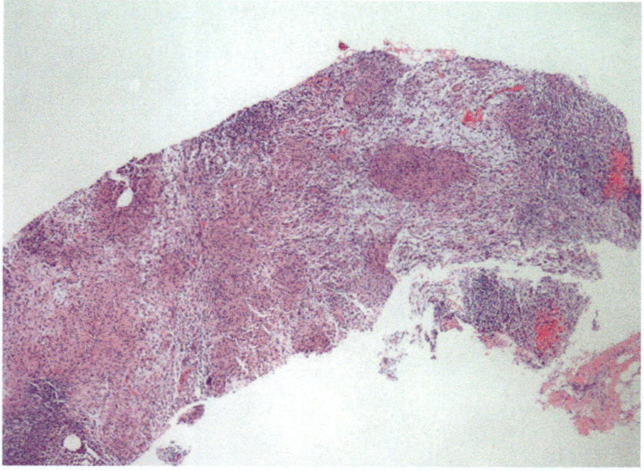

**Fig. 7.4** Core needle with cystic neutrophilic granulomatous mastitis (CNGM) showing sheets of inflammatory cells that have overrun and obliterated the background breast epithelial elements. From low power there is an alternating pattern of blue (areas of plasma cells and lymphocytes) with pink (collections of histiocytes). Note the rare microcystic spaces

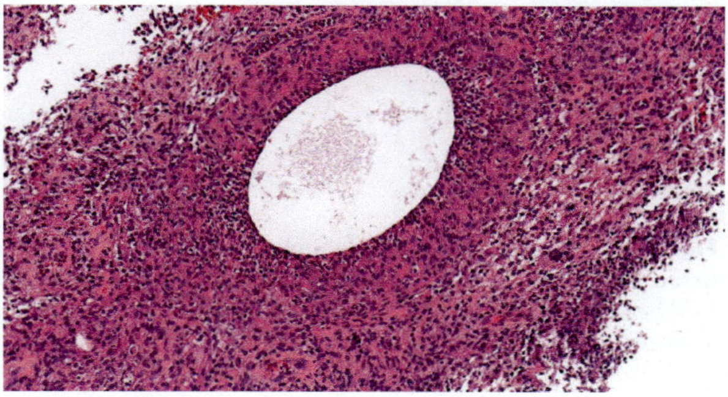

**Fig. 7.5** Typically the microcystic spaces of CNGM have cleared centers with a characteristic surrounding ring of neutrophils that are then enveloped by histiocytes. The histiocytes may have a spindled or epithelioid appearance

## Immunohistochemistry and Special Stains

No specific immunohistochemical stains are available to confirm this diagnosis. Tissue Gram stain should be employed; however, the absence of Gram-positive bacilli does not negate the diagnosis of CNGM. The microcystic spaces are variable within the tissue, and the number of organisms is typically limited, as such when the histomorphology is suggestive of this entity without definitive organisms identified, the possibility of CNMG should at least be raised.

## Molecular

Identification of the *Corynebacterium* species by polymerase chain reaction (PCR) has been unsuccessful, either due to the low numbers of the bacteria, its location within the spaces, or limits to the laboratory methodology such as retrieval methods and use of formalin-fixed, paraffin-embedded tissue sections.

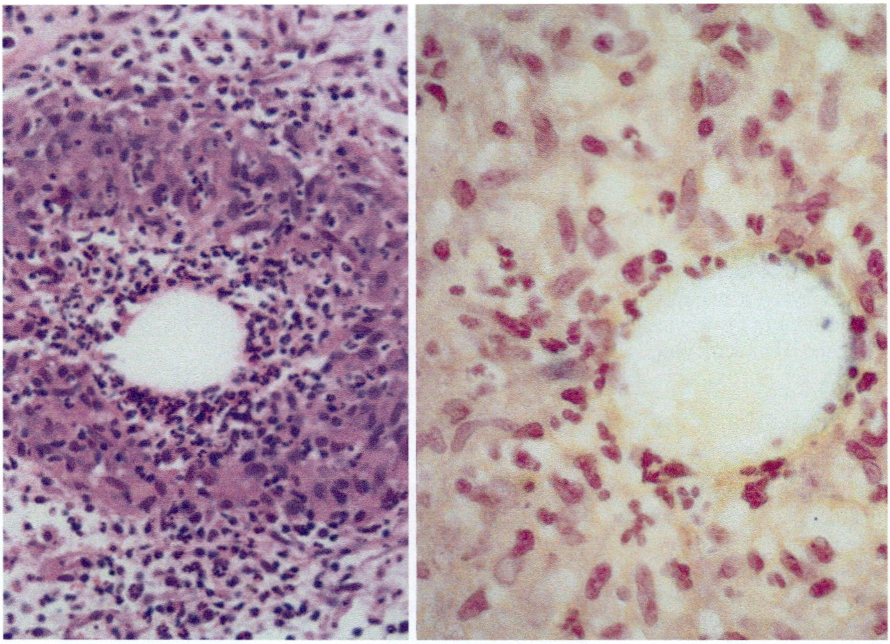

**Fig. 7.6** The panel on the left highlights the characteristic microcystic space of CNGM with the tissue Gram stain on the right highlighting rare Gram-positive structures. Most commonly, *Corynebacterium* species have been identified when these lesions are suspected and tissue culture has been performed

## Differential Diagnosis

Other inflammatory granulomatous lesions should be considered including infectious processes (fungal or mycobacterial), sarcoid-related granulomas, as well as idiopathic granulomatous mastitis. GMS and AFB stains should be performed, especially if any necrotizing granulomatous inflammation is appreciated. The singular most important entity to exclude is an invasive carcinoma, particularly the histiocytoid subtype wherein use of a cytokeratin stain can exclude an occult infiltrative epithelial process.

## Treatment and Prognosis

Treatment of this inflammatory process in the breast requires a multidisciplinary approach to diagnosis and management. Clinical history is important with knowledge of pregnancy status and history of breast feeding being valuable information. Management strategies include surgical debridement, antimicrobials (those commonly used include clarithromycin, trimethoprim-sulfamethoxazole, penicillin, doxycycline, erythromycin, clindamycin, or rifampin), as well as corticosteroids.

## Practical Tips

When faced with an inflammatory process that has worrisome imaging findings in a patient who is pregnant or lactating, CNGM should be considered. Appreciation of microcysts with the typical ring of neutrophils and envelope of histiocytes is a key histologic finding.

# Granular Cell Tumor

## Introduction

Granular cell tumor (GCT) is a mesenchymal neoplasm that arises from Schwann cells. Although GCTs are ubiquitous and have been described throughout the body, they are identified uncommonly in the breast, with GCTs in this location accounting for less than 10% of all GCTs. The vast majority of GCTs are benign; however, rare malignant cases have been identified.

## Clinical Features

In the breast, GCTs have been identified in the dermis, subcutis, the breast parenchyma itself, and very rarely within the pectoralis fascia. The age range for GCTs is broad (17–69 years), and the tumor has a predilection for non-Caucasians, particularly African-Americans. The lesions are usually solitary, but multifocality has been described in a subset of patients. As these tumors simulate invasive carcinoma by their infiltrative growth, they too can present as palpable masses.

## Imaging

By imaging, GCTs mimic invasive carcinoma as they frequently form spiculated and ill-defined masses.

## Pathologic Features

### Gross Features

On gross examination, GCT is typically an ill-defined stellate gray/tan mass that may have a gritty cut surface. The average range in size is from 5 mm up to 50 mm.

### Microscopic Features

GCTs in the breast are similar to those identified in other anatomic locations and are composed of cells that may be plump and epithelioid or subtly spindled. Abundant eosinophilic granular cytoplasm is the hallmark and is due to numerous

PAS-positive diastase-resistant secondary lysosomes. The nuclei may be small and hyperchromatic or larger with open chromatin and discernible nucleoli (Fig. 7.7). The cells may be arranged in nests, sheets, and clusters, often with intervening fibrous tissue with an overall infiltrative growth (Fig. 7.8). Perineural involvement is frequently noted. Rare examples of malignant GCT have been described, predominately in the somatic soft tissues but also rarely within the breast. In the soft tissue literature, Fanburg-Smith et al. evaluated six histologic variables within GCT that they considered potentially indicative of malignancy, including necrosis, vesicular nuclei with large nucleoli, increased mitotic rate (> 2 mitoses/10 high-power fields at 200× magnification), spindling of tumor cells, a high nuclear-to-cytoplasmic (N/C) ratio, and nuclear pleomorphism. Multivariate analysis of these histologic features showed that spindling, increased N/C ratio, and vesicular nuclei with large nucleoli were the features most related to classification as malignant GCT.

## Immunohistochemistry

S100 protein, SOX10, TFE3, and MiTF immunohistochemical stains are positive in the nuclei of granular cell tumors, while inhibin, CD68, CD57, and NSE often show cytoplasmic immunoreactivity likely owing to reactivity with the abundant

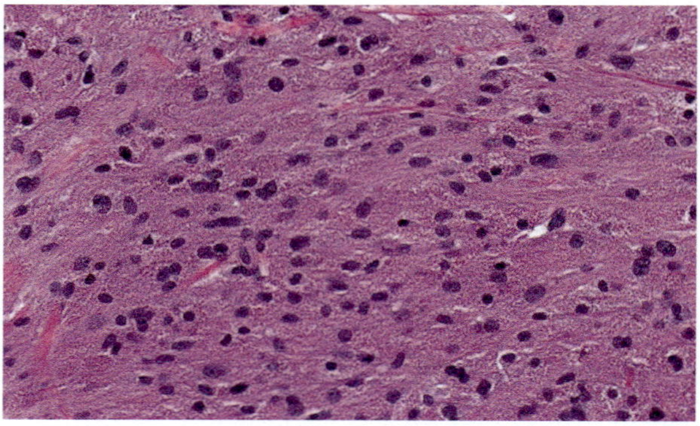

**Fig. 7.7** Granular cell tumor (GCT) with the characteristic abundant eosinophilic granular cytoplasm. The associated nuclei in this example have open chromatin and small nucleoli. There is overall uniformity of the nuclei and mitotic activity and necrosis are not apparent

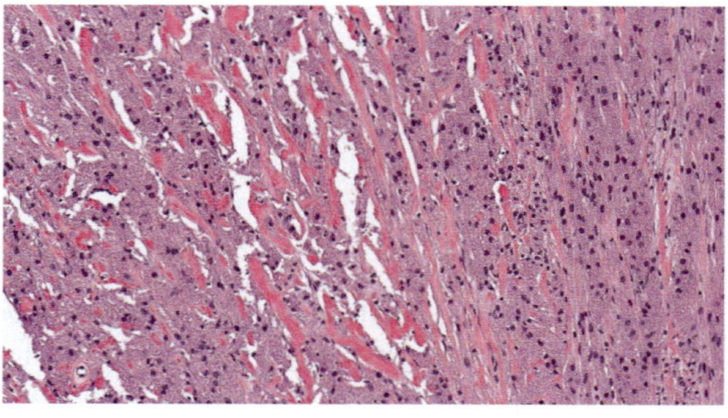

**Fig. 7.8** GCT architecturally may be arranged in sheets and clusters of cells, usually with intervening fibrous stroma imparting an infiltrative appearance to their growth

lysosomes. Melan-A, HMB45 and cytokeratins, estrogen and progesterone receptors, as well as HER2 are negative.

## Molecular

Although molecular studies for diagnosis are not needed, genetic studies have shown that the molecular underpinnings in GCT include mutations in *ATP6AP1* and *ATP6AP2*. The findings represent loss of function mutations in these two genes that encode vacuolar H + -ATPase elements that play a role in endosomal pH regulation.

## Differential Diagnosis

The differential diagnosis for GCT is somewhat dependent on the location of the lesion in the breast. Within the breast parenchyma, invasive histiocytoid carcinoma, invasive carcinoma with apocrine features, fat necrosis, as well as metastatic melanoma come into the differential. Employing a cytokeratin stain should solidify the diagnosis of invasive carcinoma, as these lesions should show strong and diffuse expression of pancytokeratin. The histiocytes of fat necrosis will be reactive for CD68; however, they will be S100 protein negative. Reliance solely on an S100 protein stain to support a diagnosis of GCT could lead to difficulties, as invasive breast carcinoma, GCT, and melanoma may all show immunoreactivity for this marker. In this instance, addition of a melanocytic marker known to be negative in GCT, such as Melan-A or HMB45, as well as a pancytokeratin, should sort out this differential. Within the dermis, melanoma, benign fibrous histiocytoma (discussed in detail in the chapter entitled "Mesenchymal Breast Tumors with Fibroblastic and Myofibroblastic Differentiation"), non-neural granular cell tumor, extension from an underlying invasive mammary carcinoma with histiocytoid or apocrine features, and cutaneous adnexal neoplasms with apocrine morphology could be considered. Cutaneous non-neural granular cell tumors have a similar morphologic appearance as the conventional GCT albeit with somewhat greater degree of cellular spindling and nuclear atypia. However, non-neural GCTs consistently lack S100 protein expression and are driven by *ALK* fusions, with resultant ALK protein expression by immunohistochemistry in the majority of cases. The differential diagnosis of GCT from invasive mammary carcinoma or skin adnexal carcinoma with apocrine features could be made by identifying cytokeratin and GATA-3 expression that would allow for separation of these carcinomas from GCT, although not from each other.

## Treatment and Prognosis

The vast majority of GTCs are benign and treatment with local excision is sufficient. Recurrences are rare and usually occur in incompletely excised tumors. However, malignant granular cell tumors have been documented, including cases arising in the breast. As mentioned above, to be considered a malignant granular cell tumor, three of the following six criteria need to be present: necrosis, spindling, vesicular nuclei with large nucleoli, mitotic rate > 2/10 high-power fields (200X magnification), high nuclear to cytoplasmic ratio, or pleomorphism. Tumors with only one or two of these features are considered atypical granular cell tumors which appear to behave in an indolent manner. By contrast, malignant granular cell tumors are aggressive neoplasms with a high rate of metastasis involving lymph nodes, lung, and bone with high rates of mortality.

## IGG4 Sclerosing Mastitis

### Introduction

IgG4 sclerosing mastitis is part of the spectrum of IgG4-related disease (IgG4-RD). This immune-mediated process leads to a fibroinflammatory response that has been shown to involve multiple organs and has been recognized as a systemic disorder. There are reports of the process involving almost every anatomic site with the sites most commonly affected being the pancreas, biliary tract, major salivary glands (submandibular, parotid), lacrimal glands, retroperitoneum, and lymph nodes. There are case reports and small series in the literature describing IgG4-RD in the breast.

There are several common features irrespective of the site of involvement that include the typical formation of tumefactive lesions by a dense lymphoplasmacytic infiltrate with prominent IgG4+ plasma cells, the presence of storiform fibrosis, and usually markedly elevated serum IgG4 concentrations. That said, normal serum IgG4 concentrations have been reported in up to 40% of patients with biopsy-proven IgG4-RD. A consensus guideline to the diagnosis of IgG4-RD was developed that offers guidance in the histologic approach to this entity, with morphology being key and tissue IgG4 counts being of secondary importance. It is important to bear in mind that simply identifying increased IgG4 plasma cells within tissue or identifying elevated serum levels of IgG4 is not diagnostic of IgG4-RD. Increased numbers of IgG4+ plasma cells have been described in a variety of inflammatory conditions, not related to IgG4-RD. As such, the diagnosis requires histologic findings in concert with the identification of increased IgG4-positive plasma cells within tissue. As with many enigmatic lesions, the histology findings may be supportive of the diagnosis, but correlation with the clinical scenario is essential for a definitive diagnosis.

### Clinical Features

In the breast, the number of cases of IgG4-RD described in the literature is limited; however, most cases have presented as painless palpable masses, either unilateral or bilateral in patients with an average age of 47.5 years. Multifocality has been described. Roughly 50% of patients have elevated serum IgG4 with the disease limited to the breast in the majority of patients and a minority showing evidence of broader systemic disease.

## Imaging

Although limited imaging is available, findings on ultrasonography have ranged from fibroadenoma-like to hypoechoic suspicious nodules with irregular margins.

## Pathologic Features

### Gross

Specific gross findings have not been well documented in the literature.

### Microscopic

The major histologic findings described in general for IgG4-RD include a dense lymphoplasmacytic infiltrate, fibrosis that at least focally develops a storiform pattern, and obliterative phlebitis. In the breast, the lesions identified to date have been composed of stromal sclerosis with spindled fibroblasts and myofibroblasts admixed with the inflammatory component in the form of irregular strands or broad fibrous bands (Fig. 7.9). The infiltrate is a lymphoplasmacytic process with small lymphocytes and plasma cells arranged in sheets or aggregates with occasional associated reactive lymphoid follicles and scattered histiocytes (Fig. 7.10). Other histologic findings that may be seen include increased numbers of eosinophils and phlebitis without luminal occlusion, although the phlebitis has not been a common finding in the breast cases described to date (Fig. 7.11).

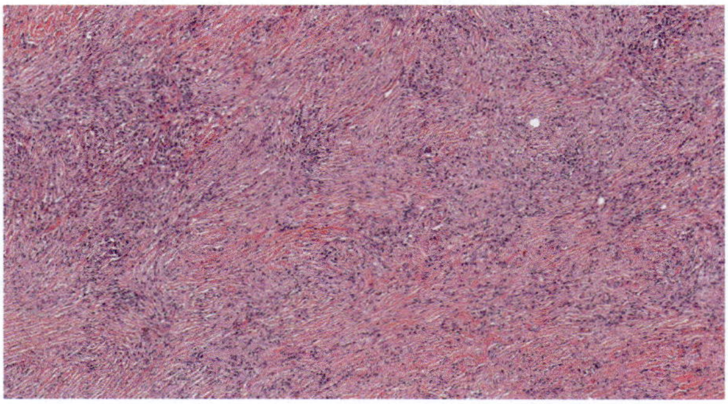

**Fig. 7.9** IgG4 sclerosing mastitis involving the breast with this scanning power showing a storiform pattern of fibrosis with an accompanying inflammatory infiltrate. The normal breast epithelial elements have been obliterated in this field

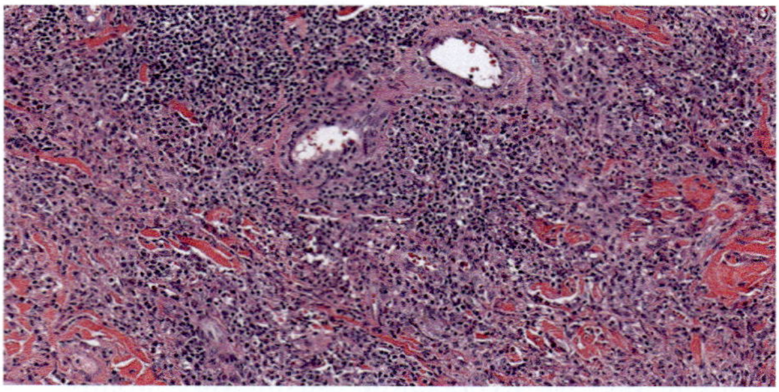

**Fig. 7.10** IgG4 sclerosing mastitis with a lymphoid aggregate identified in the upper aspect of the image and a diffuse inflammatory infiltrate composed of lymphocytes, numerous plasma cells, and eosinophils. There is a suggestion of phlebitis without luminal occlusion within the vessel in the middle of the micrograph

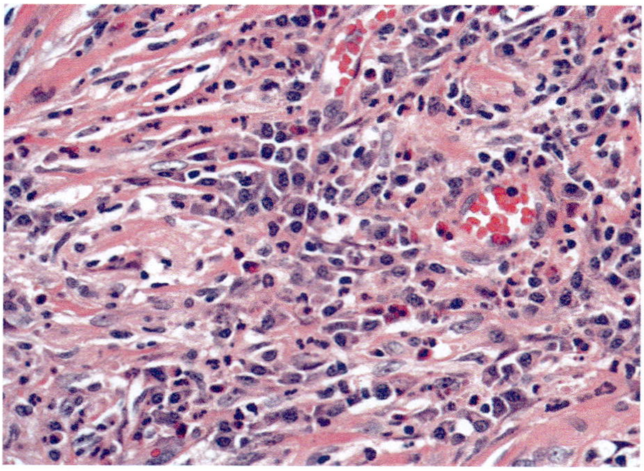

**Fig. 7.11** IgG4 sclerosing mastitis at higher magnification to highlight the admixture of prominent plasma cells, lymphocytes, and eosinophils. This patient had an elevated serum IgG4 and IgG4-positive plasma cells in tissue that were > 50/hpf

## Immunohistochemistry

In addition to identifying increased IgG4-positive plasma cells, performing an IgG immunohistochemical stain and identifying an IgG4+/IgG+ cell ratio of >40% furthers the diagnosis. The IgG4-positive plasma cell counts required for the diagnosis are organ site specific and highly variable (10 up to 200 IgG4+ plasma cells/hpf). The consensus guidelines did not offer a specific IgG4-positive plasma cell count for breast, as the number of cases described in the literature is limited. However, in the small case series, IgG4-positive plasma cells ranged from 272 to 495/high-power field with IgG4-positive plasma cells accounting for 49–85% of the total IgG+ plasma cells.

## Molecular

No specific molecular alterations have been described to date.

## Differential Diagnosis

The differential diagnosis includes hematolymphoid neoplasms as well as extranodal Rosai-Dorfman disease (RDD, discussed below) and inflammatory myofibroblastic tumor (IMT, discussed in detail in the chapter entitled "Mesenchymal Breast Tumors with Fibroblastic and Myofibroblastic Differentiation"). In IgG4-RD, CD3 and CD20 as well as kappa and lambda light chain immunohistochemical stains will show a mixed population of T and B cells without evidence of a light chain resection. RDD will also have a lymphoplasmacytic component but will also have sheets and clusters of large pale histiocytes with evidence of emperipolesis. Compounding this differential is the fact that increased numbers of IgG4+ plasma cells have been inconsistently described in the setting of RDD. However, studies have found that this finding likely represents a reflection of T-helper type 2 (Th2) cell-mediated immune response rather than a true pathogenetic relationship of RDD to IgG4+ disease. In contrast to RDD, the histiocytes in sclerosing mastitis are negative for S100 protein and OCT2. IMT also has a dense lymphoplasmacytic infiltrate and may even have areas of storiform fibrosis as well as IgG4-positive plasma cells, but the constituent spindled myofibroblasts arranged in fascicles are more prominent in IMT. Furthermore, at least in cases reported in the breast, IMTs consistently show alterations in *ALK* gene which can be identified by immunoreactivity for ALK or by appropriate molecular testing.

## Treatment and Prognosis

Speaking broadly about IgG4-RD, treatment in general is based on clinical experience and expert opinion with the site of disease taken into consideration. Treatment is not always necessary, and expectant management may be appropriate in some settings. Again, depending on the site of involvement, glucocorticoids and immunosuppression are used in cases where the disease is relapsing and remitting. In the breast, the small published series have shown that patients who underwent excision had no recurrence of disease.

## Extranodal Rosai-Dorfman Disease

### Introduction

Rosai-Dorfman disease (RDD) is an etiologically complex histiocytic disorder likely of monocytic-macrophage derivation characterized as a distinctive entity by Rosai and Dorfman in 1969, which may present as a localized or a multicentric process. The nodal form of RDD is also known as sinus histiocytosis with massive lymphadenopathy, a name that aptly reflects the clinical presentation of painless, bulky, usually cervical lymphadenopathy associated with fever, weight loss, anemia, and other systemic inflammatory symptoms, in children and young adults. The extranodal form (40% of cases) manifests as a mass lesion with or without associated lymphadenopathy, most often involving skin, subcutis, the head and neck region, bone, and CNS.

## Clinical Features

In the breast, RDD typically affects female patients in the fifth decade, although the reported age range is broad (15–84 years). In the breast, RDD presents as a mass lesion involving the parenchyma with or without ipsilateral axillary lymph node involvement that may clinically and radiologically mimic invasive breast carcinoma. In the published small series of RDD in the breast, the involvement is often multifocal and bilateral and associated with systemic involvement.

## Imaging

In the breast, RDD is most often described as a solid, high-density mass with ill-defined borders on mammography and ultrasound, closely resembling breast carcinoma. Reported size ranges from 0.4 to 6 cm.

## Pathologic Features

### Gross Features

Ill-defined, gray-tan, lobulated, variably fibrous nodule; at times, a discrete mass cannot be appreciated.

### Microscopic Features

Extranodal RDD is composed of broad syncytial layers of large pale histiocytes in association with an intervening lymphoplasmacytic infiltrate. This pattern is best appreciated at scanning magnification, as alternating pale and dark areas (Fig. 7.12). The histiocytes have round or oval vesicular nuclei with distinct nucleoli and palely eosinophilic voluminous, granular to wispy cytoplasm. The hallmark feature of RDD is *emperipolesis* – a passage of intact inflammatory cells through the cytoplasm of the histiocytes (Fig. 7.13). Prominent stromal fibrosis and conspicuous vasculature may be present, often with plasma cells seeming to line up around vessels (Fig. 7.14). The lymphoplasmacytic infiltrate is a mixture of lymphocytes, mature plasma cells, and less often, neutrophils (Fig. 7.15). Eosinophils are less common. There is no significant nuclear atypia, pleomorphism, or mitotic activity. When present in the lymph nodes, these histiocytes massively expand the sinuses.

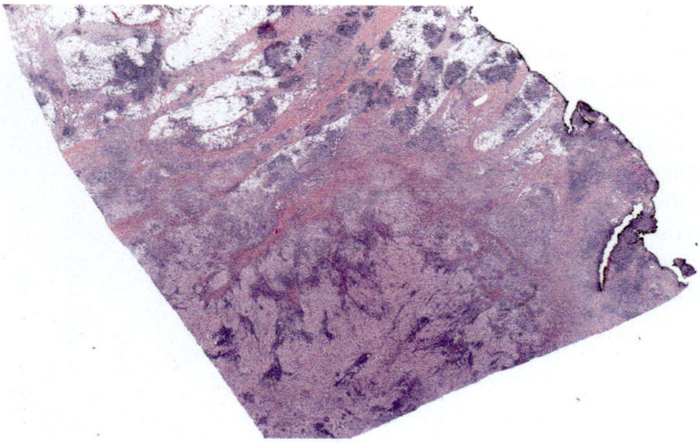

**Fig. 7.12** Extranodal Rosai-Dorfman disease at scanning magnification, presenting as an ill-defined mass composed of broad sheets of large pale histiocytes with an intervening lymphoplasmacytic infiltrate

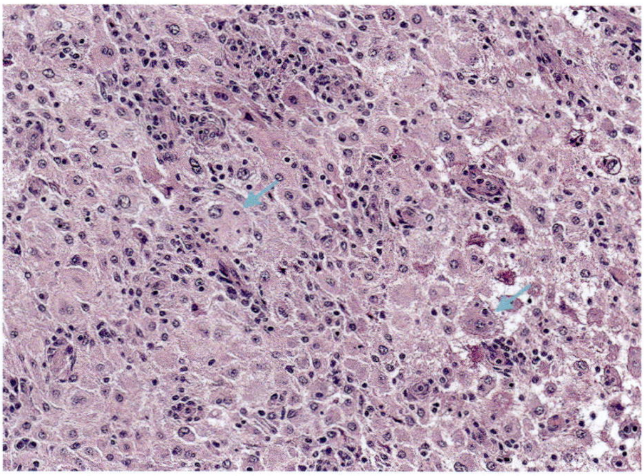

**Fig. 7.13** The histiocytes in Rosai-Dorfman disease have round or oval vesicular nuclei with distinct nucleoli and palely eosinophilic voluminous granular cytoplasm. Emperipolesis – an engulfment of intact inflammatory cells by lesional histiocytes – is indicated by the arrows

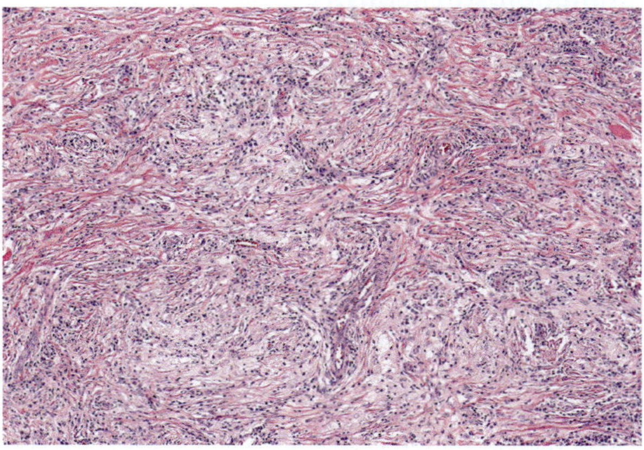

**Fig. 7.14** Prominent stromal fibrosis and conspicuous vasculature in extranodal Rosai-Dorfman disease

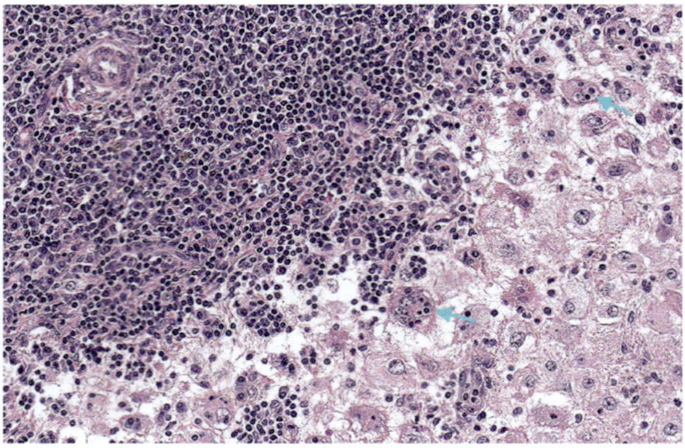

**Fig. 7.15** The lymphoplasmacytic infiltrate in Rosai-Dorfman disease contains a mixture of lymphocytes, mature plasma cells, and less often, neutrophils or eosinophils. Emperipolesis is readily identified (arrows)

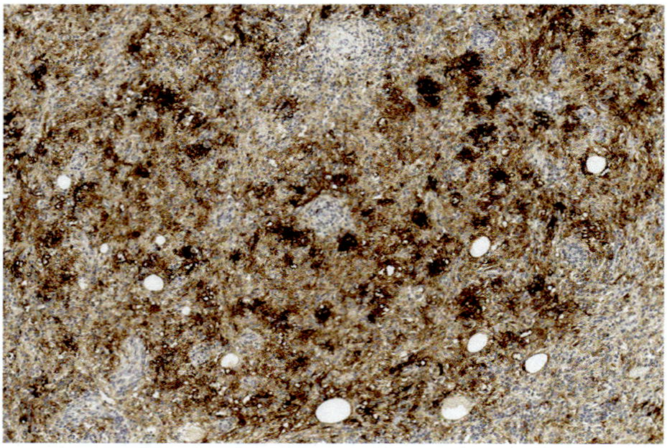

**Fig. 7.16** The histiocytes in Rosai-Dorfman disease are strongly positive for S100

## Immunohistochemistry

Histiocytes in RDD strongly and diffusely express S100 protein, which also helps to highlight engulfed inflammatory cells (Fig. 7.16), OCT2, histiocytic markers CD68 and CD163, and cyclin D1. Factor XIIIa is variably expressed. The plasma cell infiltrate in RDD may contain a population of IGg4-positive plasma cells.

## Molecular

The etiology of RDD remains uncertain, but is likely related to immune dysregulation, which leads to a non-Langerhans cell histiocytosis. Recurrent *KRAS* and *MAP2K1* mutations have been identified in approximately one-third of sporadic RDD cases, suggesting that at least a subset of these lesions are clonal proliferations. More recently, RDD has been shown to express OCT2, indicating a unique monocyte-macrophage lineage. Based on the various clinicopathologic associations, RDD is classified into sporadic classical (nodal), extranodal, neoplasia or immune disorder-associated, familial, and unclassified subtype. The presence of

IgG4(+) plasma cells in RDD led to a suggestion that it might fall within the spectrum of IgG4-related sclerosing disease, but this association has proven to be inconsistent (discussed below).

## Differential Diagnosis

Once the distinctive sheet-like arrangement of S100-positive histiocytes with emperipolesis is recognized, the diagnosis is usually straightforward. In the breast, especially in limited biopsies, RDD must be distinguished from reactive inflammatory processes, including cellular spindled histiocytic pseudotumor complicating mammary fat necrosis, idiopathic granulomatous mastitis, plasma cell mastitis, and IgG4 sclerosing mastitis. All of these can be readily distinguished by S100 and OCT2 immunostains which are diffusely positive in RDD and negative in the above mimickers as reactive histiocyte/macrophage populations do not express these markers. IgG4 sclerosing mastitis (discussed above) can present a somewhat difficult diagnostic challenge, since IgG4-positive plasma cells are present in both RDD and IgG4 sclerosing mastitis; however, a recent series by *Hoffmann* et al. documenting 22 cases of RDD in the breast demonstrated that none of the cases had a level of IgG4-positive plasma cells that met the diagnostic criteria for IgG4 sclerosing mastitis. Specifically, while a single case of mammary RDD had positive IgG4 staining in ~30% of its plasma cells, this was far below the expected level of 49–85% reported for IgG4 sclerosing mastitis. Neither storiform fibrosis nor obliterative phlebitis, both key histologic features of IgG4-RD, is seen in RDD, although, as noted above, these features are also inconsistently present in IG4-RD of the breast.

RDD has to be distinguished from other localized or systemic histiocytic proliferations, including Langerhans cell histiocytosis (LCH), Erdheim-Chester disease (ECD), juvenile xanthogranuloma, and reticulohistiocytoma. The inflammatory infiltrate in LCH often includes prominent eosinophils. The histiocytes in LCH are also S100-positive; however, morphologically LCH shows irregular, crinkled, or grooved nuclei that are eccentrically placed, and unlike RDD, are positive for CD1a and langerin while negative for CD163. OCT2 expression may be seen in rare LCH cases. Like RDD, ECD is positive for CD163 and can also be positive for S100 in 20–30% of cases, but in contrast to RDD, ECD is negative for OCT2 and is often positive for BRAF V600E, both at the immunohistochemical and genetic levels. Moreover, isolated involvement of the breast is exceptionally rare in ECD.

Both juvenile xanthogranuloma and reticulohistiocytoma are well-defined circumscribed lesions, in contrast to the ill-defined appearance of RDD. Juvenile xanthogranuloma presents as a sharply demarcated superficial papule and contains a polymorphous histiocytic population including Touton-type giant cells, which are usually not seen in RDD. Reticulohistiocytomas also tend to present as a more defined lesion composed of epithelioid histiocytes with distinctive glassy cytoplasm. Emperipolesis, a prominent plasma cell component (especially, IgG4-positive plasma cells), and S100 protein expression are not seen in juvenile xanthogranuloma or reticulohistiocytoma.

Lastly, RDD with a prominent inflammatory infiltrate can mimic cutaneous lymphomas, especially those with a polymorphous background, such as T-cell, anaplastic large cell, or Hodgkin lymphoma. These tumors invariably demonstrate cytologic atypia in the constituent lymphoid cells, and while they are often histiocyte-rich, large pale S100-positive histiocytes with emperipolesis are not identified. A prominent plasma cell component is also not characteristic. In difficult cases, a questionable atypical lymphoid population can be delineated by appropriate lymphoid immunohistochemical markers and clonality studies.

### Prognosis and Treatment

Extranodal RDD follows an indolent course. Up to a third of cases regress spontaneously while the remaining patients have chronic but stable disease. Approximately 10% of patients develop progressive disease or succumb to the mass effects of the tumor or infectious complications. Based on the limited data regarding RDD of the breast, the clinical behavior appears to be similar to that of extranodal RDD occurring elsewhere.

None of the conventional treatment modalities offer complete cure, with surgery remaining the treatment of choice for mass effect or cosmetic reasons. Identification of mutations in signaling pathways such as MAPK may open avenues for targeted therapies in the future.

## Cellular Spindled Histiocytic Pseudotumor Complicating Mammary Fat Necrosis

### Introduction

Sciallis et al. coined the term "cellular spindled histiocytic pseudotumor complicating mammary fat necrosis (CSHP)" for a lesion that can masquerade as a spindle cell lesion, mimicking fibroblastic or myofibroblastic neoplasms. True to its name, CSHP is a lesion that occurs in the setting of mammary fat necrosis and is thought to represent an exaggerated, spindled histiocytic response to this process.

### Clinical Features

Patients with CSHP span a wide age range, with a mean age of 58 years old. Similar to mammary fat necrosis, CSHP often follows an accidental trauma, surgery, or therapeutic irradiation.

## Imaging

CSHP presents as a radiologically evident single mass or multiple masses that can range in appearance from benign to that of a radiologically suspicious lesion mimicking cancer prompting a needle core biopsy. In the series by Sciallis et al., 59% of lesions had suspicious radiologic characteristics and only a third of lesions were regarded as benign by imaging. The mean size is 1.5 cm (range 0.8–2.5 cm).

## Pathologic Features

### Gross Features

Irregular, mass-like lesion variably associated with the gross findings of fat necrosis.

### Microscopic Features

Microscopically, CSHP is characteristically infiltrative in appearance and composed of a cellular spindle cell population that may be arranged in vague fascicles or occasionally have a storiform configuration (Fig. 7.17). This proliferation of spindled cells has eosinophilic, slightly granular cytoplasm and nuclear features in keeping with the histiocytic lineage of the constituent cells, including folded and grooved nuclei without hyperchromasia or distinct nucleoli (Fig. 7.18). CSHP is characteristically infiltrative in appearance with entrapment of mammary glands with a mixed chronic inflammatory cell component and often associated with multinucleated giant cells (Fig. 7.19). Conventional fat necrosis is also found at the periphery of the lesion, providing some reassurance regarding the benign nature of CSHP (Fig. 7.20). Importantly, atypical epithelial proliferative lesions or in situ carcinomas were not seen in any of the lesions described by Sciallis et al.

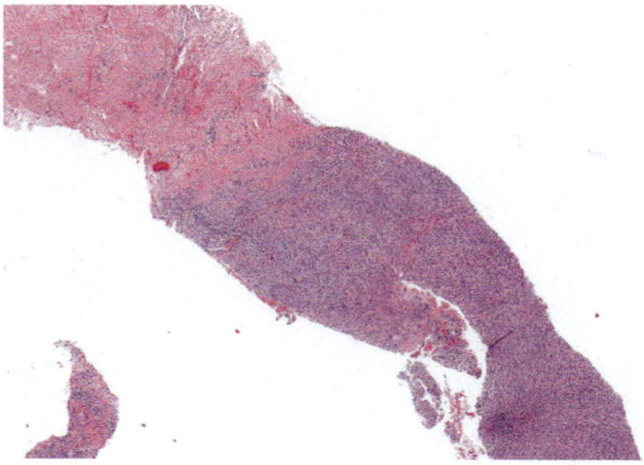

**Fig. 7.17** Cellular spindled histiocytic pseudotumor (CSHP) complicating mammary fat necrosis is a cellular, mass-like lesion with infiltrative borders at low power

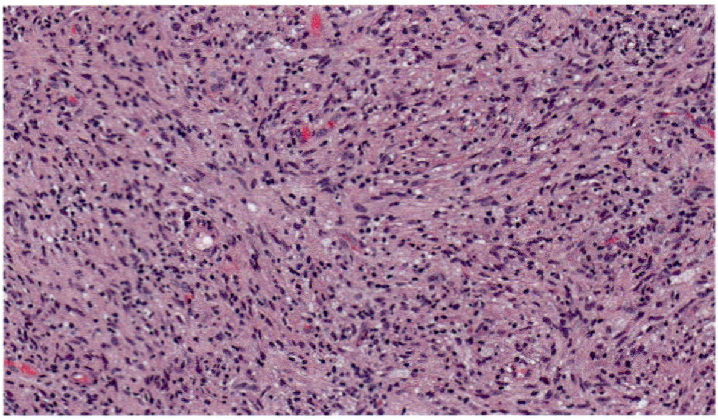

**Fig. 7.18** At high power, CSHP is recognized as a fascicular proliferation of spindled histiocytic cells with eosinophilic, slightly granular cytoplasm and irregular nuclei without hyperchromasia or prominent nucleoli

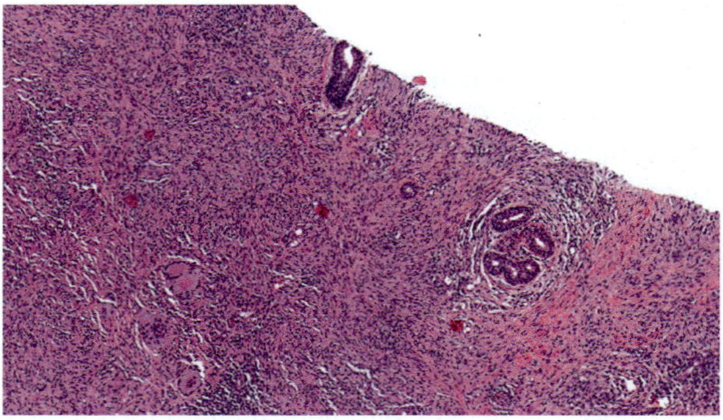

**Fig. 7.19** CSHP typically shows entrapment of mammary glands within the lesion. There is an admixed inflammatory cell component with lymphocytes and occasional foreign body giant cells can be identified

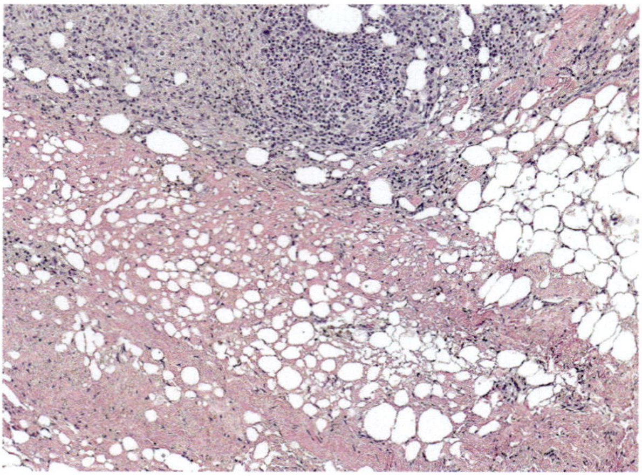

**Fig. 7.20** CSHP showing the presence of conventional fat necrosis at the edge of the spindle cell component can be a helpful histologic clue

## Immunohistochemistry

As expected, CSHP is positive for histiocytic markers, such as CD68, CD163, CD11c, and CD31 (the latter in a weak, granular cytoplasmic pattern), and is negative for multiple cytokeratins, S100, p63, beta-catenin, and fungal and mycobacterial special stains, such as GMS and AFB.

## Differential Diagnosis

The differential diagnosis of CSHP, which lends significance to this benign histiocytic proliferation, includes both benign and malignant neoplastic lesions across numerous cell lineages, as well as infectious processes. Of great importance in the breast is the similarity between CSHP and both histiocytoid invasive lobular carcinoma and low-grade fibromatosis-like metaplastic carcinoma as both of these carcinomas can present with surprisingly little nuclear atypia or mitotic activity, truly resembling the spindled histiocytes of CSHP. Fortunately, both of these carcinomas are positive for cytokeratins, while CSHP is characteristically negative allowing for their easy distinction; p63, which can be positive in spindle cell metaplastic carcinomas of the breast, is also negative in CSHP. Conversely, histiocyte-specific markers like CD163 or CD11c are positive in the latter and typically negative in breast carcinoma variants.

Inflammatory myofibroblastic tumor (IMT) closely resembles CSHP on a morphological basis, although it tends to be more circumscribed. IMT is truly a myofibroblastic lesion and, in addition to positive immunoreactivity for ALK (often accompanied by corresponding *ALK* gene rearrangements), would be expected to be positive for myofibroblastic lineage markers, such as SMA and desmin and to be negative (or only focally immunoreactive) for histiocytic markers with the exception of CD68, which is nonspecific.

Mycobacterial pseudotumor is an additional consideration, especially in the setting of severe immunocompromise, although it is more likely to involve the overlying skin rather than the breast parenchyma. Mycobacterial pseudotumors are composed of similar fascicles of spindled histiocytes and would also be positive for all of the same histiocytic immunostains as CSHP. However, by definition, mycobacterial special stains such as AFB and FITE are expected to be positive in mycobacterial pseudotumors and negative in CSHP. It is worth remembering that pseudotumors with variably spindled histiocytic and myofibroblastic phenotypes can also occur in response to bacterial infections, injected substances, ruptured silicone implants, or rarely, monoclonal immunoglobulin deposits in the setting of underlying hematolymphoid neoplasms (crystal-storing histiocytosis). All of these lesions will contain abundant CD68 and CD163-positive spindled histiocytes. The diagnosis is based largely on the careful review of the clinical presentation and identification of unique features, i.e., vacuolated, lipoblast-like histiocytes containing refractile, non-polarizable material in silicone granulomas or characteristic needle- or oval-shaped intracytoplasmic crystals in crystal-storing histiocytosis.

Finally, systemic histiocytoses, such as Rosai-Dorfman disease (RDD) or Erdheim-Chester disease (ECD), may occasionally involve the breast and also enter the differential diagnosis since they both consist of syncytial-like sheets of pale epithelioid or spindled histiocytes admixed with inflammatory cells. RDD, covered above in this text, is expected to show all of the telltale signs of RDD seen at extramammary sites, including emperipolesis and strong, diffuse immunoreactivity for S100 and OCT2, both of which are conspicuously absent in CSHP. ECD is often positive for BRAF V600E, both at the immunohistochemical and genetic levels; isolated involvement of the breast is exceptionally rare in ECD.

## Prognosis and Treatment

CSHP is an entirely benign, mass-like non-neoplastic reaction to mammary fat necrosis. In their series, Sciallis reported that all of their patients with available follow-up were alive without disease. Cases that underwent a subsequent surgical excision showed only fat necrosis. Therefore, awareness of this distinctive complication of mammary fat necrosis can help avoid overtreatment.

## Selected References

1. Adeniran A, Al-Ahmadie H, Mahoney MC, et al. Granular cell tumor of the breast: a series of 17 cases and review of the literature. Breast J. 2004;10:528–31.
2. Brown AC, Audisio RA, Regitnig P. Granular cell tumour of the breast. Surg Oncol. 2011;20:97–105.
3. Cheah AL, Billings SD, Rowe JJ. Mesenchymal tumours of the breast and their mimics: a review with approach to diagnosis. Pathology. 2016;48(5):406–24.
4. Cheuk W, Chan JK. IgG4-related sclerosing disease: a critical appraisal of an evolving clinicopathologic entity. Adv Anat Pathol. 2010;17:303–32.
5. D'Alfonso TM, et al. Cystic neutrophilic granulomatous mastitis: further characterization of a distinctive histopathologic entity not always demonstrably attributable to corynebacterium infection. Am J Surg Pathol. 2015;39:1440–7.
6. Deshpande V, Zen Y, Chan JK, et al. Consensus statement on the pathology of IgG4-related disease. Mod Pathol. 2012;25:1181–92.
7. Eusebi V, Foschini MP, Bussolati G, et al. Myoblastomatoid (histiocytoid) carcinoma of the breast. A type of apocrine carcinoma. Am J Surg Pathol. 1995;19:553–62.
8. Fanburg-Smith JC, Meis-Kindblom JM, Fante R, et al. Malignant granular cell tumor of soft tissue: diagnostic criteria and clinicopathologic correlation. Am J Surg Pathol. 1998;22:779–94.
9. Garces S, Medeiros LJ, Patel KP, et al. Mutually exclusive recurrent KRAS and MAP2K1 mutations in Rosai-Dorfman disease. Mod Pathol. 2017;30(10):1367.
10. Gautham I, Radford DM, Kovacs CS, et al. Cystic neutrophilic granulomatous mastitis: The Cleveland Clinic experience with diagnosis and management. Breast J. 2019;25(1):80–5.
11. Goyal G, Young JR, Koster MJ, et al. Mayo Clinic Histiocytosis Working Group. The Mayo Clinic Histiocytosis Working Group Consensus Statement for the Diagnosis and Evaluation of Adult Patients With Histiocytic Neoplasms: Erdheim-Chester Disease, Langerhans Cell Histiocytosis, and Rosai-Dorfman Disease. Mayo Clin Proc. 2019;94(10):2054–71. Epub 2019 Aug 28.
12. Green I, Dorfman RF, Rosai J. Breast involvement by extranodal Rosai-Dorfman disease: report of seven cases. Am J Surg Pathol. 1997;21(6):664–8.
13. Gupta D, Croitoru CM, Ayala AG, et al. E-cadherin immunohistochemical analysis of histiocytoid carcinoma of the breast. Ann Diagn Pathol. 2002;6:141–7.
14. Hamano H, Kawa S, Horiuchi A, et al. High serum IgG4 concentrations in patients with sclerosing pancreatitis. N Engl J Med. 2001;344:732–8.
15. Hoffmann JC, Lin CY, Bhattacharyya S, et al. Rosai-Dorfman disease of the breast with variable IgG4+ plasma cells: a diagnostic mimicker of other malignant and reactive entities. Am J Surg Pathol. 2019;43(12):1653–60.
16. Kamisawa T, Funata N, Hayashi Y, et al. A new clinicopathological entity of IgG4-related autoimmune disease. J Gastroenterol. 2003;38:982–4.
17. Lack EE, Worsham GF, Callihan MD, et al. Granular cell tumor: a clinicopathologic study of 110 patients. J Surg Oncol. 1980;13:301–16.

18. Liu L, Perry AM, Cao W, et al. Relationship between Rosai-Dorfman disease and IgG4-related disease: study of 32 cases. Am J Clin Pathol. 2013;140(3):395.
19. Menon MP, Evbuomwan MO, Rosai J, et al. A subset of Rosai-Dorfman disease cases show increased IgG4-positive plasma cells: another red herring or a true association with IgG4-related disease? Histopathology. 2014;64(3):455.
20. Morkowski JJ, Nguyen CV, Lin P, et al. Rosai-Dorfman disease confined to the breast. Ann Diagn Pathol. 2010;14(2):81–7.
21. Naik MA, Korlimarla A, Shetty ST, et al. Cystic neutrophilic granulomatous mastitis: a clinicopathological study with 16s rRNA sequencing for the detection of corynebacteria in formalin-fixed paraffin-embedded tissue. Int J Surg Pathol. 2020;28(4):371–81.
22. Ozkaya N, Rosenblum MK, Durham BH, et al. The histopathology of Erdheim-Chester disease: a comprehensive review of a molecularly characterized cohort. Mod Pathol. 2018;31(4):581–97. PMID: 29192649.
23. Oztekin PS, Durhan G, Nercis Kosar P, et al. Imaging Findings in Patients with Granulomatous Mastitis. Iran J Radiol. 2016;13(3):e33900.
24. Ravindran A, Goyal G, Go RS, et al. Mayo Clinic Histiocytosis working group. Rosai-Dorfman disease displays a unique monocyte-macrophage phenotype characterized by expression of OCT2. Am J Surg Pathol. 2021;45(1):35–44.
25. Shimizu S, Kitamura H, Ito T, et al. Histiocytoid breast carcinoma: histological, immunohistochemical, ultrastructural, cytological and clinicopathological studies. Pathol Int. 1998;48:549–56.
26. Stone JH, Zen Y, Deshpande V. IgG4-related disease. N Engl J Med. 2012;366:539–51.
27. Tan PH, Harada O, Thike AA, et al. Histiocytoid breast carcinoma: an enigmatic lobular entity. J Clin Pathol. 2011;64:654–9.
28. Vargas AC, Lakhani SR, Simpson PT. Pleomorphic lobular carcinoma of the breast: molecular pathology and clinical impact. Future Oncol. 2009;5(2):233–43.
29. Wu JM, Turashvili G. Cystic neutrophilic granulomatous mastitis: an update. J Clin Pathol. 2020;73:445–53.

# Miscellaneous Mesenchymal Tumors of the Breast

# 8

Darya Buehler and Paul Weisman

## Contents



D. Buehler (✉) · P. Weisman
Department of Pathology and Laboratory Medicine, School of Medicine and Public Health, University of Wisconsin-Madison, Madison, WI, USA
e-mail: buehler2@wisc.edu



J. J. Rowe, E. Downs-Kelly (eds.), *Mesenchymal Tumors of the Breast and Their Mimics*, https://doi.org/10.1007/978-3-030-74474-8_8

## Solitary Fibrous Tumor

### Clinical Features

Solitary fibrous tumors (SFTs), originally described in the pleura, may be found at any anatomic site. The use of a historic term "hemangiopericytoma" is no longer recommended as these tumors are now incorporated into the SFT category. SFTs most often affect middle-aged or older adults of both sexes with a predilection for body cavities, viscera, head and neck, deep soft tissues of the trunk and extremities, intracranial locations, and, uncommonly, breast parenchyma. Primary SFTs of the breast parenchyma usually present as slow growing, well-circumscribed non-tender palpable masses in adults in their fourth through sixth decade (reported age range 33–81), with a slight female predilection. The average size is 3.5 cm (range 0.6–19 cm). Very small tumors may be discovered incidentally.

### Imaging

Well-circumscribed solid mass, with or without calcification; well-circumscribed hypoechoic mass with increased vascularity by ultrasonography.

### Pathologic Features

#### Gross Features

Well-circumscribed, homogenous, variably fibrous white-tan mass; malignant examples have a fleshy appearance and may show areas of hemorrhage or necrosis.

#### Microscopic Features

SFTs have a broad spectrum of histologic features. They are generally circumscribed and unencapsulated (Fig. 8.1) and show variable proportions of more cellular and less cellular fibrous or myxoid zones, usually in a somewhat alternating configuration. Numerous branching staghorn-like vessels are present (Fig. 8.2). The

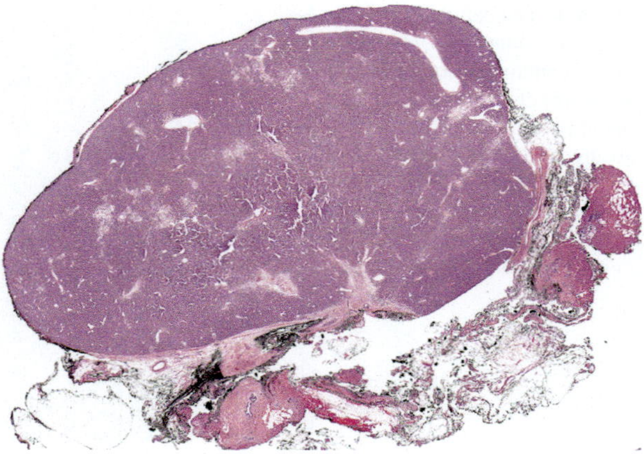

**Fig. 8.1** Solitary fibrous tumor of the breast presenting as a circumscribed unencapsulated mass with a pushing border

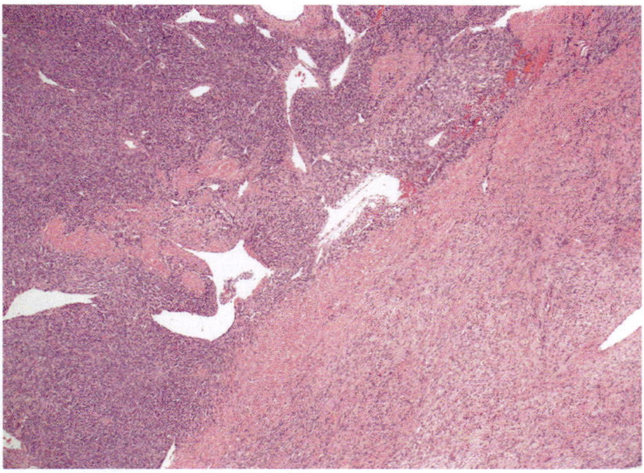

**Fig. 8.2** Solitary fibrous tumor showing alternating more cellular and less cellular fibrous zones. Numerous branching staghorn-like vessels are present

cellular zones contain monotonous short spindle cells arranged in a vaguely fascicular pattern commonly referred to as a "patternless pattern" with minimal intervening collagenous stroma. The cells contain uniform round to oval nuclei with vesicular chromatin and usually have inconspicuous nucleoli and amphophilic or basophilic cytoplasm (Fig. 8.3). In the fibrous zones, the cells are separated by a large amount of collagenous stroma, which may contain keloidal or ropey-type collagen fibers resembling myofibroblastoma (Figs. 8.4 and 8.5). The vessels in the less cellular zones are larger and more dilated, often with hyalinized walls or intraluminal fibrin. Myxoid stroma, microcystic changes, stromal hyalinization, inflammatory and mast cells, clear cell changes, and pseudovascular spaces lined by multinucleated giant cells are often present (Figs. 8.6 and 8.7). A lipomatous or fat-forming variant has been characterized (Fig. 8.8). Hypercellularity, cytologic atypia, necrosis, and increased mitotic activity within a conventional SFT warrant closer assessment, although the most robust predictors of malignant behavior in SFTs are size, mitotic

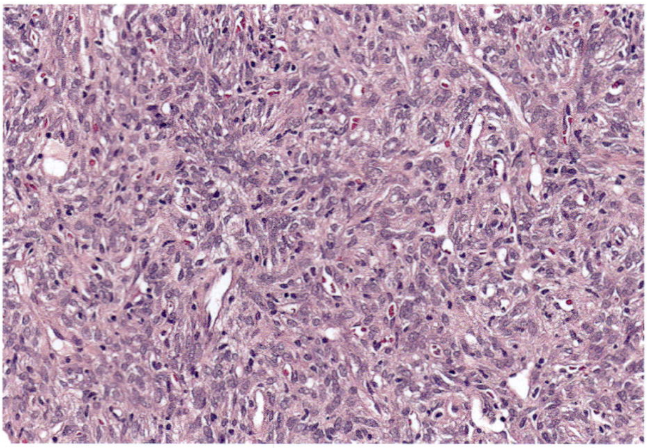

**Fig. 8.3** The cellular zones in solitary fibrous tumor contain monotonous short spindle cells with bland nuclear features, arranged in a "patternless pattern" with minimal intervening collagenous stroma

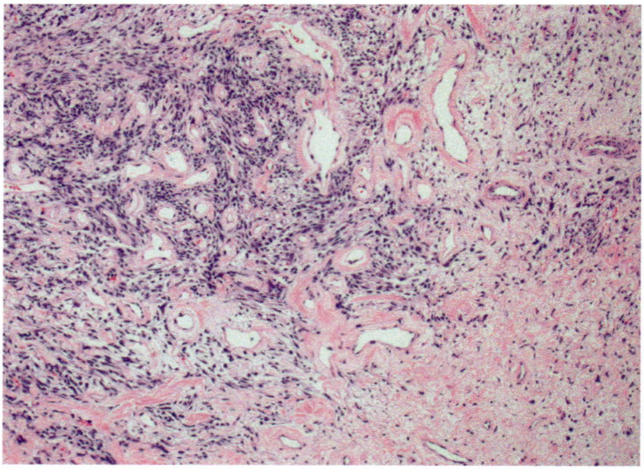

**Fig. 8.4** Hypocellular zones in solitary fibrous tumor containing hyalinized vasculature

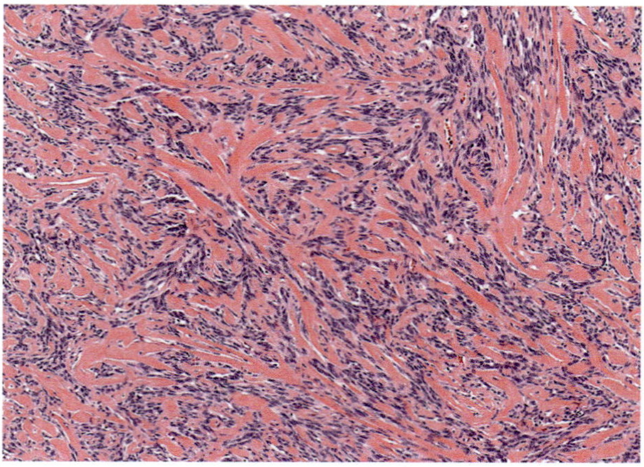

**Fig. 8.5** Solitary fibrous tumor with prominent ropey-type collagen fibers resembling myofibroblastoma

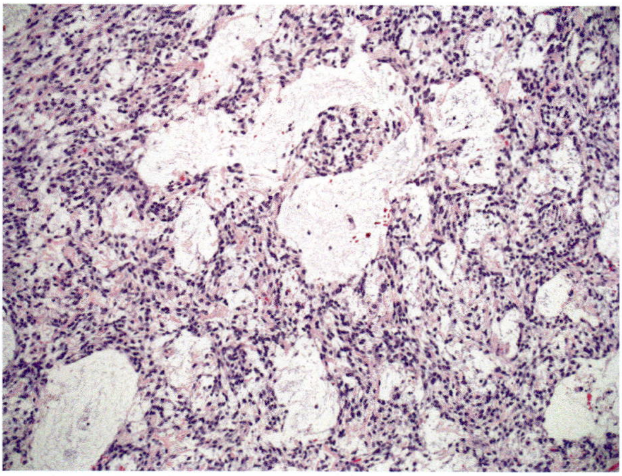

**Fig. 8.6** Solitary fibrous tumor with myxoid stroma and microcystic changes

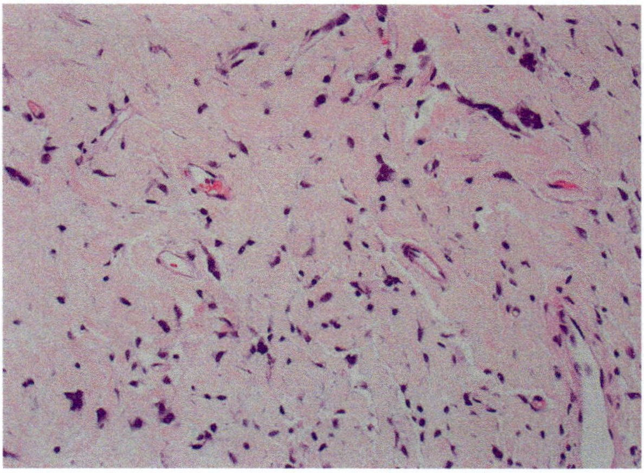

**Fig. 8.7** Solitary fibrous tumor with pseudovascular spaces lined by multinucleated giant cells (a histologic pattern originally described as "giant cell angiofibroma")

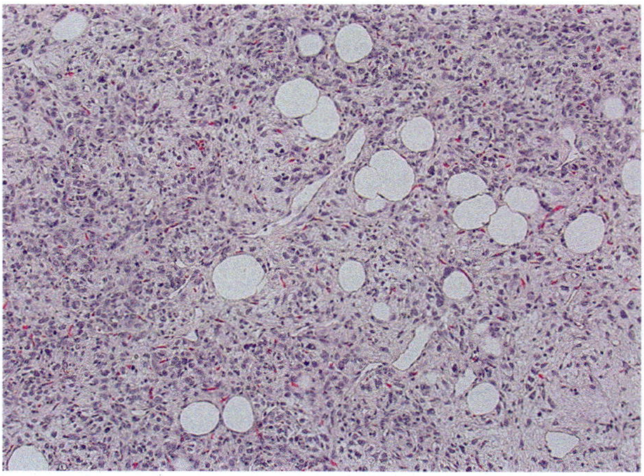

**Fig. 8.8** A lipomatous or fat-forming variant of solitary fibrous tumor with myxoid stroma, mature adipocytes, and prominent vasculature

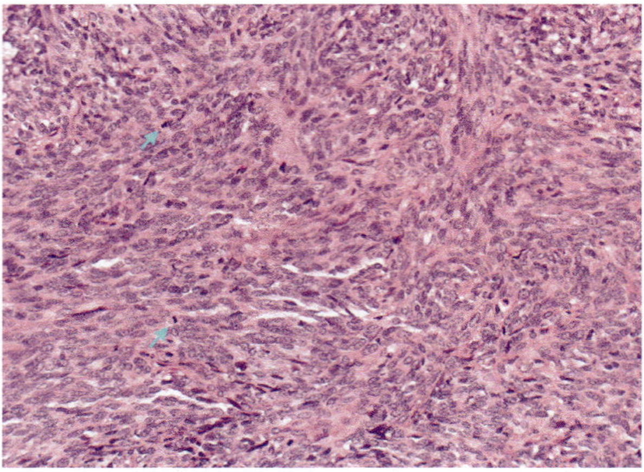

**Fig. 8.9** High-risk solitary fibrous tumor with increased cellularity, fascicular growth pattern, and frequent mitotic figures (arrows)

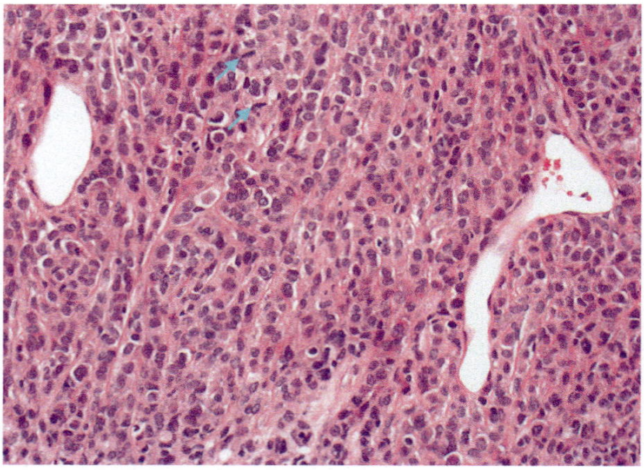

**Fig. 8.10** Another example of high-risk solitary fibrous tumor with increased cellularity, diffuse nuclear atypia, and frequent mitotic figures (arrows)

activity, and necrosis (Figs. 8.9 and 8.10), discussed in detail below. Dedifferentiated SFTs usually show areas of anaplasia or an abrupt transition to a high-grade spindle cell or pleomorphic sarcoma, but dedifferentiation toward other lineages, such as rhabdomyosarcoma and osteosarcoma, has been reported. While malignant SFTs in the breast have been reported, dedifferentiation to a high-grade sarcoma has not yet been described in SFTs of the breast.

## Immunohistochemistry

Strong diffuse expression of CD34 is seen in most classic SFTs and in the above-mentioned variants, but this marker lacks specificity and may be lost in approximately 10% of cases, especially in histologically malignant examples.

Genetically, SFTs show a paracentric inversion within chromosome 12q resulting in pathognomonic *NAB2-STAT6* gene fusion as a driver event. This results in nuclear expression of the STAT6 protein, which can be detected immunohistochemically in SFTs from all sites and is a highly sensitive diagnostic test with a near 100% specificity for SFT using a rabbit monoclonal antibody. STAT6 expression may be lost in dedifferentiated SFTs. SFTs variably express CD99, bcl-2, SMA, EMA, beta-catenin, GFAP, and GRIA2, but these markers lack specificity and their use for diagnosis of SFT is discouraged. Expression of estrogen receptor is variable and inconsistent.

## Molecular

SFTs show a paracentric inversion within chromosome 12q resulting in a pathognomonic *NAB2-STAT6* gene fusion.

## Differential Diagnosis

The most important diagnostic pitfall in the context of breast location are the CD34-positive superficial mesenchymal tumors with bland fibroblastic morphology. Myofibroblastoma is characterized by *RB1* deletion on 13q and is especially similar to SFT, being composed of short and bland CD34-positive spindle cells arranged in a whorled or vaguely fascicular pattern in a fibrous background containing mast cells and hyalinized vessels. However, a prominent staghorn-like vascular pattern is not a typical feature. STAT6 is not expressed in this tumor, and conversely, *RB1* and *FOXO1A* gene deletions and the loss of Rb expression by IHC do not occur in SFTs. Another important diagnostic mimic, particularly in younger patients, is dermatofibrosarcoma protuberans (DFSP), which enters the differential diagnosis based on the whorled arrangement of the monotonous short spindle cells with bland nuclei and diffuse CD34 expression. Keloidal collagen fibers and ectatic hyalinized staghorn vessels of SFTs are not typical of DFSP, but the most reliable features to exclude the latter are diffuse infiltration of the subcutis in a "honeycomb" pattern and entrapment of adnexal structures. DFSP is negative for STAT6 expression and may be confirmed by FISH for *PDGFB* gene rearrangement, which is not seen in SFTs.

Soft tissue perineuriomas and hybrid schwannomas/perineuriomas are well-circumscribed, often subcutaneous, tumors composed of cytologically bland spindle cells with slender bipolar processes arranged in a whorled growth pattern in a collagenous background and are often CD34-positive. These tumors can resemble cellular SFTs, although they typically lack the distinctive staghorn vessels and perivascular hyalinization. The slender bipolar processes that typify perineurial cells are not seen in SFTs, although this feature may be difficult to appreciate in perineuriomas as well without the use of IHC. A helpful IHC combination in this context would include EMA and/or GLUT1 to highlight the bipolar processes in perineurioma and STAT6, which would be positive in SFTs, but negative in perineuriomas.

Low-grade fibromyxoid sarcoma, additionally discussed in the myofibroblastic tumor chapter, can be distinguished from SFT based on MUC4 expression and negative CD34 and STAT6 immunostains. In ambiguous cases (such as MUC4-negative examples of LGFMS with *YAP1* fusion), confirmatory testing for rearrangements involving *FUS*, *EWSR1*, or *YAP1* genes may be required to diagnose LGFMS, but this is rarely necessary as the above immunohistochemical stains are very specific in this context.

Lastly, cellular SFTs with fascicular architecture as well as hypercellular and cytologically atypical SFTs may closely resemble monophasic synovial sarcoma, low-grade fibromatosis-like metaplastic carcinoma, fibrosarcomatous DFSP, and, in cases with greater nuclear atypia, malignant phyllodes tumor with sarcomatous stromal overgrowth. CD34 immunostain in this context may be unreliable as its expression in malignant SFT, fibrosarcomatous DFSP, and the stromal component of PT is highly variable and may be negative. However, all of the above mimickers are consistently negative for STAT6 expression.

## Treatment and Prognosis

The behavior of SFTs has been extensively studied over the years. Most extracranial SFTs with typical morphologic features tend to behave in an indolent fashion, with a small overall risk of systemic metastasis (5–10%) which can occur even in seemingly the most banal-looking SFTs, leading to the classification as a tumor of intermediate malignant potential. Overtly histologically malignant SFTs metastasize in up to 30% of cases. A small subset of SFTs may undergo dedifferentiation into a high-grade sarcoma, and these tumors behave comparably to other soft tissue sarcomas. But predicting the behavior in ordinary SFTs that lack overt sarcomatoid or anaplastic features is notoriously difficult. Traditional histologic criteria for malignancy in SFTs such as cytologic atypia, nuclear pleomorphism, necrosis, hypercellularity, and mitotic activity >4/10 HPF have been inconsistently associated with adverse outcomes.

In the last few years, a number of multivariate risk stratification models for development of metastasis in SFT were put forth, of which the most popular is a four-variable model by Demicco et al. In this model, a score is assigned based on the patient's age, tumor size, mitotic count, and presence of necrosis, and the overall risk (low, intermediate, or high) is calculated based on the total score (Table 8.1). In the validation studies using this system, SFTs classified as low-risk showed essentially no metastasis, whereas SFTs classified as intermediate- and high-risk were associated with approximately 10% and 70% risk of metastasis, respectively. Whether the above risk-assessment system is applicable to SFTs arising in the breast requires further study.

**Table 8.1** Modified four-variable risk stratification model for development of metastasis in solitary fibrous tumors by Demicco et al.

| *Risk factor* | *Score* |
|---|---|
| Age | |
| <55 | 0 |
| ≥55 | 1 |
| Tumor size (cm) | |
| <5 | 0 |
| 5 to 10 | 1 |
| 10 to 15 | 2 |
| ≥15 | 3 |
| Mitotic count (/10 high-power fields) | |
| 0 | 0 |
| 1–3 | 1 |
| ≥4 | 2 |
| Tumor necrosis | |
| <10% | 0 |
| ≥10% | 1 |
| *Risk class* | *Total score* |
| Low | 0–3 |
| Intermediate | 4–5 |
| High | 6–7 |

Reproduced with permission from: Demicco et al. [31]

Treatment of benign SFTs at all sites is best accomplished by a complete surgical excision whenever possible, to minimize the risk of local recurrence. Malignant SFTs at all sites are best treated by a multimodal approach similar to other sarcomas.

## Ossifying Fibromyxoid Tumor

### Clinical Features

Ossifying fibromyxoid tumor (OFMT) is a distinctive, translocation-associated mesenchymal neoplasm which occurs mostly in middle-aged adults (age range 10–88 years), with a slight predilection for male patients. Most are solitary, well-circumscribed painless masses involving the superficial tissues of the lower limbs, but OFMTs may present anywhere including the upper limbs, trunk, head and neck, and unusual locations like the skeletal muscle, mediastinum, retroperitoneum, thyroid gland, and breast. The median size is 3–4 cm, although some tumors can be quite large (up to 21 cm).

## Imaging

Mammographic and ultrasonographic findings show a solid circumscribed mass with peripheral calcifications, suggestive of calcified fibroadenoma. OFMTs detected in soft tissues by other imaging modalities demonstrate similar findings. Superficial OFMTs typically involve the subcutis and may not be imaged.

## Pathologic Features

### Gross Features

Well-circumscribed fibrous or somewhat fleshy tan-white mass with calcifications.

### Microscopic Features

OFMT is circumscribed and has a fibrous pseudocapsule. However, focal infiltrative growth and microscopic satellite nodules may be seen. The classic telltale histological feature of OFMT is a peripheral shell of mature lamellar bone (Fig. 8.11), but this feature is variably present (40–85% of cases). The remaining examples represent the so-called non-ossifying variant of OFMT (Fig. 8.12). Both variants are variably cellular and are composed of epithelioid or spindled cells arranged in corded, nested, trabecular, or sheet-like patterns. The stroma shows variable proportions of myxoid, fibrous, densely hyalinized, and chondroid zones (Figs. 8.13, 8.14, 8.15, and 8.16) and may show deposits of woven bone without embedded tumor cells. Many cases show prominent vessels. Microcystic changes, spindle cell areas with or without fascicle formation, and rhabdoid-like morphology may rarely occur. This morphologic diversity may occasionally be present within a single case.

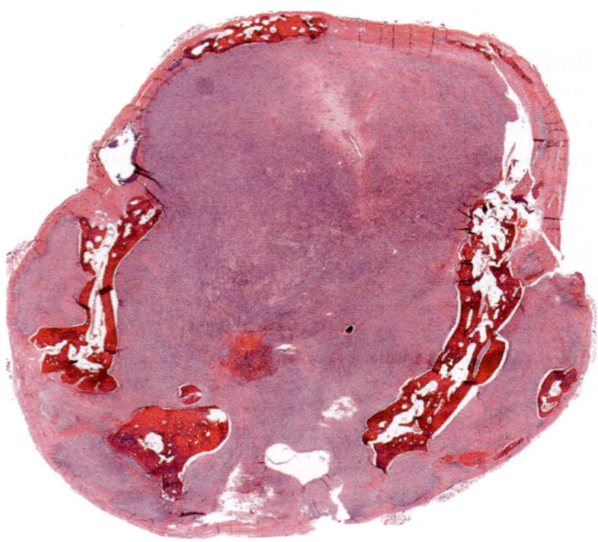

**Fig. 8.11** Ossifying fibromyxoid tumor (OFMT) presenting as a circumscribed mass with a peripheral shell of mature lamellar bone

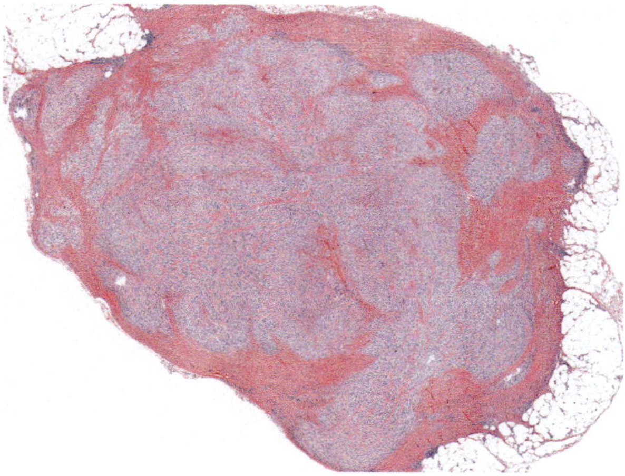

**Fig. 8.12** Non-ossifying variant of OFMT with a fibrous pseudocapsule

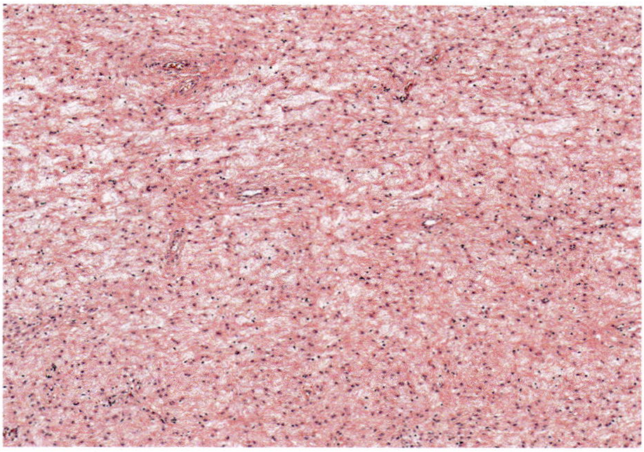

**Fig. 8.13** OFMT with a corded growth pattern in a fibromyxoid stroma

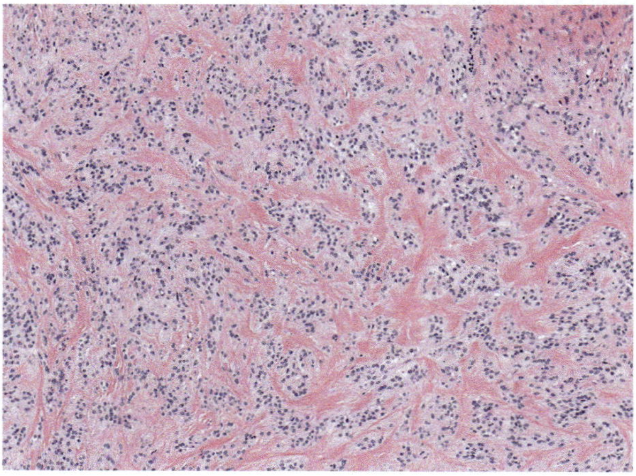

**Fig. 8.14** OFMT with a nested arrangement in a collagenous stroma

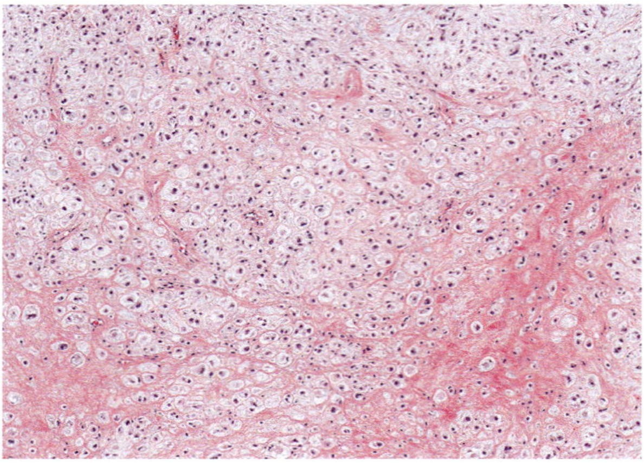

**Fig. 8.15** OFMT with chondroid zones

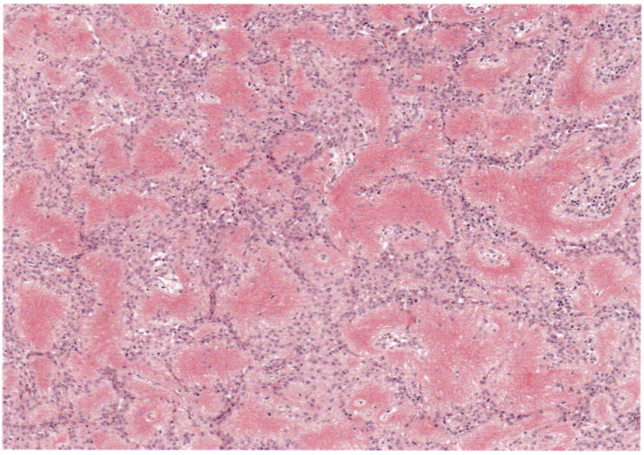

**Fig. 8.16** OFMT showing a sheet-like growth pattern with intervening broad collagen bands

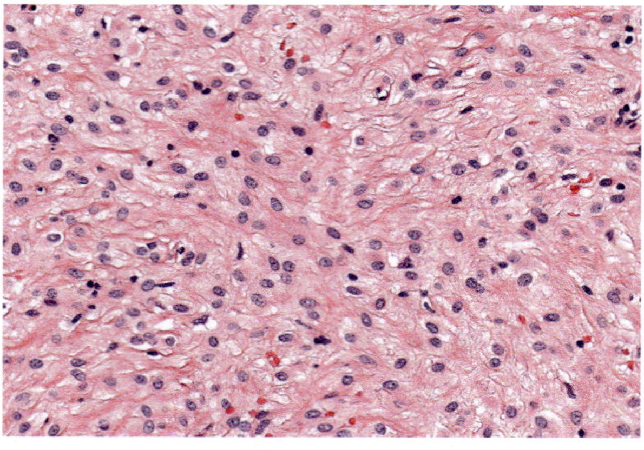

**Fig. 8.17** Typical OFMTs show very uniform oval nuclei with fine chromatin and delicate pinpoint nucleoli, without significant nuclear atypia

Irrespective of the growth pattern, all OFMTs show strikingly similar, uniform oval nuclei with fine chromatin and delicate pinpoint nucleoli (Fig. 8.17). These nuclear features are one of the most helpful clues for identifying OFMT. In most cases, the nuclei are banal and there is virtually no mitotic activity. Scattered nuclear atypia of degenerative type may be present.

More worrisome histologic features including diffuse nuclear atypia, high cellularity, necrosis, or increased mitotic activity can be associated with aggressive behavior. Folpe and Weiss proposed an outcome-based risk stratification system dividing OFMTs into typical, atypical, and malignant forms. Malignant OFMT is defined as having high nuclear grade (Figs. 8.18 and 8.19) or a combination of high cellularity and a mitotic count of >2/50 HPF (Fig. 8.20). Cases having at least one atypical feature such as a mitotic count of >2/50 HPF alone or high cellularity or moderate nuclear atypia with a mitotic count of ≤2/50 HPF are considered atypical OFMTs. Some malignant OFMTs arise de novo, whereas others progress from a more typical benign OFMT precursor.

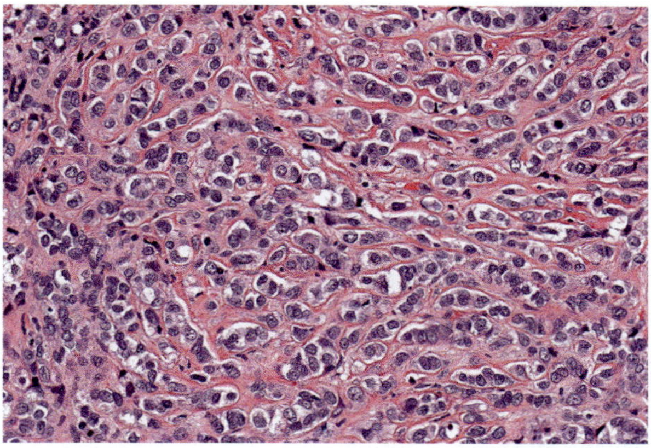

**Fig. 8.18** Malignant OFMT showing a high-grade nuclear atypia

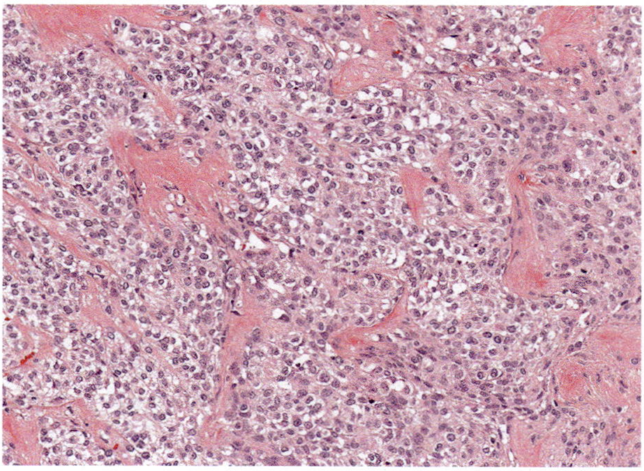

**Fig. 8.19** Malignant OFMT showing clear cell change

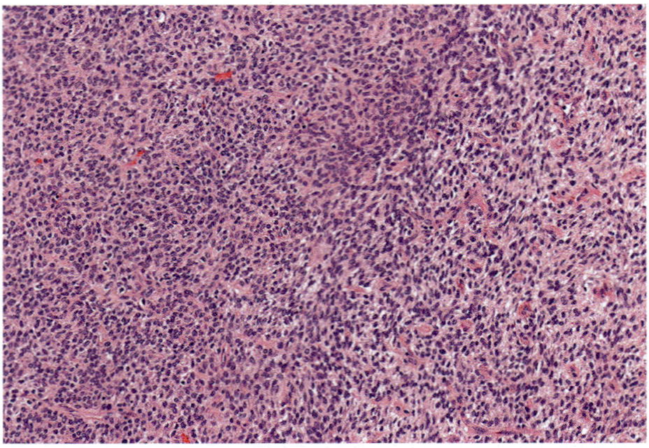

**Fig. 8.20** Malignant OFMT with a combination of high cellularity and a mitotic count of >2/50 HPF

## Immunohistochemistry

As is often the case with translocation-driven neoplasms, OFMT has a complex immunophenotype. S100 protein is expressed in approximately 70–90% of cases, but expression can be focal. Desmin is expressed in 10–40% of cases. OFMTs show inconsistent immunoreactivity for SMA, p63, GFAP, CD10, ER, and PR. EMA and cytokeratins may show focal expression, although only in a minority of cases and more often in malignant OFMT. OFMTs are negative for melanocytic markers, CD34 and CD31. SOX10 expression is noted in only 4% of the tumors. Approximately a quarter of cases express MUC4 due to upregulation of this protein. TFE3 is expressed by IHC in *TFE3*-rearranged OFMTs. Mosaic loss of INI1 expression can be observed in a subset of cases due to hemizygous deletions of *SMARCB1*.

## Molecular

Up to 85% of OFMTs (including typical, atypical, and malignant cases) have recurrent gene rearrangements, most commonly involving *PHF1* on 6p21 with fusion partners that include *EP400*, *MEAF6*, and *EPC1*. Less common variant fusions include *ZC3H7B-BCOR, CREBBP-BCOR1*, and *KDMA2-WWTR1*. Most recently, *PHF1-TFE3* fusions have been reported in five non-ossifying OFMTs; these tumors are diffusely positive for TFE3 by IHC. Most of the above genes participate in epigenetic regulation and histone modification. More data is needed to correlate the type of fusion with the clinical behavior, but it appears that OFMTs with variant non-*PHF1* fusions and those with *PHF1-TFE3* fusion behave more aggressively. FISH to detect *PHF1* rearrangements is a useful ancillary diagnostic technique in difficult cases. Commercially available next-generation sarcoma fusion panels typically include *PHF1* as well as some of the above variant fusion partners, which can help to identify non-*PHF1* rearranged OFMTs.

## Differential Diagnosis

Given the variety of growth patterns and the lack of a peripheral shell of bone in many cases, it is not surprising that OFMTs often are mistaken for other mesenchymal neoplasms including myoepithelioma and myoepithelial carcinoma. Like OFMT, myoepithelioma consists of epithelioid or spindled cells arranged in various combinations of reticular, trabecular, and nested patterns, within a fibromyxoid stroma. Cartilaginous and osseous differentiation may occur in myoepithelial tumors, although it rarely takes the form of a peripheral rim of mature lamellar bone as seen in OFMT. Markers of myoepithelial differentiation such as p63, SMA, and particularly S100 protein are of limited value, because they are also expressed in OFMT. However, strong diffuse expression of keratins, EMA, and SOX10 would favor a myoepithelial tumor since these markers are expressed in only a small percentage of OFMT and usually only focally. *PHF1* gene rearrangement has not been observed in myoepithelial tumors, which, in contrast, may demonstrate rearrangements of *EWSR1* (~80% of cases), *FUS*, and *PLAG1*. Since the array of gene fusions in both neoplasms is quite broad, a commercially available sarcoma fusion assay will likely surpass individual FISH probes for an accurate diagnostic classification.

In the context of primary breast tumors, OFMT has the greatest degree of morphological overlap with low-grade spindle cell metaplastic carcinomas, such as the so-called low-grade fibromatosis-like metaplastic carcinoma. The presence of small clusters of epithelioid cells and diffuse expression of keratins, especially high molecular weight cytokeratins, can distinguish this particular variant of metaplastic carcinoma from OFMT. Another primary mammary spindle cell lesion that frequently enters the differential diagnosis is myofibroblastoma, both conventional and epithelioid, which can be differentiated from OFMT by the frequent expression of estrogen receptor and CD34 and the lack of Rb expression. Heterologous cartilage and bone formation has been described in myofibroblastoma, but it rarely takes the form of a peripheral shell of mature lamellar bone as seen in OFMT.

Epithelioid schwannomas resemble OFMT, because they are also composed of epithelioid cells arranged in a nested or trabecular pattern, have hyalinized or myxoid stroma, and often lack Antoni A areas. Both tumors can be positive for S100 and show inactivation of SMARCB1/INI1, which is seen in 42% of epithelioid schwannomas. However, the nuclei in epithelioid schwannomas are more irregular and reniform in appearance, and metaplastic ossification or desmin expression is entirely uncharacteristic. The presence of a conventional schwannoma component with hyalinized vasculature, a true capsule with EMA or GLUT1-positive perineurial cells, and very strong, diffuse immunoreactivity for SOX10 favors epithelioid schwannoma.

Malignant OFMT may be confused with epithelioid MPNSTs, which are often superficial. Although separating these two entities might be virtually impossible in some cases without ancillary testing, epithelioid MPNSTs typically lack desmin immunoreactivity and show strong and diffuse S100 and SOX10 expression. Homozygous SMARCB1/INI loss is characteristic of epithelioid MPNSTs, while INI1 is usually retained or lost in a mosaic pattern in OFMT.

OFMTs with a collagenous stroma may resemble low-grade fibromyxoid sarcoma (LGFMS), which also often presents as a well-circumscribed firm tumor in the subcutis. A prominent whorled/storiform arrangement of constitutive tumor cells and characteristic arcades of vessels in myxoid zones favor a diagnosis of LGFMS. OFMTs with particularly densely hyalinized stroma and cord-like arrangement of lesional cells can be confused with sclerosing epithelioid fibrosarcoma (SEF). By immunohistochemistry, both LGFMS and SEF are more often positive for EMA and negative for S100. MUC4, a sensitive and specific marker of both LGFMS and SEF, can be positive in 20–30% of OFMT, although the staining is usually focal and weak. Diagnostically challenging cases of LGFMS and SEF can be distinguished from OFMT by testing for *FUS*, *EWSR1*, and *YAP1* rearrangements (present in both LGFMS and SEF) and/or *PFH1* rearrangements. A commercially available sarcoma fusion assay will detect most variant fusions present in both tumors allowing for an accurate classification. Low-grade fibromyxoid sarcoma is discussed further in the myofibroblastic tumor chapter.

Although the hallmark feature of OFMT is a well-formed shell of lamellar bone at the tumor periphery, some cases show a more diffuse, lace-like, or random pattern of woven bone deposition. If coupled with atypical or malignant cytology, such cases may be mistaken for a metaplastic breast carcinoma with mesenchymal differentiation (in the form of osteosarcomatous differentiation) or true primary osteosarcoma of the breast. Matrix-producing metaplastic carcinoma may also resemble malignant OFMT due to corded or nested growth pattern in myxohyaline stroma. Marked atypia and nuclear pleomorphism would favor metaplastic carcinoma or primary osteosarcoma as these features are not typical of OFMT, even in malignant cases. The presence of DCIS and the diffuse expression of cytokeratins would provide further support for a metaplastic carcinoma. It is worth remembering that malignant OFMTs may show cytokeratin expression in approximately 10% of cases, and rare examples can also express p63, although expression of these markers does not reach the extent seen in metaplastic carcinomas of the breast.

## Treatment and Prognosis

If graded according to the proposed risk stratification by Folpe and Weiss, malignant OFMTs show local recurrence in 22% and metastasis in 12.5% of cases, while typical OFMTs recur or metastasize very rarely (0–4% and 0–6%, respectively, based on various series). Because adverse events were reported even in cases with the typical low-grade morphology, all OFMTs at present are regarded as neoplasms of uncertain malignant behavior. The treatment for typical OFMTs is a complete surgical resection with a negative margin. Malignant OFMTs, which behave rather aggressively, are best managed by a multidisciplinary sarcoma team with a combination of surgery and radiation therapy. The data on chemotherapy use in OFMT is very sparse.

## Synovial Sarcoma

### Clinical Features

Synovial sarcoma is an uncommon translocation-associated malignant mesenchymal neoplasm with partial epithelial differentiation and pathognomonic *SS18-SSX1/2/4* gene fusions. The typical presentation is an extremity-based periarticular soft tissue tumor in adolescents or young adults (median age 39 years), but SS spans a broad age range (from infancy to 85 years) and may occur at virtually any anatomic site; the breast, although uncommon, is no exception. In the breast and elsewhere, synovial sarcomas present as an asymptomatic or tender mass or swelling. The tumors range in size from minute to over 10 cm in greatest dimension.

### Imaging

Ultrasonographic findings are often of a solid, variably hypoechoic soft tissue mass or complex cyst with irregular margins. Mammography shows a solid mass or cyst which may contain punctate calcifications. At soft tissue sites, the MRI features of synovial sarcoma are well characterized, showing heterogeneously enhancing multilobulated soft tissue mass, which may contain cystic changes, areas of hemorrhage, and calcifications.

### Pathologic Features

Histologically, synovial sarcomas are broadly divided into three main subtypes: monophasic (pure spindle cell), biphasic (spindle cell and epithelial component), and poorly differentiated subtype with round cell morphology. The monophasic spindle cell variant is composed of monotonous fascicles of basophilic spindle cells arranged in a so-called "herringbone" pattern (Fig. 8.21). The spindle cells show uniform elongated vesicular nuclei with evenly distributed chromatin, scant cytoplasm, and indistinct cell borders (Fig. 8.22). Nuclear pleomorphism is not characteristic of treatment-naïve SS. The stroma usually demonstrates delicate wiry collagen fibers or little intervening collagen, but in other examples the stroma can be markedly fibrous, hyalinized, or myxoid (Figs. 8.23 and 8.24). Cystic changes, areas of hemorrhage, and mast cells are common. Many spindle cell synovial sarcomas have prominent branching staghorn-like vessels like those seen in SFTs (Figs. 8.25 and 8.26).

Biphasic synovial sarcoma is composed of an admixture of a monotonous spindle cell component and epithelial cells forming elaborate glandular structures and papillary projections lined by cuboidal or columnar cells with similar nuclear features (Fig. 8.27). Pure monophasic epithelial tumors are very rare (<1%). As mentioned above, calcifications are common (approximately 30%)

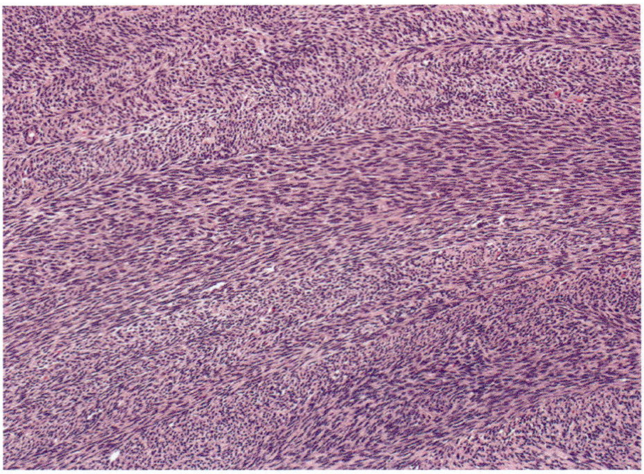

**Fig. 8.21** Monophasic spindle cell synovial sarcoma composed of monotonous fascicles of basophilic spindle cells

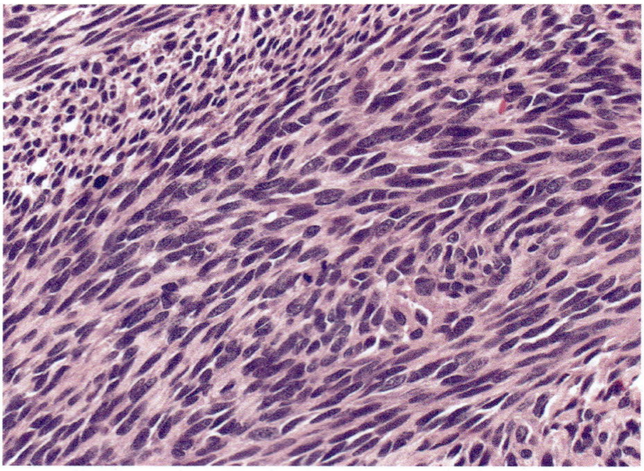

**Fig. 8.22** Monophasic spindle cell synovial sarcoma showing uniform elongated vesicular nuclei with evenly distributed chromatin, scant cytoplasm, and indistinct cell borders

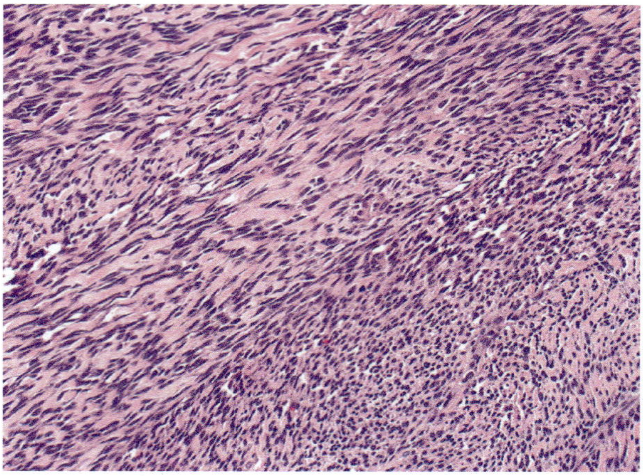

**Fig. 8.23** Delicate wiry collagen fibers separating individual tumor cells in spindle cell synovial sarcoma

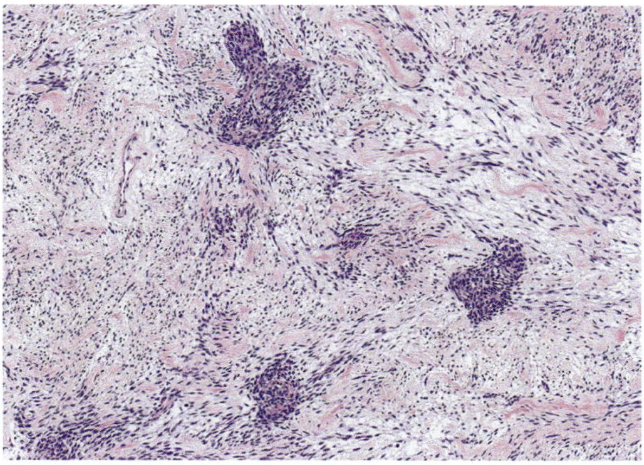

**Fig. 8.24** Monophasic spindle cell synovial sarcoma with prominent myxoid stroma

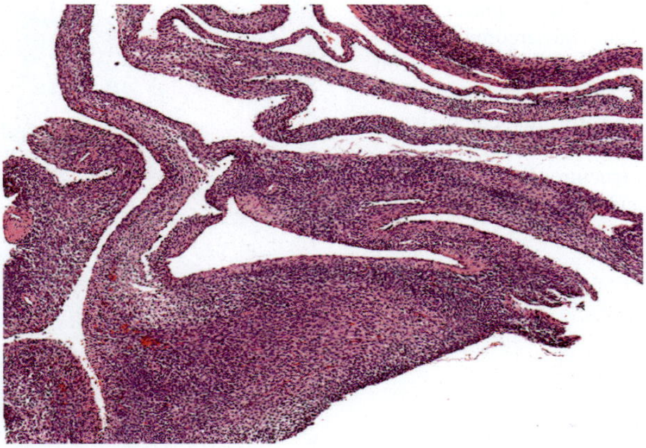

**Fig. 8.25** Monophasic synovial sarcoma with cystic changes

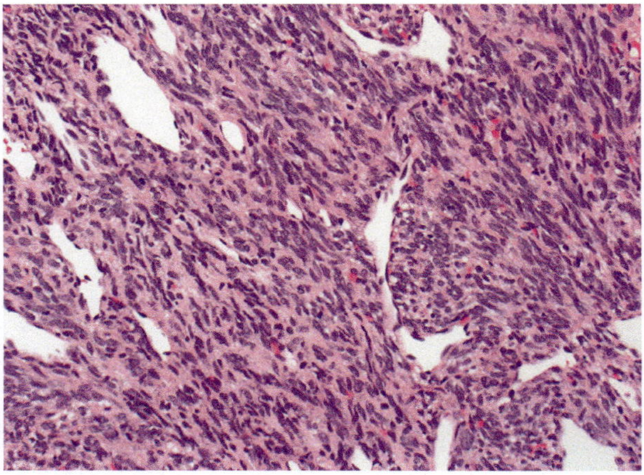

**Fig. 8.26** Many spindle cell synovial sarcomas have prominent branching staghorn-like vessels like those seen in SFTs

and can occur in both subtypes. Extensive calcifications in synovial sarcoma replacing glandular structures or associated with hyalinized fibrous stroma and cytologically low-grade spindle cells are referred to as calcifying synovial sarcoma (Fig. 8.28). This variant tends to occur in lower limbs and can be associated with improved outcome. Less common features include squamous metaplasia, ossification, rhabdoid features, granular cell change, and primary intraneural location.

Conventional monophasic or biphasic synovial sarcomas are graded according to the FNCLCC grading system. Poorly differentiated synovial sarcoma occurs in conjunction with either the epithelioid or biphasic subtype and is composed of sheets of ovoid cells with rounded atypical nuclei, scant cytoplasm, variably prominent nucleoli, frequent mitotic figures, and areas of necrosis resembling an undifferentiated round cell sarcoma (Fig. 8.29). Synovial sarcoma with rhabdoid morphology is also best considered to be poorly differentiated.

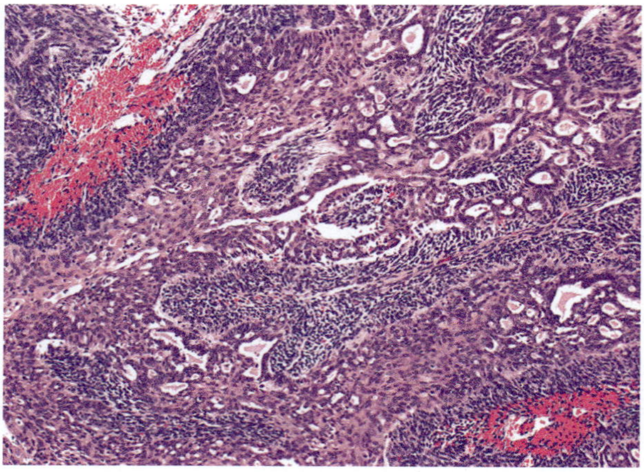

**Fig. 8.27** Biphasic synovial sarcoma composed of a spindle cell component and epithelial cells forming elaborate glandular and papillary structures lined by cuboidal or columnar cells

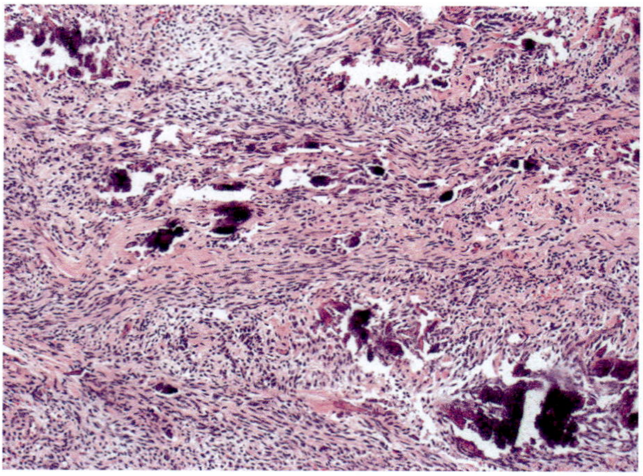

**Fig. 8.28** Calcifying synovial sarcoma with cytologically low-grade nuclear features and extensive calcifications

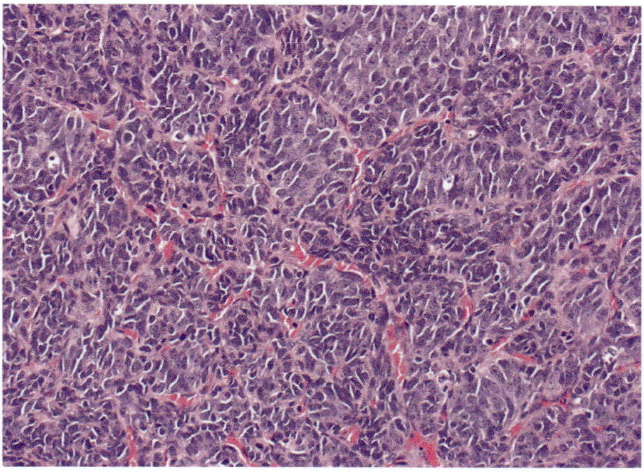

**Fig. 8.29** Poorly differentiated synovial sarcoma composed of sheets of ovoid cells with rounded atypical nuclei, scant cytoplasm, variably prominent nucleoli, and frequent mitotic figures resembling an undifferentiated round cell sarcoma

## Immunohistochemistry

Both monophasic and biphasic synovial sarcomas express variable combinations of epithelial markers including cytokeratins and EMA, but these markers may be only focally expressed. CD34 is reliably negative. CD99 is seen in approximately 70% of synovial sarcoma emphasizing the poor specificity of this marker in the context of mesenchymal spindle cell neoplasms. A third of cases may express S100. P63 expression has been observed in synovial sarcoma, an important point when metaplastic breast carcinoma is considered in the differential diagnosis. Nuclear expression of TLE1 has excellent sensitivity for the diagnosis of synovial sarcoma; however, this antibody has fallen out of use due to difficulties with optimization and reduced specificity.

## Molecular

Genetically, synovial sarcoma (SS) is defined by a reciprocal t(X;18)(p11.2;q11.2), with pathognomonic *SS18-SSX1*, *SS18-SSX2*, or, rarely, *SS18-SSX4* or cryptic gene fusions, with downstream effects on SWI/SNF chromatin remodeling complexes. FISH for *SS18* gene rearrangement and RT-PCR for synovial sarcoma fusion transcripts, which has greater sensitivity compared to FISH, are the most useful and practical diagnostic tests to objectively confirm the diagnosis, although it appears that the novel fusion-specific antibodies might at one point surpass FISH testing for the diagnosis of synovial sarcoma. There is no prognostic correlation with monophasic vs. biphasic histology or the type of fusion transcript.

More recently, two groups demonstrated excellent results with novel fusion-specific antibodies, an SS18-SSX fusion-specific antibody (E9X9V) and an SSX-specific antibody (E5A2C, directed at the C-terminus of SSX). These were tested on 139 genetically confirmed synovial sarcoma samples and 880 histologic mimics and demonstrated nuclear expression. SS19-SSX antibody demonstrated 87–95% sensitivity and 100% specificity for synovial sarcoma, whereas SSX-C-terminus antibody showed 92–100% sensitivity and 93–96% specificity. False-negative staining was associated with small biopsies and decalcified samples.

## Differential Diagnosis

In the breast, the most important diagnostic consideration is spindle cell metaplastic carcinoma and borderline/malignant phyllodes. Differentiating spindle cell metaplastic carcinoma from synovial sarcoma is not trivial, as cytokeratins may be variably expressed in both tumors, and p63 can be variably expressed in synovial sarcoma. In fact, in the absence of clear-cut DCIS or conventional invasive ductal carcinoma, FISH or RT-PCR testing for the diagnostic gene fusions may be the only reliable way to differentiate these two entities. The novel fusion-specific antibodies have been tested on a small number of sarcomatoid carcinomas but have not yet been systematically evaluated in metaplastic breast carcinomas.

Biphasic synovial sarcoma may cause considerable diagnostic difficulty with borderline/malignant phyllodes tumors, since both have malignant-appearing spindle cells interdigitating with low-grade glandular elements. Again, ancillary molecular testing and/or fusion-specific antibodies for synovial sarcoma may be the only way to establish a definitive diagnosis in difficult cases.

Additional differential diagnostic considerations include malignant spindle cell tumors arising from the overlying skin (i.e., spindle cell melanoma or fibrosarcomatous DFSP), conventional MPNST, and solitary fibrous tumor (SFT). Spindle cell melanoma affects an older patient population and morphologically may display a focally nested growth pattern and a junctional component. S100 protein can be positive in both tumors and therefore is of limited value in this context, although strong, diffuse expression would favor spindle cell melanoma. SOX10 is a very helpful marker because it is positive in most melanomas, including the spindle cell subtypes, and is usually negative in synovial sarcoma, being observed only in primary intraneural examples of this entity. The fascicular and monotonous growth pattern of fibrosarcomatous DFSP can mimic synovial sarcoma. The most helpful histologic clue is identification of a conventional DFSP component. CD34 can serve as a quick screening tool as it is variably positive in fibrosarcomatous DFSP, but consistently negative in synovial sarcoma. Synovial sarcoma with prominent collagenous stroma and staghorn vessels can be mistaken for SFT, and the malignant examples of the latter can show a fascicular growth pattern and greater nuclear crowding and atypia. STAT6 expression can readily distinguish SFT from synovial sarcoma. MPNSTs and synovial sarcoma synovial sarcoma may be virtually identical histologically, especially in poorly differentiated tumors, and both tumors can express S100. Unlike synovial sarcoma, MPNSTs are more often positive for SOX10 and about 75% of cases show loss of H3K27me3 by immunohistochemistry. In all of these scenarios, FISH and RT-PCR for synovial sarcoma gene fusions are extremely helpful, as these tests are universally negative in the histologic mimics of synovial sarcoma. The abovementioned fusion-specific SS19-SSX and SSX-CT antibodies were negative in over 90% of reported MPNSTs.

## Treatment and Prognosis

Synovial sarcoma may have a protracted clinical course, but ultimately behaves aggressively with late local recurrences and systemic metastases, most commonly to the lungs, lymph nodes, and bones and less commonly to the breast. Synovial sarcoma has an overall approximately 60% 5-year survival. Adverse clinical parameters include large tumor size (>5 cm), visceral location, and poorly differentiated tumor morphology, while the most favorable outcomes are observed in small fibrous and extensively calcified synovial sarcoma of hands and feet, as they are amenable to complete excision. Although cases are very limited, patients with breast parenchymal synovial sarcomas were free of disease on surveillance 1 and 4 years after completion of multimodal therapy.

For localized disease, surgical excision is the treatment of choice, while a multimodal approach, including radiation therapy, conventional chemotherapy, tyrosine kinase inhibitors (imatinib, pazopanib), or immunotherapy targeting NY-ESO-1 and other biomarkers, can be used for locally advanced and metastatic disease.

# Perivascular Epithelioid Cell Tumor (PEComa)

## Clinical Features

Perivascular epithelioid cell tumors (PEComas) are a diverse family of mesenchymal neoplasms characterized by epithelioid tumor cells that co-express smooth muscle and melanocytic markers. PEComas can occur at virtually any site including the skin, soft tissues, bone, and viscera. Formerly distinct clinicopathologic entities such as lymphangioleiomyomatosis, renal and hepatic angiomyolipoma, epithelioid angiomyolipoma, clear cell "sugar" tumor of the lung, clear cell myomelanocytic tumor of the falciform ligament/ligamentum teres, and abdominopelvic sarcoma are also now considered to be a part of the PEComa family of tumors.

In the breast, one can encounter either cutaneous PEComas, which account for approximately 8% of all PEComas, or exceptionally rare primary breast parenchymal PEComas. Both visceral and cutaneous PEComas typically affect young or middle-aged adults, with a striking female predilection. Cutaneous tumors usually appear on the legs, arms, or trunk as firm, tan, or pink-colored small (<2 cm) cutaneous nodules or plaques and are clinically reminiscent of fibrous histiocytoma. Primary breast parenchymal PEComas reported so far presented in young females (mean age 19 years) as non-tender firm palpable masses mimicking fibroadenoma.

## Imaging

Breast PEComas show mammographic and ultrasonographic findings that mimic fibroadenoma, although the data is limited.

## Pathologic Features

### Gross Features

Soft tissue and breast parenchymal PEComas are well-circumscribed, solid, brown to pale fibrous, or fleshy masses. Cutaneous PEComas present as variably tan dermal-based nodules with focal subcutaneous extension, resembling benign fibrous histiocytomas.

### Microscopic Features

Primary breast and cutaneous PEComas are composed of nests, sheets, or cords of epithelioid, polygonal, or less often, spindled cells with abundant clear or granular eosinophilic cytoplasm surrounded by delicate capillary vessels. The cells have round, vesicular nuclei with small but very distinct nucleoli (Figs. 8.30, 8.31, 8.32, and 8.33). Perivascular growth pattern, with the tumor cells abutting the overlying endothelium, is characteristic, although this feature is easier to appreciate in cases with a more fibrous background. The appearance of *TFE3*-rearranged PEComas is similar to other Xp11.2-rearranged malignancies, with nested or alveolar architecture, pure epithelioid cytomorphology, and focal melanin deposition in some cases. The sclerosing variant of PEComa, composed of cords of relatively uniform epithelioid cells with clear cytoplasm in a densely collagenized stroma, has not yet been characterized in the skin or the breast parenchyma. Most visceral and breast parenchymal PEComas are well-circumscribed with a pushing border. Cutaneous PEComas on the other hand typically have a somewhat

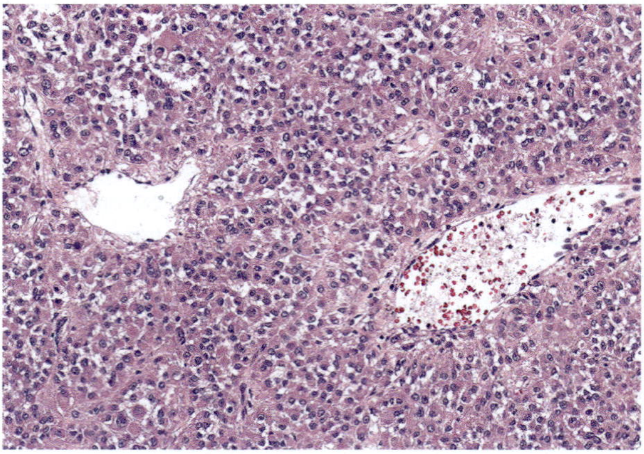

**Fig. 8.30** Perivascular epithelioid cell tumor (PEComa) composed of nests of epithelioid tumor cells with eosinophilic granular cytoplasm surrounded by delicate capillary vessels

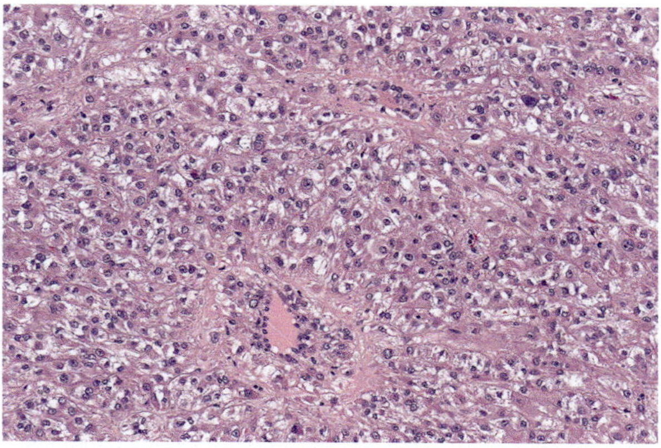

**Fig. 8.31** Another PEComa containing polygonal cells with abundant clear cytoplasm, round, vesicular nuclei, and small distinct nucleoli. Perivascular growth pattern, with the tumor cells abutting the overlying endothelium, is characteristic

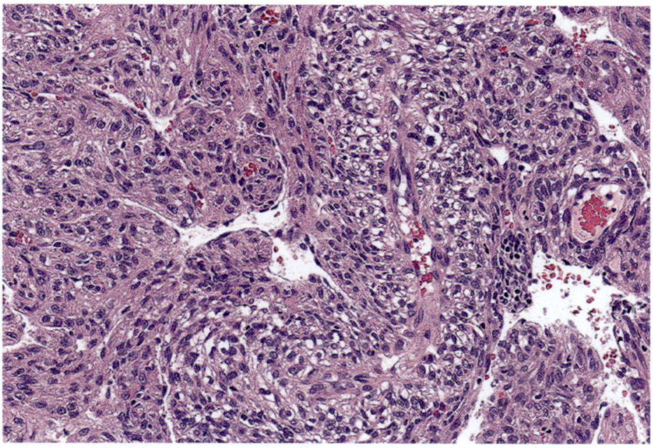

**Fig. 8.32** PEComa with spindle cell growth pattern and an accentuated perivascular arrangement of the lesional cells

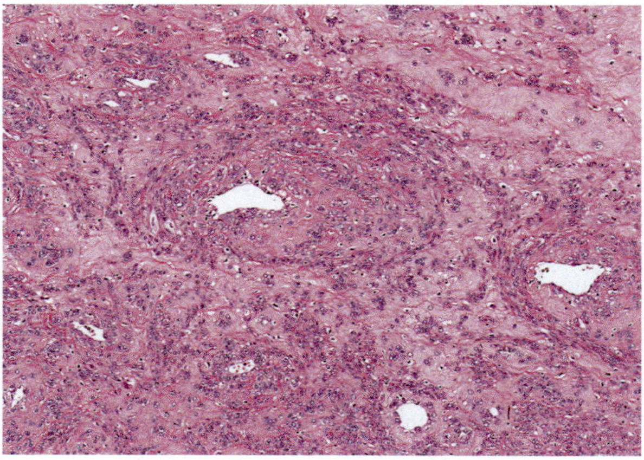

**Fig. 8.33** Sclerosing variant of PEComa composed of nests and cords of monomorphic tumor cells embedded in a hyalinized stroma containing numerous vessels

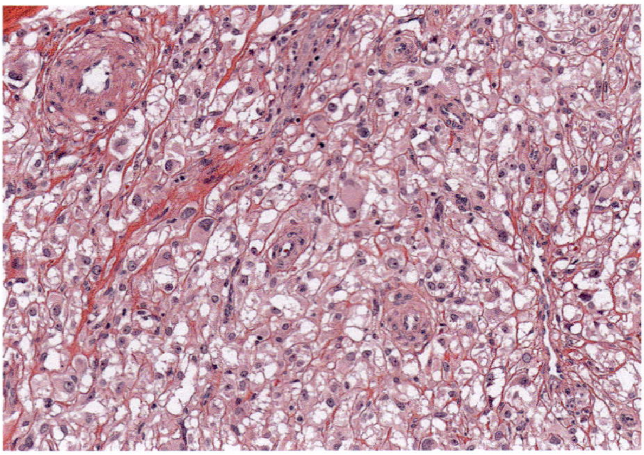

**Fig. 8.34** Cutaneous PEComa composed of nests of large polygonal tumor cells with clear or palely eosinophilic cytoplasm, round nuclei, and distinct nucleoli, percolating between dermal collagen

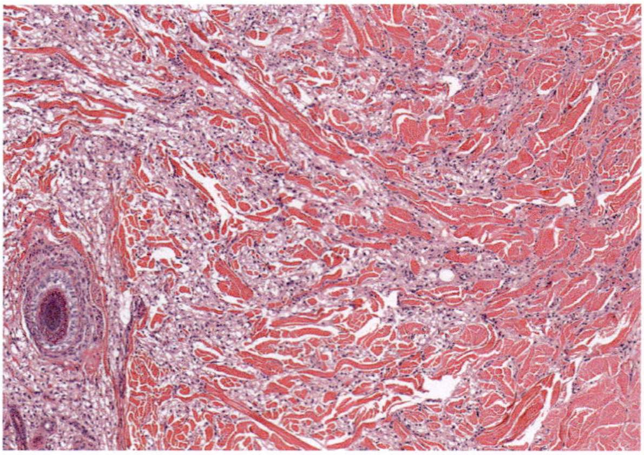

**Fig. 8.35** The tumor edge in cutaneous PEComas is somewhat infiltrative and often shows collagen trapping at the periphery, reminiscent of benign fibrous histiocytoma

infiltrative edge and often show dermal collagen trapping at the periphery, reminiscent of benign fibrous histiocytoma (Figs. 8.34 and 8.35). A mild degree of cellular pleomorphism is typical of PEComas at all sites, and multinucleated wreath-like giant cells with peripherally located nuclei can be seen. The mitotic count is typically very low (<1/10 HPF).

The proposed histological criteria for malignancy in deep soft tissue PEComas include size >5 cm, an infiltrative growth pattern, high nuclear grade, mitotic activity >1/50 HPF, necrosis, and vascular invasion (Figs. 8.36 and 8.37). PEComas lacking any of these features are classified as benign, those with 2 or more features as malignant, and those with only nuclear pleomorphism/giant cells (so-called symplastic PEComas) or size >5 cm as having uncertain malignant potential. It remains unclear whether this classification scheme is equally applicable to cutaneous and breast PEComas due to the scarcity of published cases.

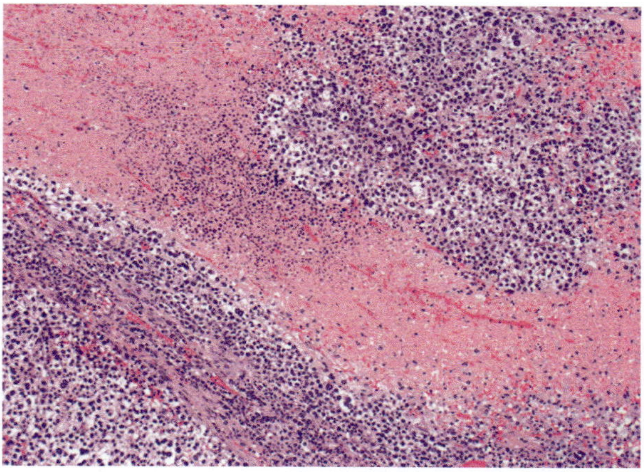

**Fig. 8.36** Malignant PEComa showing geographic areas of necrosis

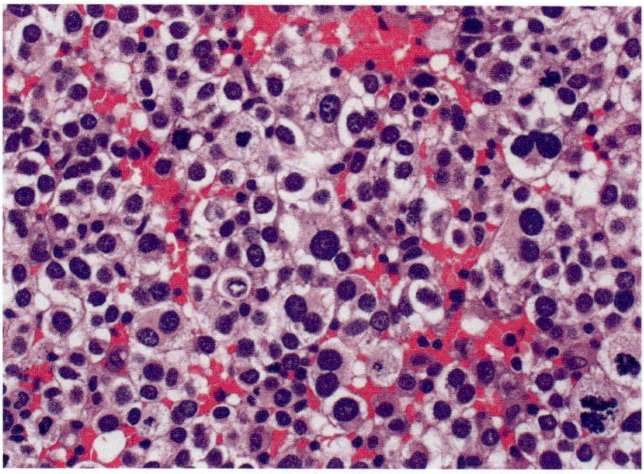

**Fig. 8.37** Malignant PEComa showing an overtly malignant high-grade cytology and increased mitotic figures

## Immunohistochemistry

By definition, PEComas demonstrate variable co-expression of melanocytic markers (HMB45, MITF, NKI/C3, Melan-A, PNL2, and S100) and markers of smooth muscle differentiation (desmin, SMA, caldesmon, and calponin) and also express cathepsin K. HMB45 and MITF are the most sensitive melanocytic markers in cutaneous and soft tissue/visceral PEComas; however, MiTF and Melan-A expression can be focal or negative in PEComas with *TFE3* fusions. Instead, *TFE3*-rearranged PEComas show diffuse nuclear expression of TFE3. S100 protein expression is seen focally in a minority of cases and SOX10 is universally negative. Generally speaking, PEComas with epithelioid morphology, including the *TFE3*-rearranged cases, tend to show a more diffuse expression of HMB45, whereas expression of muscle

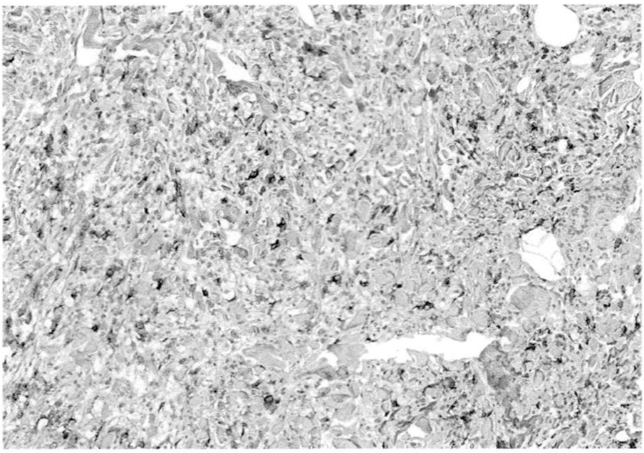

**Fig. 8.38** Cutaneous PEComa showing the typical scattered staining pattern with HMB-45

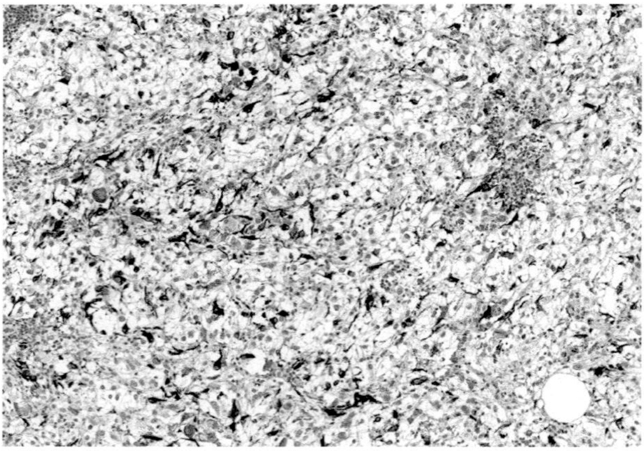

**Fig. 8.39** Cutaneous PEComa showing expression of desmin, which appears to have greater sensitivity than SMA in this setting

markers can be very focal or negative. In the cutaneous examples, desmin appears to have greater sensitivity than SMA (Figs. 8.38 and 8.39). Cytokeratins and EMA are negative in PEComas. Estrogen (ER) and progesterone receptor (PR) expression has been demonstrated in over 50% of PEComas of the gynecologic tract. Interestingly, both parenchymal PEComas of the breast reported so far expressed PR but were negative for ER. Hormone receptor expression in cutaneous PEComas is unknown.

## Molecular

Most sporadic and tuberous sclerosis complex (TSC)-associated visceral and soft tissue PEComas are associated with *TSC1* (9q34) or *TSC2* (16p13.3) alterations, the most common being loss of heterozygosity in the *TSC2* locus. This results in a downstream upregulation of the mammalian target of rapamycin (mTOR) pathway.

A smaller subset of PEComas harbors oncogenic fusions of the *TFE3* (Xp11.2) gene, a member of MiT family, with a variety of partners. *TFE3*-rearranged and *TSC1/2* mutations in PEComas appear to be mutually exclusive. Of the two reported breast parenchymal PEComas, one expressed TFE3 by immunohistochemistry.

Primary cutaneous PEComas do not seem to be associated with *TSC* mutations. However, expression of 4E-binding protein (4EBP1), a downstream target in the mTOR pathway, has been observed in cutaneous PEComas. Likewise, cutaneous PEComas typically lack *TFE3* rearrangements.

## Differential Diagnosis

PEComas need to be distinguished from a variety of tumors with clear or granular cytoplasm. Unlike PEComas, mammary granular cell tumors demonstrate a more syncytial arrangement of constituent cells, the absence of a prominent vasculature, and a lack of nucleoli. That being said, an uncommon clear cell variant of granular cell tumor can be more difficult to distinguish from PEComa, because it has very similar cytologic characteristics. However, both conventional and clear cell granular cell tumors are negative for HMB45, Melan-A, desmin, and SMA and are uniformly strongly positive for S100 protein and SOX10; inhibin has also been shown to be positive in granular cell tumors. Myoepitheliomas with clear cell morphology have a somewhat overlapping immunophenotype because the markers of myoepithelial differentiation S100, SMA, and calponin can also be expressed in cutaneous PEComas. However, myoepithelial tumors can be ready distinguished from PEComas by co-expression of cytokeratins and EMA and lack of HMB-45 or MiTF immunoreactivity. Cutaneous PEComa and benign fibrous histiocytoma can look strikingly similar, especially at scanning magnification, but the latter can be readily distinguished by lack of expression of melanocytic markers.

Of the malignant primary breast tumors with clear cytoplasm, the tumor with the most histological overlap with PEComa is the so-called glycogen-rich invasive breast carcinoma which, unlike PEComa, would be expected to be diffusely positive for cytokeratin.

Rare metastases to the breast, most notably metastatic renal cell or hepatocellular carcinoma, can be separated from PEComa based on cytokeratin and EMA immunoreactivity and lack of melanocytic and smooth muscle marker expression.

## Treatment and Prognosis

Breast parenchymal PEComas reported to date displayed no histologic features of malignancy and showed no recurrence or metastasis. Most cutaneous PEComas also behave in a benign fashion, with only four reported cases of lymph node or systemic metastases (one in a pregnant patient), and one case that met histologic criteria for malignancy but did not recur or metastasize after a complete excision. Large studies detailing the behavior of histologically malignant cutaneous PEComa are currently lacking. Based on this limited data, complete excision at both cutaneous and breast sites would be recommended for histologically benign PEComas. Malignant PEComas at all sites are best treated by a multidisciplinary sarcoma team, with a combination of surgery, radiation, and chemotherapy, including possible use of mTOR pathway inhibitors.

## Pleomorphic Hyalinizing Angiectatic Tumor

### Clinical Features

Pleomorphic hyalinizing angiectatic tumor (PHAT) is a distinctive slow-growing subcutaneous neoplasm of adults with the potential for local recurrence and, in rare cases, progression to a higher-grade sarcoma. PHAT has a predilection for the lower extremities but can also occur at other sites such as the arm, thigh, buttocks, or trunk and has been reported in the male breast. The median size of a typical lesion is approximately 6 cm. Because ectatic, hyalinized vessels are a prominent feature, PHAT may be clinically mistaken for a hematoma or a vascular neoplasm.

### Imaging

Well-circumscribed high-density somewhat lobulated mass without calcifications; ultrasound shows a hypoechoic lesion with an irregular margin and prominent vascularity.

### Pathologic Features

#### Gross Features

A well-circumscribed but unencapsulated lobulated mass, which may contain areas of hemorrhage.

#### Microscopic Features

PHAT is a vaguely circumscribed mass composed of spindled or pleomorphic cells surrounding clusters of thin-walled, hyalinized, ectatic vessels with subendothelial and intraluminal fibrin deposits (Figs. 8.40 and 8.41). Although PHAT may seem circumscribed at low power, the margin is usually infiltrative. Constituent tumor cells range from hyperchromatic and spindled to strikingly pleomorphic and may show frequent intranuclear inclusions (Fig. 8.42). The mitotic activity in PHAT is characteristically very low (0–1/50 HPF). Hemosiderin deposits can be seen in macrophages or in the cytoplasm of the lesional cells. Scattered inflammatory cells are usually present. At their periphery, PHATs may show areas reminiscent of the tumor known as hemosiderotic fibrolipomatous tumor (HFLT). These areas are composed

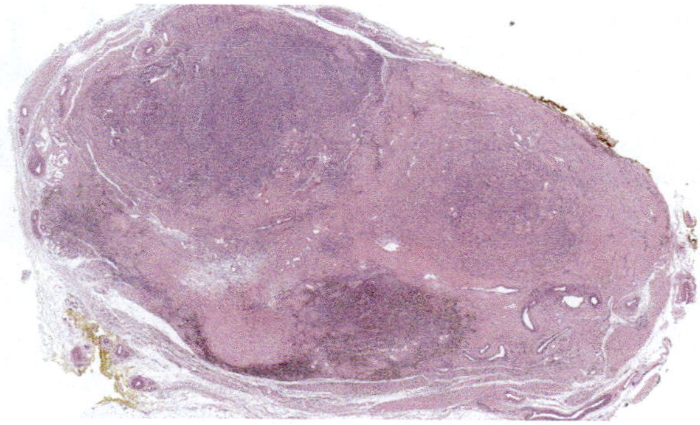

**Fig. 8.40** Pleomorphic hyalinizing angiectatic tumor (PHAT) presenting as a circumscribed mass with a focally infiltrative edge and numerous hemosiderin deposits

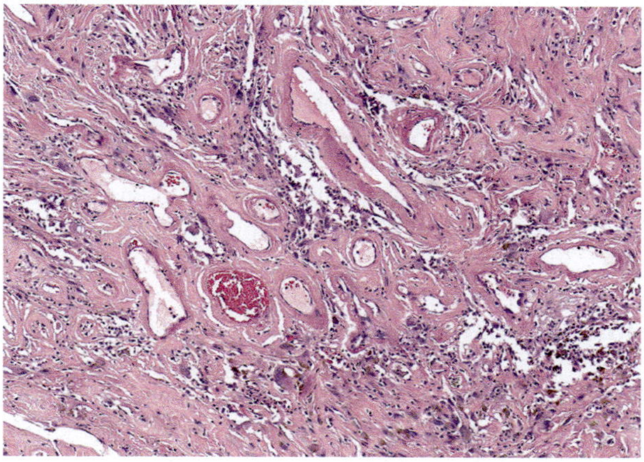

**Fig. 8.41** PHAT composed of spindled or pleomorphic cells surrounding clusters of thin-walled, hyalinized, ectatic vessels with subendothelial and intraluminal fibrin deposits

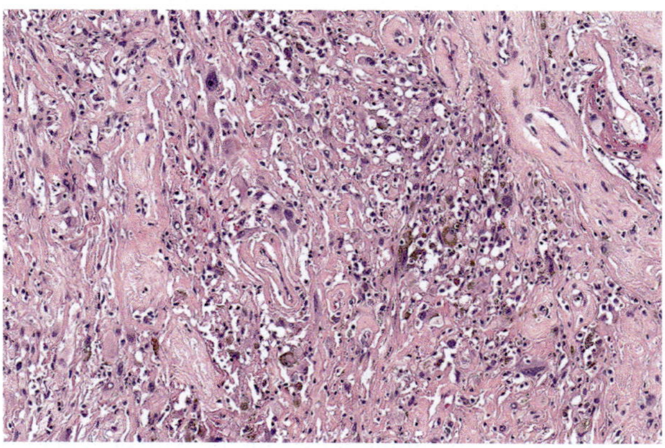

**Fig. 8.42** PHAT showing spindled to pleomorphic hyperchromatic cells with intranuclear inclusions and intracytoplasmic hemosiderin deposits. The mitotic activity in PHAT is characteristically inconspicuous

of cytologically banal spindle cells with intracytoplasmic hemosiderin deposits, which infiltrate between the adipocytes in a manner resembling lipofibromatosis or DFSP (Fig. 8.43). This finding can be of diagnostic utility and also provides support for the notion that these two tumors are closely related.

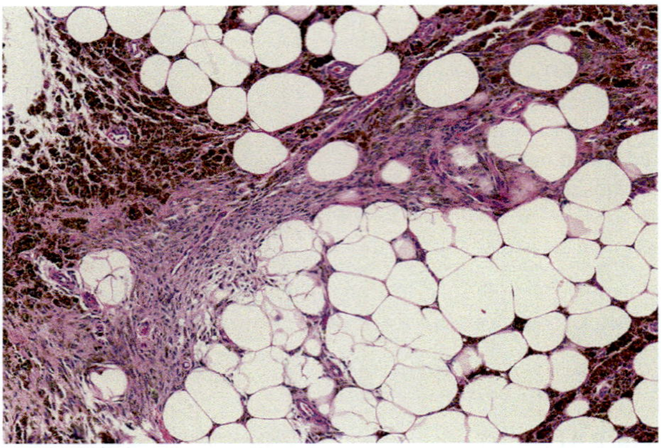

**Fig. 8.43** Hemosiderotic fibrolipomatous tumor (HFLT)-like areas in PHAT composed of cytologically banal spindle cells with intracytoplasmic hemosiderin deposits, which infiltrate between the adipocytes in a diffuse manner resembling lipofibromatosis or DFSP

Rarely, PHAT may progress to a sarcoma of higher histologic grade, especially in the setting of local recurrence. The sarcomatous components associated with PHAT often have myxoid stroma and a prominent inflammatory infiltrate resembling myxoinflammatory fibroblastic sarcoma (MIFS) or myxofibrosarcoma. Solid, undifferentiated spindle cell sarcoma-like morphology can also occur.

## Immunohistochemistry

Most PHATs are positive for CD34 and negative for S100 protein, SMA, desmin, and vascular markers CD31 and ERG.

## Molecular

*TGFBR3* and *OGA* (*MGEA5)* gene rearrangements have been found in tumors showing mixed features of PHAT and HFLT and, less consistently, in classic PHAT – a finding that provides further support for the relatedness of these two tumors. FISH testing for *TGFBR3* and *MGEA5* rearrangements can be used in diagnostically challenging cases, but most cases can be confidently diagnosed by careful histologic examination.

## Differential Diagnosis

PHAT can closely mimic schwannoma with degenerative ("ancient") change, which often contains clusters of hyalinized vessels, inflammatory aggregates, and pleomorphic Schwann cells. In contrast to PHAT, schwannomas are well-circumscribed and encapsulated lesions without a HFLT-like component at the periphery. S100 and SOX10 proteins are diffusely expressed in schwannomas and are consistently negative in PHAT.

Owing to the striking degree of nuclear atypia and pleomorphism often seen in PHAT, it can be misdiagnosed as undifferentiated pleomorphic sarcoma; however, a lack of mitotic activity would favor the former over the latter. By contrast, identification of a bona fide spindle cell sarcoma with myxoid stroma in association with a recognizable classic PHAT may indicate sarcomatous progression. As with many of the tumors in this chapter, both metaplastic breast carcinomas and malignant phyllodes tumors enter the diagnosis with PHAT. The presence of DCIS, foci of conventional invasive ductal carcinoma, and diffuse cytokeratin expression all favor metaplastic breast carcinoma, while finding a biphasic, intracanalicular growth pattern would favor a phyllodes tumor. In both of these tumors, the degree of nuclear atypia and mitotic activity are proportional, in contrast to the strikingly pleomorphic yet mitotically quiescent PHAT. In rare difficult cases, FISH for *TGFBR3* and *MGEA5* rearrangements may be used.

### Treatment and Prognosis

Because of its infiltrative nature, PHAT is associated with a significant (30–50%) risk of local recurrence and is therefore considered to represent a tumor of intermediate malignant potential. Limited studies indicate that PHAT may undergo transformation to a higher-grade sarcoma and acquire metastatic potential. The optimal treatment approach is complete surgical excision with tumor-free margins.

## Giant Cell Tumor of Soft Tissue

### Clinical Features

Giant cell tumor of soft tissue (GCT-ST) is a distinctive, mostly superficial mesenchymal neoplasm morphologically identical, but pathogenetically unrelated to giant cell tumor of bone. GCT-ST usually affects adult patients and presents as a painless slowly growing subcutaneous or deep-seated nodule, most often in the distal limbs followed by the trunk and head and neck region. Mean size is 3 cm. These tumors are rare in the breast, chest wall, or axilla but the diagnostic awareness of this lesion among breast pathologists is important for two reasons: firstly, GCT-ST can be mistaken for breast carcinoma with osteoclast-like stromal giant cells, extraskeletal osteosarcoma, or undifferentiated pleomorphic sarcoma; secondly, GCT-ST has a tendency for local recurrence and therefore is ideally treated by complete excision as exceptionally rare metastases have been documented. In the breast, GCT-ST presents as a palpable, firm, non-tender mass.

## Imaging

Mammography shows a well-demarcated solid and cystic mass, which has mixed echogenicity by ultrasound. Giant cell tumor of soft tissue with metaplastic bone formation may show calcifications on imaging.

## Pathologic Features

### Gross Features

Giant cell tumor of soft tissue is a well-demarcated, unencapsulated multinodular mass with gray-tan cut surfaces and frequent cystic and hemorrhagic spaces; cases with metaplastic bone formation may show gritty calcifications.

### Microscopic Features

At scanning magnification, giant cell tumor of soft tissue presents as multiple circumscribed nodules separated by thick fibrous bands (Fig. 8.44). These nodules are composed of numerous osteoclast-type giant cells and mononuclear round, plasmacytoid, or spindled cells with amphophilic cytoplasm, vesicular nuclei, and small nucleoli, packed in a richly vascularized stroma (Fig. 8.45). The mononuclear cells are the neoplastic component in this tumor, which induce osteoclast recruitment by a RANKL-dependent mechanism. Peripheral metaplastic bone formation, aneurysmal bone cyst-like changes, extravasated red blood cells, stromal fibrosis, and hemosiderin deposits are often present (Fig. 8.46). In the breast parenchyma, the tumor can be observed spreading into the breast ducts. Vascular invasion can be present in up to a third of giant cell tumors of soft tissue, but as is the case with giant cell tumors of bone, vascular invasion is not predictive of aggressive behavior.

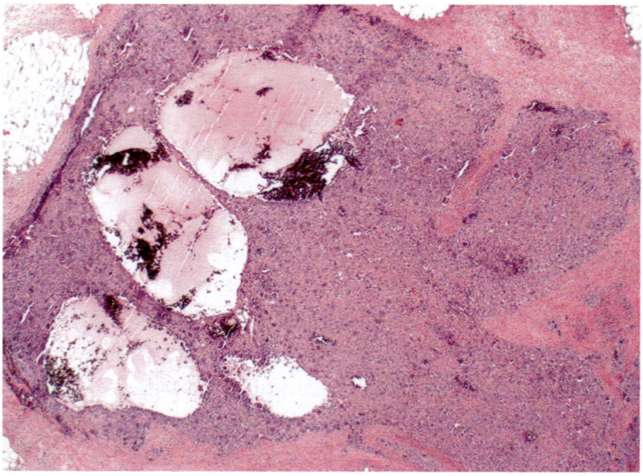

**Fig. 8.44** Giant cell tumor of soft tissue composed of multiple nodules separated by thick fibrous bands

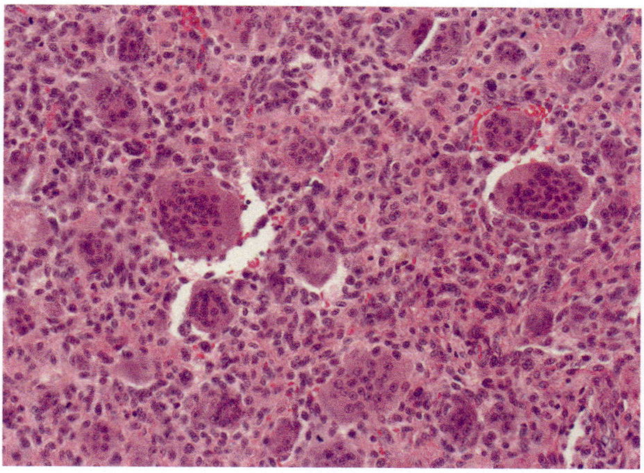

**Fig. 8.45** Giant cell tumor of soft tissue showing numerous osteoclast-type giant cells and mononuclear round, plasmacytoid, or spindled cells with amphophilic cytoplasm, vesicular nuclei, and small nucleoli, packed in a richly vascularized stroma

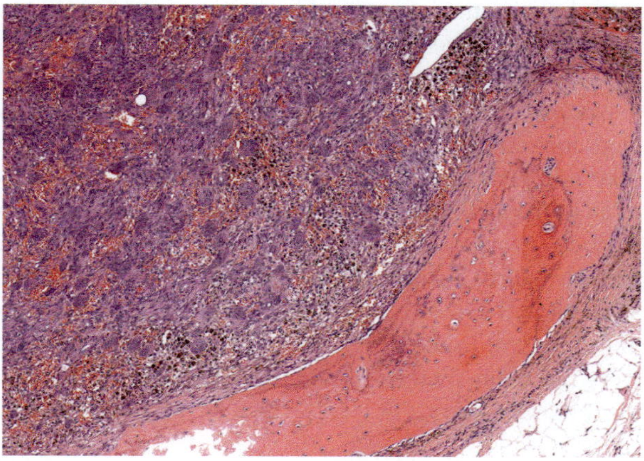

**Fig. 8.46** Peripheral metaplastic bone formation, hemorrhage, and hemosiderin deposits in giant cell tumor of soft tissue

Mitotic activity in giant cell tumor of soft tissue is often quite brisk, but as a general rule, atypical mitotic figures, significant nuclear atypia, and pleomorphism are uncharacteristic and, when present, should raise suspicion for a sarcoma or carcinoma rich in osteoclast-type giant cells.

## Immunohistochemistry

Giant cell tumor of soft tissue can be variably and usually focally immunoreactive for S100, SMA, SATB2, and p63, while osteoclast-type giant cells pick up CD68. This immunoprofile is usually unhelpful. GCT-ST is consistently negative for cytokeratins, melanocytic markers, and estrogen and progesterone receptor expression.

## Molecular

In contrast to giant cell tumors of bone characterized by *H3F3A* G34W mutation, GCT-ST does not show this or other histone 3 alterations, suggesting that they represent a pathogenetically distinct tumor type. Unfortunately, for the same reason, H3F3A immunostain, often used as a diagnostic adjunct in giant cell tumors of bone, is unhelpful in giant cell tumor of soft tissue.

## Differential Diagnosis

Breast carcinoma with osteoclast-like stromal giant cells, extraskeletal osteosarcoma, and undifferentiated pleomorphic sarcoma are the most significant diagnostic mimickers. As a general rule, all of the above can be readily distinguished from giant cell tumor of soft tissue based on the overtly malignant nuclear characteristics and the presence of atypical mitotic figures. In addition to cytomorphology, breast carcinoma can be ruled out by identifying an epithelial component or DCIS and by demonstrating immunoreactivity for cytokeratins. Similar to giant cell tumor of soft tissue, extraskeletal osteosarcoma often develops aneurysmal bone cyst-like changes and contains numerous osteoclast-type giant cells. However, the presence of lace-like immature osteoid deposits intimately associated with the tumor cells (in contrast to the well-developed rim of mature metaplastic bone in giant cell tumor of soft tissue) favors osteosarcoma. The diagnosis of undifferentiated pleomorphic sarcoma requires a rigorous exclusion of other lineages, most notably metaplastic carcinoma and osteosarcoma. Theoretically, one also needs to differentiate giant cell tumor of soft tissue from a metastatic giant cell tumor of bone; the latter scenario is very rare in its own right, and furthermore, such cases have not yet been reported in the breast region.

## Treatment and Prognosis

Approximately 10% of GCT-ST locally recur, including some cases reported in the breast, and therefore, complete surgical excision is a preferred treatment option. Metastases are exceedingly rare and do not justify regarding giant cell tumor of soft tissue as a malignant neoplasm. No single histologic feature is predictive of behavior as tumors with overtly malignant nuclear features are classified as other tumor types.

# Extraskeletal Osteosarcoma

## Clinical Features

Extraskeletal osteosarcoma is defined as a primary malignant bone-forming neoplasm arising without connection to the skeletal system. Extraskeletal osteosarcoma arising in the breast is very uncommon, comprising <0.005% of all breast malignant neoplasms and approximately 5% of all primary breast sarcomas based on various published series. When making the diagnosis of breast osteosarcoma, meticulous exclusion of matrix-producing metaplastic carcinoma with heterologous osteosarcomatous differentiation, sarcomatous overgrowth of malignant phyllodes tumor, and primary chest wall or metastatic osteosarcoma is essential as all of the above are more common than primary breast osteosarcoma. The risk factors for breast osteosarcoma are similar to those at other locations including genetic predisposition syndromes like Li-Fraumeni or prior radiation therapy. Clinically, mammary osteosarcomas present as a rapidly enlarging breast mass in older female patients (median age 64.5 years, range 27–89), with a mean size of 4.6 cm (range 1.4–13 cm). In contrast to breast carcinomas, axillary lymphadenopathy is uncharacteristic.

## Imaging

Mammographic findings are those of a large, high-density coarsely calcified mass; cases with lobulated border may be mistaken for a calcified fibroadenoma, whereas those with irregular margins are more suspicious of malignancy. Ultrasonography shows an irregular hypoechoic mass with shadowing calcifications. CT scan may be recommended to delineate the extent of mineralization and ensure that the lesion does not represent an extension from a bone or soft tissue osteosarcoma of the chest wall. The appearance on CT scan is often of a well-circumscribed, heterogeneous ring-enhancing mass with central hypodense non-enhancing areas. Importantly, skeletal scintigraphy with Tc-99 m, if performed, will show an avid uptake highly suggestive of a bone-forming neoplasm; however, this modality will not distinguish between a primary breast osteosarcoma and its bone-forming mimics mentioned above. Axillary lymph nodes are usually not involved.

## Pathologic Features

### Gross Features

Primary breast osteosarcoma can range from a densely calcified, well-circumscribed, and lobulated mass to a more irregular fleshy, necrotic, and hemorrhagic appearance; the cartilaginous component may stand out as somewhat blue-gray, glossy areas.

### Microscopic Features

Breast osteosarcomas show the same histologic patterns seen in skeletal and extraskeletal osteosarcomas at other sites. Conventional osteoblastic osteosarcomas are composed of polygonal osteoblastic stromal cells with overt nuclear atypia and pleomorphism, intimately associated with lace-like immature neoplastic osteoid deposits with a variable degree of maturation and mineralization (Figs. 8.47, 8.48, and 8.49). Telangiectatic osteosarcomas tend to show large, aneurysmal bone cyst-like spaces and contain numerous osteoclast-type giant cells; the osteoid formation

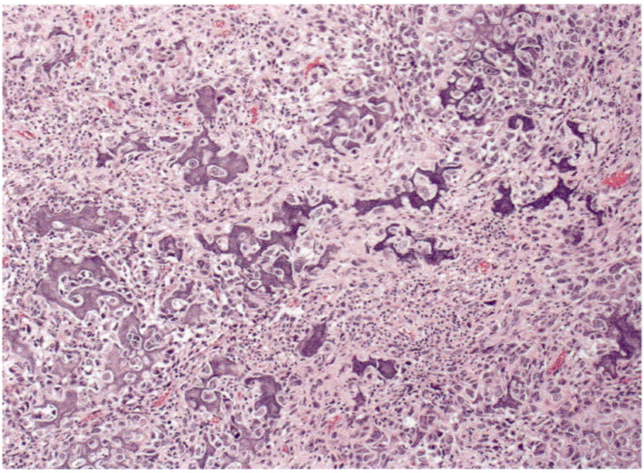

**Fig. 8.47** Osteoblastic osteosarcoma of the breast composed of sheets of polygonal osteoblastic stromal cells intimately associated with lace-like immature neoplastic osteoid deposits

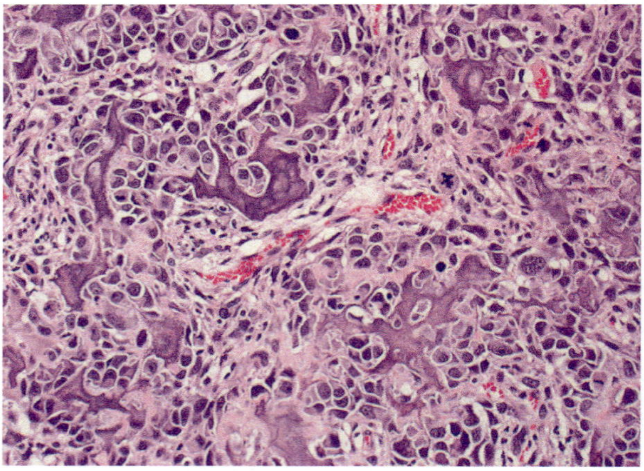

**Fig. 8.48** At high power, the malignant cells in osteoblastic osteosarcoma show overt nuclear atypia and brisk mitotic activity, including atypical forms

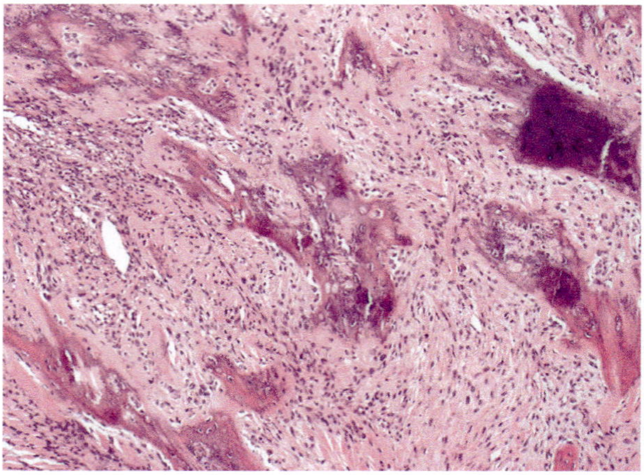

**Fig. 8.49** Osteoblastic osteosarcoma containing relatively mature osteoid deposits and low- to intermediate-grade atypical spindle cells

in this subtype is often limited to the walls of the cystic spaces (Figs. 8.50, 8.51, and 8.52). Chondroblastic osteosarcoma shows sheets of neoplastic cartilage with high-grade nuclear atypia, admixed with the osteoblastic or spindle cell component (Fig. 8.53). Fibroblastic osteosarcomas are composed of sheets or intersecting fascicles of undifferentiated pleomorphic or spindle cells resembling an undifferentiated spindle cell or pleomorphic sarcoma; the osteoid deposits in this subtype can be focal and may require a careful search (Fig. 8.54). While the conventional osteoblastic subtype appears to be the most common subtype among all extraskeletal osteosarcomas, the largest single well-characterized series of breast osteosarcomas by Silver and Tavassoli showed a predominance of the fibroblastic pattern. The overwhelming majority of extraskeletal osteosarcomas, including those arising in the breast, are of high nuclear grade.

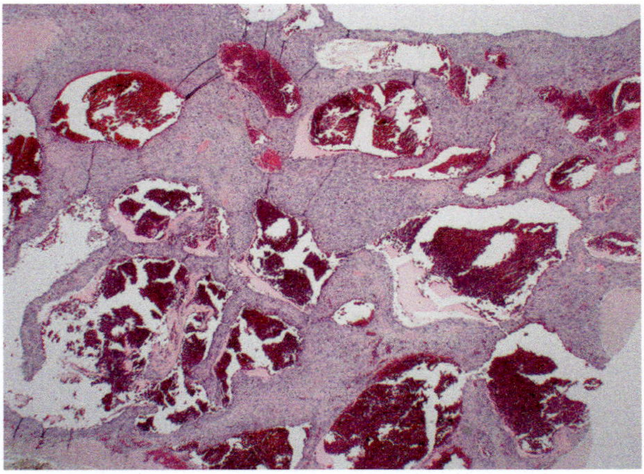

**Fig. 8.50** Extraskeletal telangiectatic osteosarcoma showing large, aneurysmal bone cyst-like spaces at scanning magnification

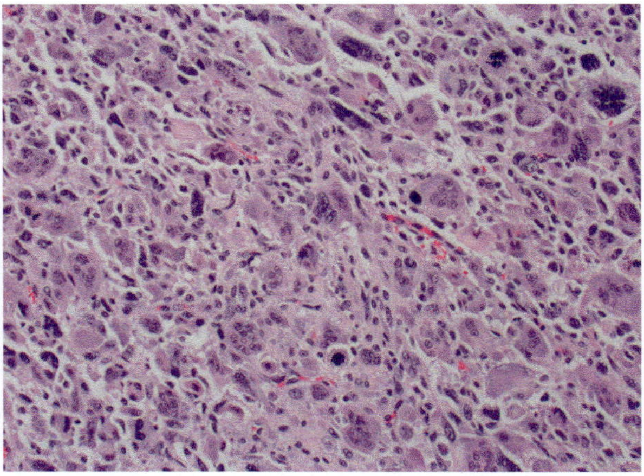

**Fig. 8.51** Telangiectatic osteosarcoma showing an admixture of overtly malignant pleomorphic tumor cells and osteoclast-type giant cells

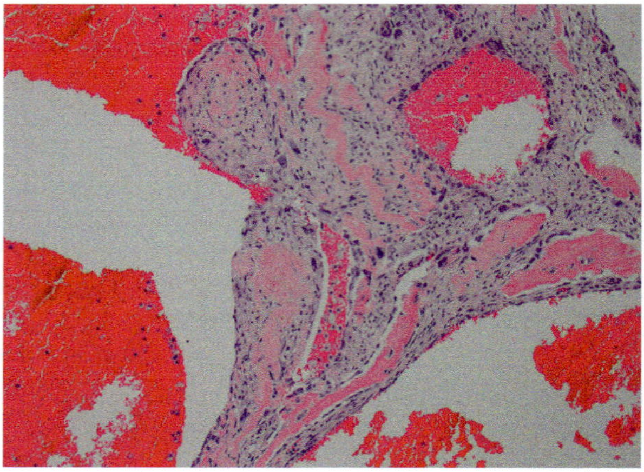

**Fig. 8.52** The osteoid formation in telangiectatic osteosarcoma is often limited to the walls of the cystic spaces

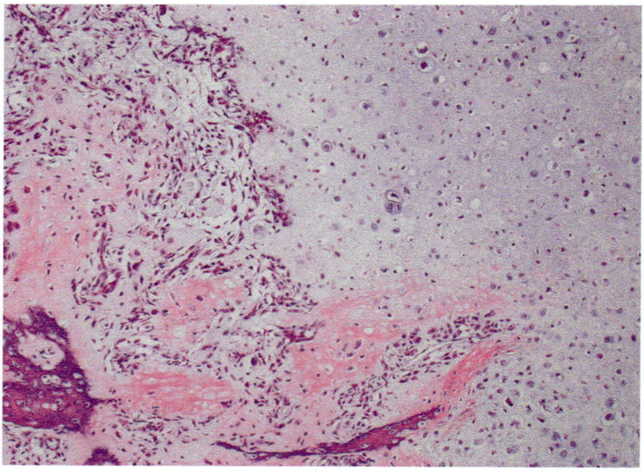

**Fig. 8.53** Chondroblastic osteosarcoma showing sheets of neoplastic cartilage with high-grade nuclear atypia, admixed with the osteoblastic component

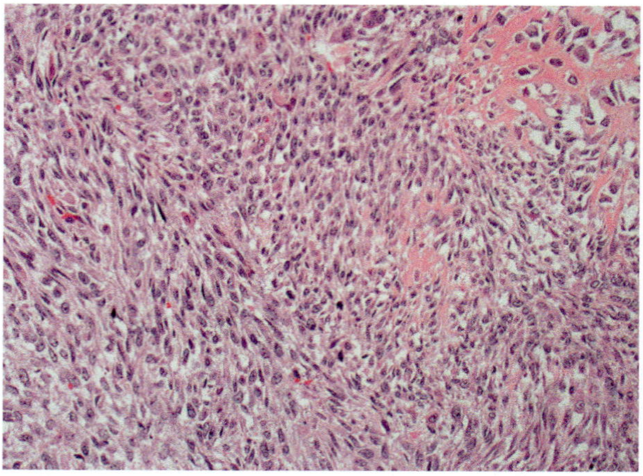

**Fig. 8.54** Fibroblastic osteosarcoma composed of sheets or intersecting fascicles of undifferentiated spindle cells with only focal osteoid deposits

## Immunohistochemistry

SATB2 expression can confirm that the neoplastic cells are osteoid producing, which can help in situations where there is a dispute between immature osteoid deposits and sclerotic collagen. Of note, SATB2 immunopositivity does not discriminate between a primary osteosarcoma and tumors with heterologous osteosarcomatous differentiation. Immunostains are extremely important when breast osteosarcoma is considered in order to rule out metaplastic carcinomas. Primary osteosarcomas are generally negative for cytokeratins, S100, SOX10, melanocytic markers, and markers of smooth and skeletal muscle differentiation (desmin, h-caldesmon, smooth muscle myosin heavy chain, myogenin, Myo-D1), although cytokeratin and EMA may be expressed in extraskeletal osteosarcomas. Focal membranous expression of SMA or desmin in fibroblastic osteosarcomas is indicative of fibroblastic/myofibroblastic differentiation and should not deter one from making the diagnosis. A more significant caveat is that up to a third of osteosarcomas can show nuclear expression of p63 severely limiting the utility of this stain in distinguishing between osteosarcoma and metaplastic carcinoma.

## Molecular

Osteosarcomas demonstrate complex clonal genetic alterations involving *TP53, PIK3CA, PTEN, CDKN2A, WNT*/beta-catenin, and other common pathways. No single genetic alteration in high-grade osteosarcoma is specific or diagnostically useful. Low-grade central and parosteal osteosarcomas arising in the bone and their rare soft tissue equivalents are associated with *MDM2* and *CDK4* gene amplification.

## Differential Diagnosis

The most challenging differential diagnosis in the breast is with metaplastic breast carcinoma with heterologous osteosarcomatous differentiation, which requires extensive sampling to identify an epithelial precursor or an in situ component. The presence of diffuse cytokeratin expression, especially high molecular weight cytokeratins (34ßE12, CK5/6) in this context, would favor metaplastic carcinoma. However, osteosarcomas may show focal cytokeratin immunostaining. As mentioned above, p63 must be used with extreme caution due to its relatively frequent expression in the stromal component of osteosarcoma. The simultaneous presence of several heterologous metaplastic elements (e.g., osteosarcomatous and rhabdomyosarcomatous elements) would favor metaplastic carcinoma. In core biopsies, the distinction between metaplastic breast carcinoma with heterologous osteosarcomatous differentiation and primary osteosarcoma may be impossible, and a descriptive diagnosis including the differential diagnosis is warranted.

Of the benign tumors, primary breast osteosarcoma needs to be distinguished from myositis ossificans, a self-limited neoplasm on a histologic spectrum with nodular fasciitis and aneurysmal bone cyst that may occasionally occur in the breast parenchyma or chest wall. Histologically, myositis ossificans is characterized by a central fasciitis-like proliferation of mitotically active myofibroblastic cells transitioning to a zonal pattern of new bone formation with prominent osteoblastic rimming and gradual maturation toward a well-formed lamellar bone at the periphery (Figs. 8.55, 8.56, and 8.57). In contrast, the neoplastic osteoid deposits in osteosarcoma are haphazardly distributed and rarely exhibit significant maturation or a zonal distribution. Cytologically, the spindle cells and the plump osteoblasts that form myositis ossificans do not show the degree of nuclear anaplasia and pleomorphism typical of osteosarcoma. In challenging cases, FISH or molecular testing for *USP6* gene rearrangement, which is a defining genetic alteration in myositis ossificans and the closely related aneurysmal bone cyst and nodular fasciitis, may be utilized.

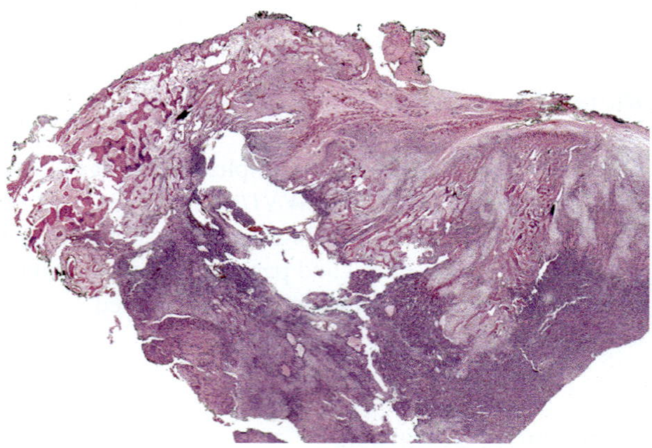

**Fig. 8.55** Myositis ossificans: a well-circumscribed cellular mass with a rim of new bone formation at the periphery

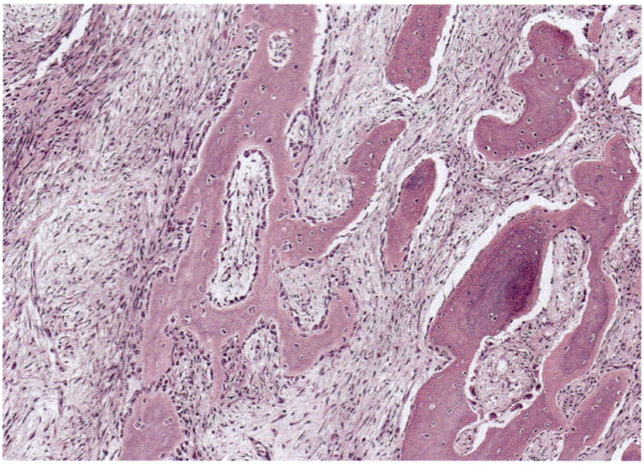

**Fig. 8.56** The osteoid deposits in myositis ossificans show a prominent osteoblastic rimming and gradual maturation toward a well-formed lamellar bone at the periphery. Nuclear atypia or pleomorphism is not characteristic of either osteoblastic or myofibroblastic spindle cell component

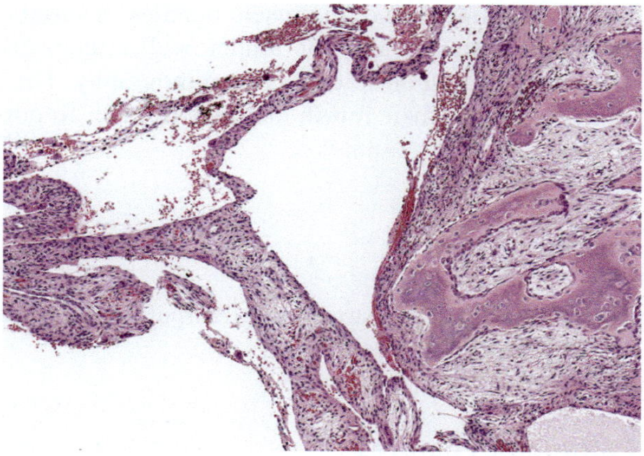

**Fig. 8.57** Aneurysmal bone cyst-like changes in myositis ossificans, in keeping with the genetic and histologic relatedness of these two lesions

Primary osteosarcoma with a telangiectatic pattern may need to be distinguished from giant cell tumor of soft tissue (GCT-ST, discussed above). The most helpful histologic features in this context are lack of significant nuclear atypia and atypical mitotic figures in GCT-ST. The bone formation in both lesions is focal and generally confined to the fibrous septa. In contrast to osteosarcoma, the bone in GCT-ST is metaplastic, with a lamellar or mature woven quality, and is not intimately associated with neoplastic tumor cells. This principle is also helpful in distinguishing osteosarcoma from other breast tumors that may have metaplastic ossifications such as benign fibroepithelial tumors, myofibroblastoma, and OFMT.

## Treatment and Prognosis

Extraskeletal osteosarcomas at all sites have a substantially worse prognosis compared to primary osteosarcomas of bone. The reported overall 5-year survival is 37–77% for all and 38% for primary breast extraskeletal osteosarcomas, with 28% rate of local recurrence and 40% rate of metastasis based on the largest series by Silver and Tavassoli. The optimal treatment strategy for extraosseous soft tissue sarcoma is not standardized. Treatment generally follows NCCN guidelines for soft tissue sarcomas with a combination of oncologic resection with or without radiation. The benefit of adjuvant or neoadjuvant chemotherapy for extraosseous osteosarcoma is unproven although some studies suggest that multiagent chemotherapy similar to skeletal osteosarcomas may result in comparable outcomes.

# Myoid Hamartoma

## Clinical Features

Myoid hamartoma is a rare benign mesenchymal lesion composed of breast parenchymal elements (breast ducts and lobules, stroma, and adipose tissue) as well as prominent smooth muscle bundles in variable proportions. Myoid hamartoma may present as a non-tender, well-circumscribed palpable mass or as an incidental finding on screening mammography. The lesions most often occur in adult women in their fourth and fifth decade. Reported sizes vary widely from <1 cm to 11 cm.

## Imaging

Mammography demonstrates a well-circumscribed high-density mass most suggestive of a fibroadenoma.

## Pathologic Features

### Gross Features

A well-circumscribed fibrofatty mass.

### Microscopic Features

Myoid hamartoma is a well-circumscribed mass with a pushing border. It is composed of an admixture of ductal and lobular structures with features of adenosis, mature fibrofatty stroma, and benign-appearing fascicles of smooth muscle surrounding glandular structures (Figs. 8.58, 8.59, and 8.60). There is no significant atypia or mitotic activity.

## Immunohistochemistry

As expected, the smooth muscle component in myoid hamartomas is diffusely positive for muscle markers (desmin, SMA, h-caldesmon, smooth muscle myosin) and estrogen and progesterone receptors. CD34 expression may be present in some cases, suggesting an overlap with leiomyomatous myofibroblastomas.

## Molecular

A recent genetic study demonstrated a t(5;12)(p13;q14) translocation in a case of myoid hamartoma, with a corresponding *HMGA2* (12q14) gene rearrangement, lending further support to the hypothesis that myoid hamartomas are similar to hamartomas in the breast and other sites and likely originate from a pluripotent mesenchymal precursor.

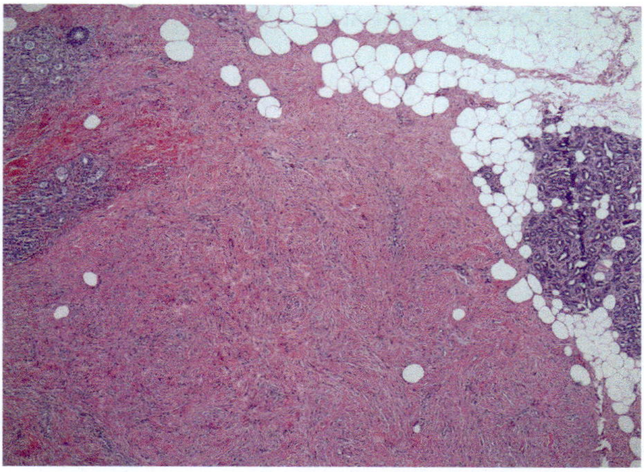

**Fig. 8.58** Myoid hamartoma is a well-circumscribed mass with a pushing border composed of mammary glands with features of adenosis and fibrofatty stroma

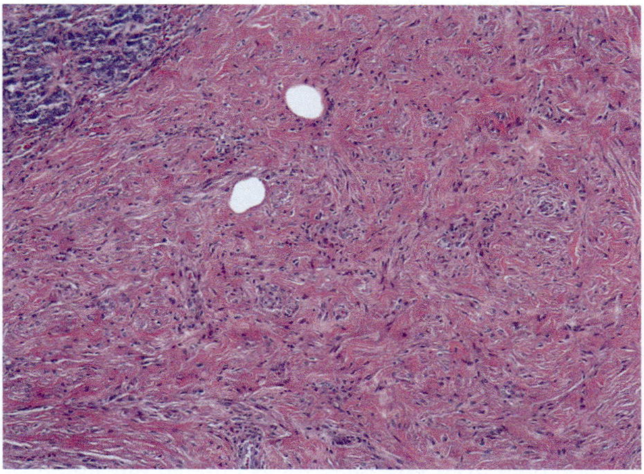

**Fig. 8.59** The fibrous stroma in myoid hamartoma contains fascicles of cytologically benign smooth muscle cells surrounding glandular structures

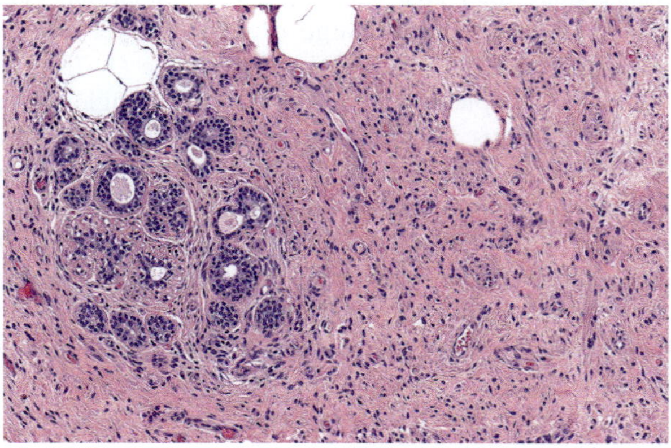

**Fig. 8.60** Another example of myoid hamartoma with prominent fascicles of benign smooth muscle cells surrounding breast glands

## Differential Diagnosis

The differential diagnosis of myoid hamartoma includes breast lesions with a prominent smooth muscle component including the leiomyomatous variant of myofibroblastoma, myoid stroma in fibroepithelial lesions, and leiomyoma of the breast parenchyma and nipple. Myofibroblastoma, by definition, does not contain intratumoral breast glands and will contain areas with a more conventional fibroblastic CD34-positive spindle cell component admixed with collagen fibers. Rb1 immunohistochemistry or *RB1/FOX01* deletions by FISH can objectively confirm the diagnosis of myofibroblastoma. Fibroadenomas can be readily separated by recognition of either an intracanalicular or pericanalicular growth pattern. Pure benign smooth muscle tumors lack fibrofatty and glandular elements.

## Treatment and Prognosis

Myoid hamartomas behave in a benign fashion and can be treated by simple excision or observed. Recurrences are exceptionally rare.

# Leiomyoma of the Nipple/Areola and Breast

## Clinical Features

As mammary parenchyma normally lacks native smooth muscle elements, most leiomyomas encountered in the breast region represent either genital-type leiomyomas originating from the smooth muscle of the nipple-areola complex or cutaneous leiomyomas arising from the arrector pili muscle. Leiomyomas of the breast parenchyma are rare. Clinically, nipple and cutaneous leiomyomas present as slightly protuberant, well-circumscribed, pinkish-tan nodules in adults, usually less than 2 cm in size. They are characteristically tender or (in the case of nipple leiomyoma) can change their size with hormonal fluctuations related to the menstrual cycle. There is no nipple discharge or skin change. Nipple leiomyomas have a slight female predilection and a broad age range (1–75 years, mean age approximately 48 years). Nipple leiomyomas are usually single but in male patients can be bilateral. Cutaneous leiomyomas are often multiple occurring in crops. The clinical importance of recognizing multiple leiomyomas is in their association with the hereditary leiomyomatosis and renal cell carcinoma syndrome (HLRCC), an autosomal dominant disorder due to germline mutations of the fumarate hydratase (*FH*) gene characterized by multiple cutaneous and uterine leiomyomas, renal cell carcinoma, and a variety of other tumors.

Reported primary breast parenchymal leiomyomas presented as a palpable mass or were discovered incidentally by screening mammography. They almost always occur in adult female patients (mean age 47.6 years) and range from 0.5 to 13 cm in size.

## Imaging

Nipple leiomyomas can present as hypoechoic lesions on ultrasound, although these are rarely imaged. Deep breast leiomyomas present as a moderate- or high-density well-circumscribed mass without calcifications. By ultrasound, these are solid, hypoechoic, well-circumscribed homogenous lesions.

## Pathologic Findings

### Gross Findings

Cutaneous and nipple leiomyomas are somewhat ill-defined, pink-tan dermal nodules; in contrast, parenchymal leiomyomas are well-circumscribed. Like all smooth muscle tumors, parenchymal leiomyomas are firm, white-tan lesions with a rubbery cut surface.

### Microscopic Findings

Cutaneous and nipple leiomyomas are composed of short, disorganized bundles of benign smooth muscle that fill the reticular dermis. Pilar leiomyomas have a somewhat infiltrative edge, percolating between dermal collagen fibers, whereas nipple leiomyomas can be either circumscribed or more infiltrative, in which case they are essentially indistinguishable from pilar leiomyomas (Figs. 8.61 and 8.62). In contrast, deep-seated leiomyomas are always well-circumscribed and are composed of dense intersecting fascicles or whorls of smooth muscle cells. Cytologically, the tumor cells have elongated, blunt-ended nuclei, uniformly distributed chromatin and brightly eosinophilic cytoplasm with crisp cytoplasmic membranes, and the occasional presence of perinuclear cytoplasmic vacuoles (Figs. 8.63 and 8.64). The vasculature is inconspicuous. Both superficial and deep leiomyomas show essentially no cytologic atypia or pleomorphism, and mitotic figures are very rare. That

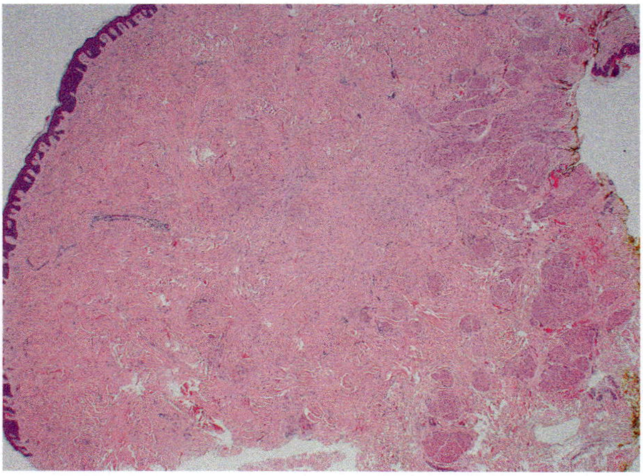

**Fig. 8.61** Low-power image of a nipple leiomyoma wherein the dermis is expanded by an unencapsulated hypocellular spindle cell process arranged in intersecting fascicles. There is a subepithelial grenz zone that is not involved by the dermal spindle cell lesion

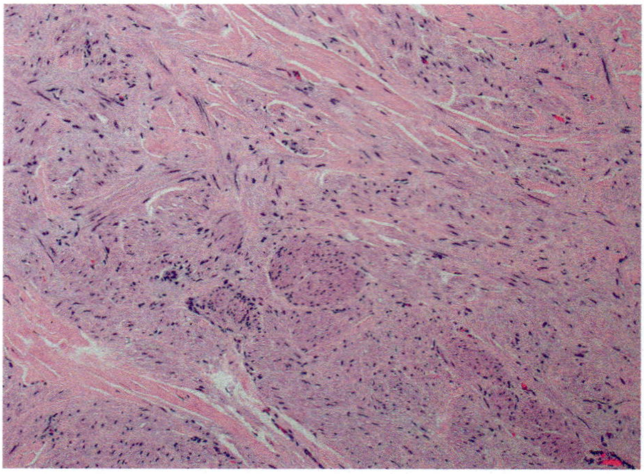

**Fig. 8.62** Nipple leiomyoma showing the typical morphology of benign smooth muscle cells is appreciated with elongated nuclei with blunt ends and prominent eosinophilic cytoplasm

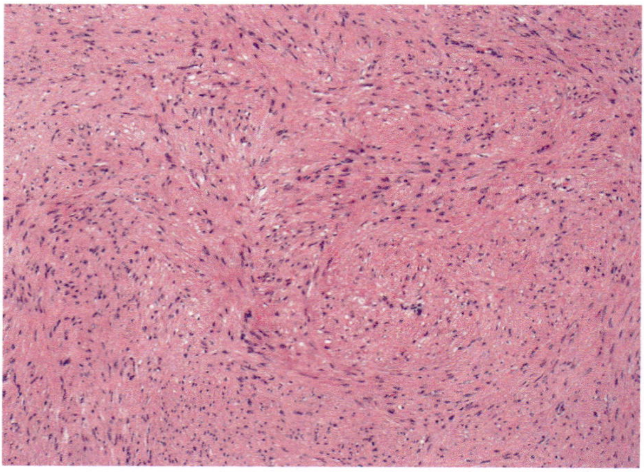

**Fig. 8.63** Leiomyoma composed of dense intersecting fascicles or whorls of smooth muscle cells

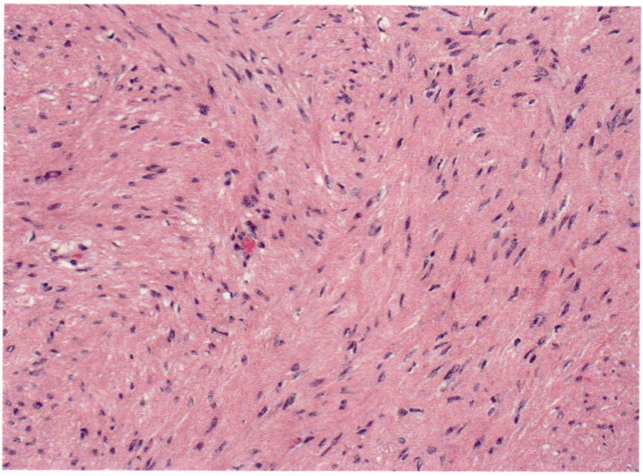

**Fig. 8.64** The tumor cells in leiomyoma have elongated, blunt-ended nuclei, uniformly distributed chromatin, and brightly eosinophilic cytoplasm with crisp cytoplasmic borders. There is no nuclear atypia or mitotic activity

being said, cutaneous leiomyomas associated with HLRCC syndrome can show a somewhat increased degree of nuclear atypia or symplastic change. Prominent nucleoli observed in HLRCC-associated uterine leiomyomas are not typical in the cutaneous and nipple lesions. Cutaneous leiomyomas typically do not extend beyond the dermis. As with smooth muscle tumors in other locations, edema, stromal fibrosis, and dystrophic calcifications may be present, although they are much more common in deep examples.

## Immunohistochemistry

Benign smooth muscle tumors are diffusely positive for SMA, desmin, h-caldesmon, and smooth muscle myosin heavy chain. Nipple leiomyomas may somewhat inconsistently express estrogen (ER) and progesterone (PR) receptors, while pilar leiomyomas are reliably negative for these markers, which can be helpful diagnostically. Loss of FH expression by immunohistochemistry can be used as a quick screen to identify patients possibly affected by HLRCC and has a sensitivity of approximately 80%. Cytokeratin expression can occasionally be observed. SOX10, S100, melanocytic markers, and CD34 are reliably negative.

## Molecular

Currently leiomyoma does not have a molecular signature.

## Differential Diagnosis

The principal differential diagnosis of cutaneous and nipple leiomyomas is with cutaneous leiomyosarcoma and the terminologically related atypical intradermal smooth muscle neoplasm (discussed in the next section). The differential diagnosis of a parenchymal leiomyoma is with the aforementioned myoid hamartoma and leiomyomatous myofibroblastoma. Desmoid-type fibromatosis can be distinguished by its markedly infiltrative edge, the slender fibroblastic appearance of its lesional cells, its densely collagenous stroma, the uniformly distributed slit-like or gaping vessels, and its focal, membranous staining pattern with muscle markers like desmin and SMA. Molecular testing for mutations in exon 3 of *CTNNB1* (beta-catenin) or nuclear expression of beta-catenin by immunohistochemistry can be used in problematic cases.

The most helpful histologic clues for distinguishing leiomyomas from leiomyosarcoma are cytologic atypia and hyperchromasia, which can be appreciated at scanning magnification even in low-grade leiomyosarcomas. Increased cellularity, mitotic activity, necrosis, vascular invasion, and, in case of the superficial lesions, substantial involvement of the subcutis would also favor leiomyosarcoma (discussed below). In core biopsies, the possibility of smooth muscle metaplasia in phyllodes tumor or metaplastic breast carcinoma needs to be considered.

### Treatment and Prognosis

Cutaneous, nipple, and breast parenchymal leiomyomas are benign and are treated by simple excision.

## Leiomyosarcoma

Several types of leiomyosarcomas can be encountered in the breast region: these include cutaneous leiomyosarcomas that originate in the dermis and subcutis, rare primary breast parenchymal leiomyosarcomas that arise from vascular smooth muscle and are similar to their deep soft tissue and visceral and retroperitoneal counterparts, and metastases from other sites. Rarely, breast leiomyosarcomas have been described in the setting of prior radiation.

Cutaneous leiomyosarcomas present in older adults, with predilection for male patients, as solitary, somewhat lobulated protuberant tan-red nodules, usually less than 2 cm in size (range 0.3–5 cm), which, just like pilar leiomyomas, can be painful. Primary breast leiomyosarcomas present as a slow-growing palpable mass or mastalgia in adult, predominantly female patients (median age 56 years, range 24–83). Reported cases range from 1.5 to 9 cm in size. Subcutaneous and chest wall leiomyosarcomas have clinical findings similar to their somatic soft tissue counterparts at other sites.

### Imaging

Cutaneous leiomyosarcomas are not imaged. Parenchymal leiomyosarcomas present as an irregular mass without calcifications on mammogram, with non-homogenous echogenicity on the corresponding ultrasound.

### Pathologic Features

#### Gross Features

Breast parenchymal leiomyosarcomas present as well-circumscribed, gray-tan fleshy masses which may contain areas of necrosis, cystic change, or hemorrhage. Nipple and cutaneous leiomyosarcomas are small, slightly lobulated dermal nodules with irregular margins.

#### Microscopic Features

Microscopically, leiomyosarcomas are composed of cellular intersecting fascicles of smooth muscle cells with blunt-ended hyperchromatic nuclei and brightly eosinophilic cytoplasm with well-defined cell borders and occasional perinuclear vacuoles (Fig. 8.65 and 8.66). Increased cellularity and nuclear atypia and hyperchromasia are defining features of leiomyosarcoma, along with mitotic activity, necrosis, and vascular invasion (Fig. 8.67). Frank pleomorphism, dystrophic calcifications, and stromal hyalinization can be observed.

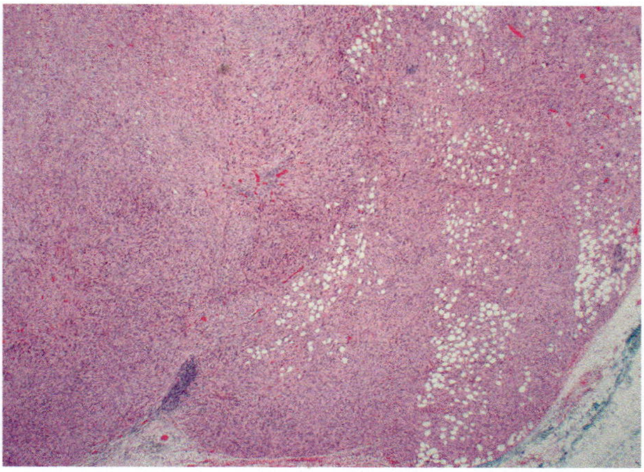

**Fig. 8.65** Leiomyosarcoma presenting as a circumscribed mass with infiltration of the subcutaneous soft tissue

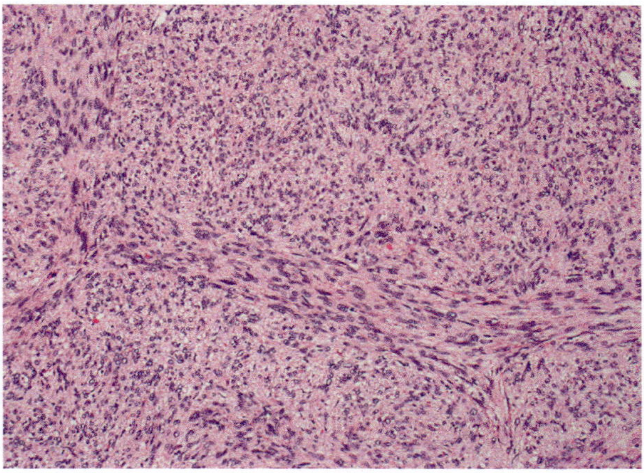

**Fig. 8.66** Leiomyosarcoma composed of cellular intersecting fascicles of smooth muscle cells with blunt-ended nuclei, brightly eosinophilic cytoplasm, well-defined cell borders, and occasional perinuclear vacuoles

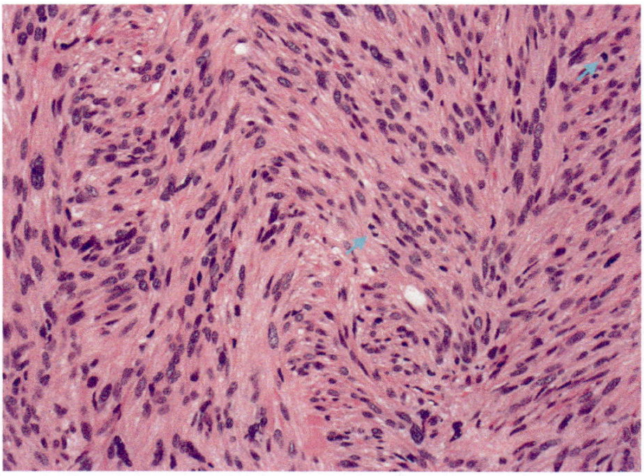

**Fig. 8.67** Leiomyosarcoma characteristically showing an increase in cellularity, nuclear hyperchromasia, and mitotic activity

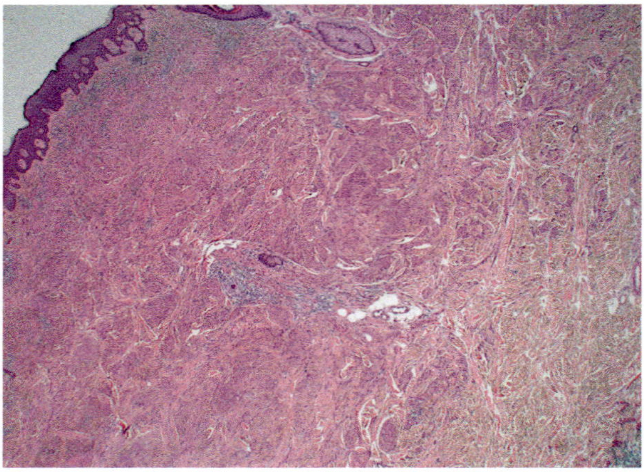

**Fig. 8.68** Cutaneous leiomyosarcoma (also referred to as atypical intradermal smooth muscle neoplasm) is confined to the dermis with no or only minimal involvement of the subcutis

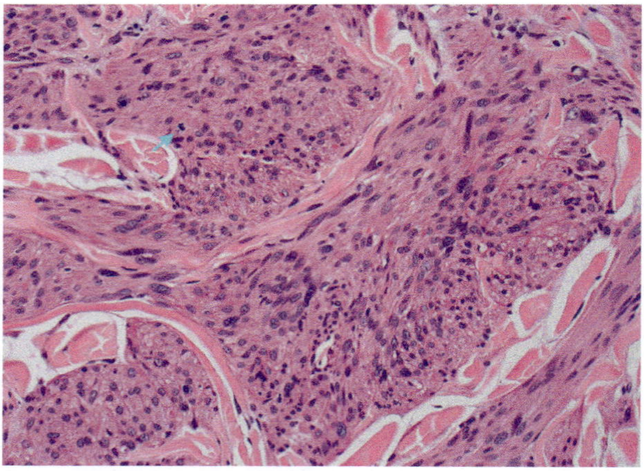

**Fig. 8.69** Cutaneous leiomyosarcoma composed of bundles of smooth muscle cells infiltrating derma collagen, with overt nuclear atypia and mitotic activity (arrows)

Breast parenchymal leiomyosarcomas and leiomyosarcomas centered on the subcutis are comparable in every way to their somatic soft tissue counterparts and should be graded according to the FNCLCC grading system. However, cutaneous leiomyosarcomas of lower nuclear grade that are completely confined to the dermis or show only very minimal involvement of the subcutis and no vascular invasion tend to behave substantially better than their deep-seated counterparts (Figs. 8.68 and 8.69). For these lesions, a designation as "atypical intradermal smooth muscle neoplasm" has been proposed, provided that the interface with the subcutis can be adequately examined.

## Immunohistochemistry

Leiomyosarcomas are variably positive for SMA, desmin, h-caldesmon, and smooth muscle myosin heavy chain, and the extent and intensity of immunostaining generally correlates with the degree of differentiation. Inconsistent expression of estrogen and progesterone receptor can occur. Importantly, approximately 40–50% of leiomyosarcomas can be positive for cytokeratins.

## Molecular

Currently leiomyosarcoma does not have a molecular signature.

## Differential Diagnosis

Metaplastic carcinoma, malignant phyllodes tumor with heterologous leiomyosarcomatous differentiation and metastatic leiomyosarcoma must be carefully excluded, which requires extensive sampling to identify an epithelial precursor or an in situ component. As mentioned above, the diagnostic utility of cytokeratins in this context is limited. If the origin is suspected to be the chest wall, adult pleomorphic rhabdomyosarcoma and dedifferentiated liposarcoma with heterologous smooth muscle differentiation may also be considered; helpful diagnostic tools in this context include markers of skeletal muscle differentiation like myogenin and Myo-D1 (rhabdomyosarcoma) and FISH testing for *MDM2* gene amplification (dedifferentiated liposarcoma). Identification of multiple lines of differentiation, such as smooth muscle, skeletal muscle, or osteosarcomatous differentiation, within the same tumor would favor metaplastic carcinoma or dedifferentiated liposarcoma over a primary leiomyosarcoma of the breast.

The differential diagnosis with benign smooth muscle lesions of the breast is discussed in the previous section.

## Treatment and Prognosis

Primary breast and subcutaneous leiomyosarcomas are aggressive and behave similarly to their somatic soft tissue counterparts, with tumor size, grade, and completeness of surgical resection determining the outcomes. Reported primary breast leiomyosarcomas are associated with approximately 25% risk of hematogenous metastases, sometimes years after the original diagnosis.

In contrast, the prognosis of cutaneous leiomyosarcomas tends to be much more favorable due to the smaller size, superficial location, and resectability of these tumors. In a large series by Kraft and Fletcher, atypical smooth muscle tumors strictly confined to the dermis or with only very limited subcutaneous involvement demonstrated a 35% risk of local recurrence but no metastases. Based on these observations, the term "atypical intradermal smooth muscle neoplasm" was proposed for these lesions, emphasizing the need for complete surgical excision to minimize the risk of local recurrence while avoiding potential overtreatment. Other large studies, however, showed a small risk of systemic metastasis even from dermal-only cutaneous leiomyosarcomas or those with minimal subcutaneous extension (approximately 5%), suggesting that the term "cutaneous leiomyosarcoma" should be retained.

Whatever the preferred terminology, it appears that the best treatment strategy for dermal-based cutaneous leiomyosarcomas is complete surgical excision with negative margins, whereas breast parenchymal, subcutaneous, and chest wall leiomyosarcomas should be treated by a multimodality approach.

## Rhabdomyosarcoma

Breast parenchymal rhabdomyosarcomas are very rare, comprising 0.2%–6% of all rhabdomyosarcomas based on various published series, and are encountered in adolescent female patients, most often in the metastatic setting. Chest wall rhabdomyosarcomas can also occur in both pediatric and adult patients. Rhabdomyosarcomas are subdivided based on the histopathologic features into embryonal, alveolar, spindle cell/sclerosing, and (adult) pleomorphic subtypes. While these rubrics are maintained in the 2020 WHO classification of soft tissue and bone tumors, recent advances in molecular genetics led to identification of clinically and prognostically relevant molecular subsets of rhabdomyosarcoma, which are briefly reviewed here in the context of the morphologic findings. All four major histologic types of rhabdomyosarcoma have been reported in the breast, with the alveolar subtype comprising the majority (86–100%). Epithelioid and spindle cell rhabdomyosarcoma with *EWSR1/FUS-TFCP2* fusion and other emerging rhabdomyosarcoma subtypes that have not yet been reported in the breast are only briefly mentioned here. For a comprehensive review of this topic, the reader is referred to the corresponding soft tissue pathology literature.

### Clinical Features

Both primary and metastatic breast rhabdomyosarcomas are almost always encountered in young female patients (mean age 15 years). Metastatic rhabdomyosarcoma presents as either isolated breast involvement or in combination with other metastatic sites such as the lung or bone. Primary breast rhabdomyosarcomas present as a relatively large mass (range 3–21 cm), with or without regional axillary lymphadenopathy. Bilateral disease is reported in both the primary and metastatic settings.

### Imaging

On mammography, breast rhabdomyosarcomas present as a large, ill-defined heterogeneously enhancing mass with malignant characteristics with or without corresponding axillary lymphadenopathy. The CT and MRI findings are similar to those reported at other sites.

## Pathologic Features

### Gross Features

Ill-defined, multinodular fleshy mass with areas of necrosis and hemorrhage.

### Microscopic Features

Embryonal rhabdomyosarcoma (ERMS) consists of uniform mesenchymal spindled to round cells with hyperchromatic nuclei and scant basophilic cytoplasm, growing loosely within a myxoid stroma and resembling primitive skeletal muscle. Admixed with the spindle cells are variable numbers of spindled to polygonal rhabdomyoblasts with brightly eosinophilic cytoplasm and occasional striations (Figs. 8.70 and 8.71), but rhabdomyoblasts can be entirely absent in this subtype. Solid and nested growth with round cell morphology resembling alveolar rhabdomyosarcoma can also be seen. Scattered or diffuse anaplasia can occur in approximately 10% of ERMS defined by the presence of bizarre multinucleated tumor cells

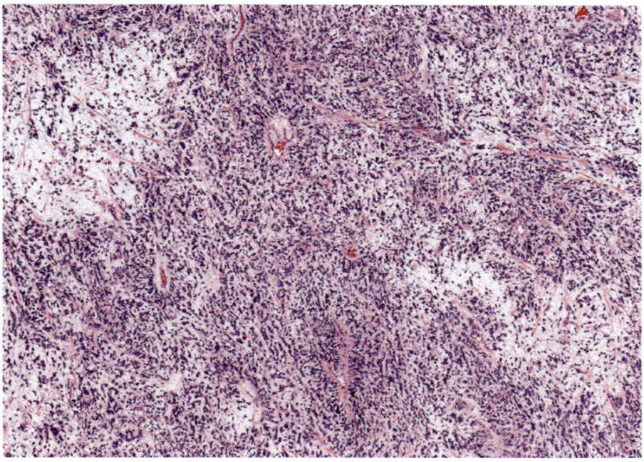

**Fig. 8.70** Embryonal rhabdomyosarcoma (RMS) composed of primitive round to spindle cells growing loosely within a myxoid stroma

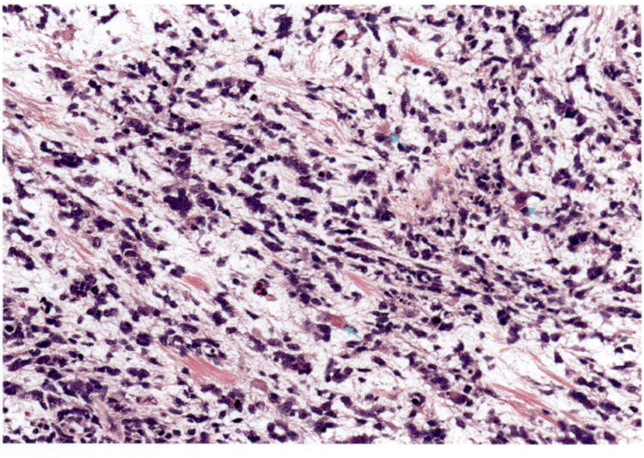

**Fig. 8.71** The cells in embryonal RMS demonstrate hyperchromatic nuclei and scant basophilic cytoplasm resembling primitive skeletal muscle. Spindled to polygonal rhabdomyoblasts with brightly eosinophilic cytoplasm and occasional striations are variably present (arrows)

and frankly atypical multipolar mitotic figures (Fig. 8.72). Rarely, foci of neuroectodermal or other mesenchymal (usually, cartilaginous) differentiation may be seen.

Alveolar rhabdomyosarcoma (ARMS) is composed of nests or solid sheets of undifferentiated round cells separated by fibrous septa. The alveolar appearance is the result of cellular dishesion in the center of the nests, although many examples of the ARMS are essentially completely solid (Figs. 8.73 and 8.74). Plump epithelioid rhabdomyoblasts are variably present (Fig. 8.75), and in some cases, distinctive multinucleated wreath-like giant cells may be observed. In contrast to the ERMS, the stroma is usually inconspicuous. Treated ARMS can demonstrate striking maturation in the form of sheets of epithelioid rhabdomyoblasts.

Spindle cell rhabdomyosarcoma is characteristically composed of cellular monotonous eosinophilic fascicles of spindle cells in a fibrosarcoma-like growth pattern mimicking leiomyosarcoma, nodular fasciitis, spindle cell metaplastic breast carcinoma or malignant phyllodes tumor with stromal overgrowth, and other

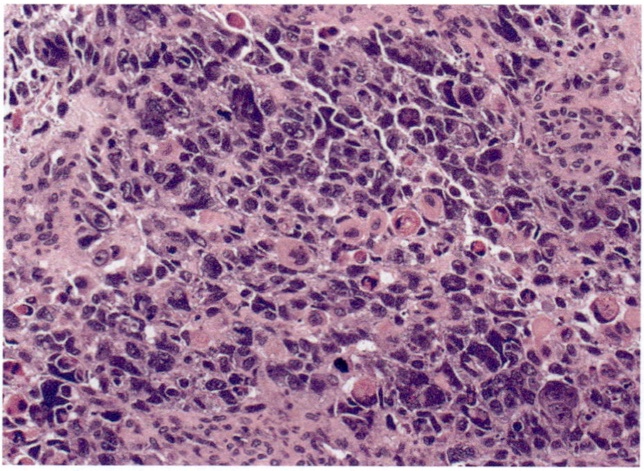

**Fig. 8.72** Embryonal RMS with diffuse anaplasia defined by the presence of bizarre multinucleated tumor cells and frankly atypical multipolar mitotic figures; numerous rhabdomyoblasts with brightly eosinophilic cytoplasm are also present

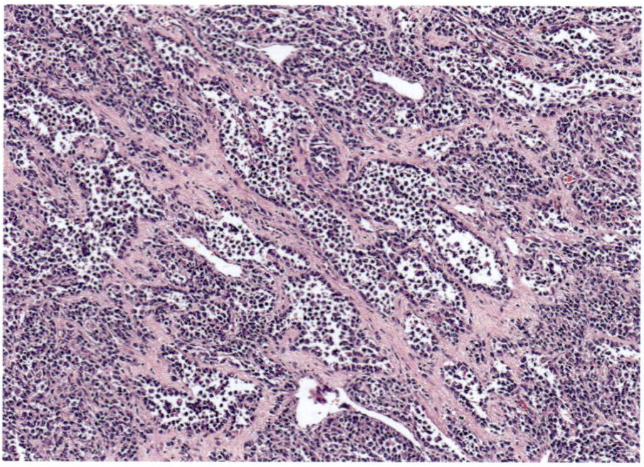

**Fig. 8.73** Alveolar RMS composed of nests or sheets of undifferentiated round cells separated by fibrous septa

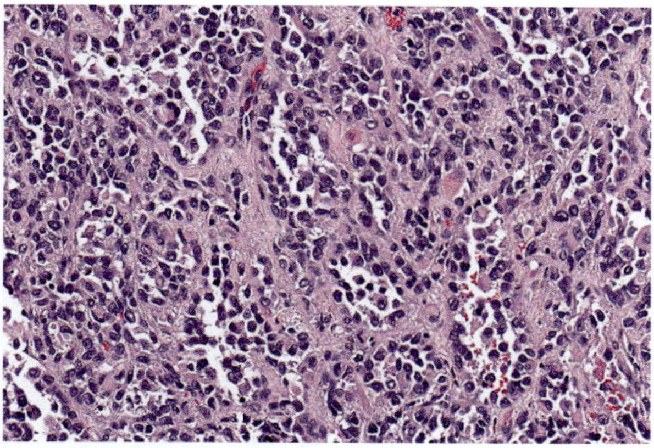

**Fig. 8.74** Alveolar RMS: cellular dishesion in the center of the tumor nests produces the characteristic alveolar appearance

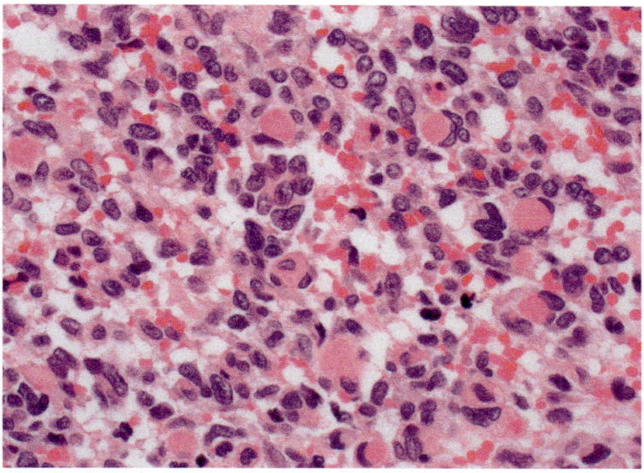

**Fig. 8.75** Alveolar RMS with plump epithelioid rhabdomyoblasts and enlarged, hyperchromatic nuclei with variably prominent nucleoli

fascicular spindle cell neoplasms (Fig. 8.76). Cytologically, the tumor cells show elongated nuclei with vesicular chromatin and small nucleoli. The degree of nuclear atypia is highly variable, and some spindle cell rhabdomyosarcomas can be surprisingly banal in appearance (Figs. 8.77 and 8.78). Spindled rhabdomyoblasts with hyperchromatic nuclei and brightly eosinophilic cytoplasm can be variably present (Fig. 8.79), but this feature is often inconspicuous. Occasional cases show a primitive mesenchymal component with myxoid background reminiscent of ERMS. Mitotic activity is usually brisk, and atypical mitotic figures may be seen. A variant morphology with densely sclerotic stroma containing nests and cords of tumor cells and imparting a pseudoangiomatous appearance has been referred to as sclerosing rhabdomyosarcoma (Fig. 8.80); this pattern is usually seen in spindle cell rhabdomyosarcomas associated with *MYOD1* mutations (more on that below).

Pleomorphic (adult) rhabdomyosarcoma (RMS) is, by definition, a high-grade pleomorphic sarcoma composed of sheets of undifferentiated pleomorphic or spindle cells with overt nuclear atypia and mitotic activity, admixed with brightly eosinophilic pleomorphic rhabdomyoblasts (Figs. 8.81 and 8.82).

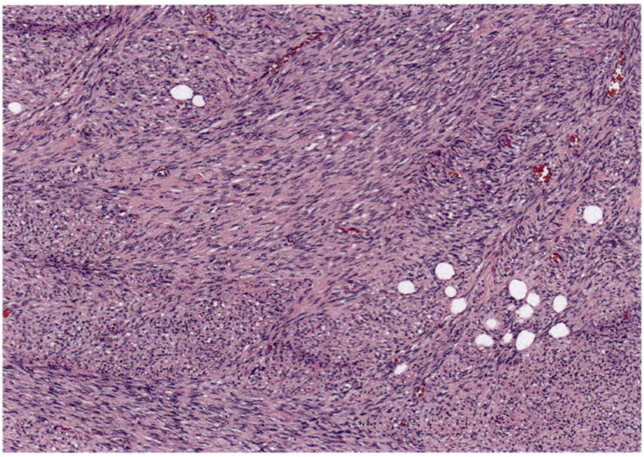

**Fig. 8.76** Spindle cell RMS composed of intersecting fascicles of eosinophilic spindle cells

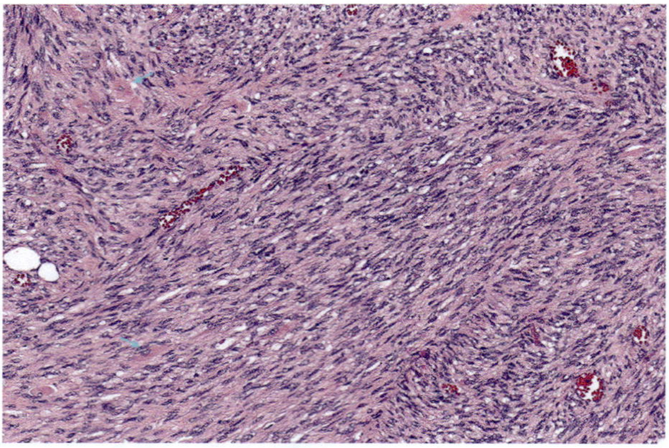

**Fig. 8.77** The tumor cells in spindle cell RMS show elongated nuclei with vesicular chromatin, small nucleoli, and mitotic figures

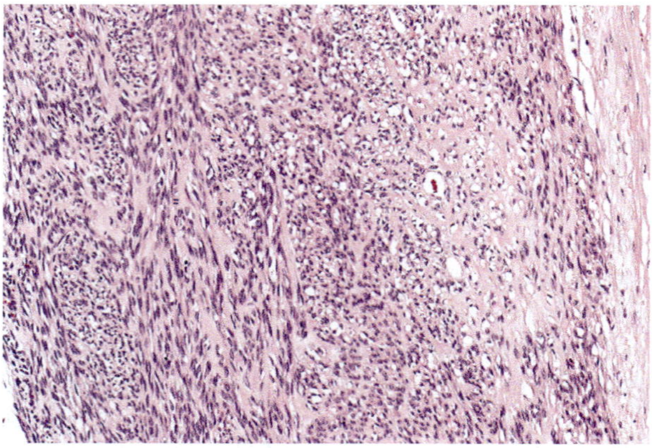

**Fig. 8.78** Another example of spindle cell RMS; the tumor cells can show a range of nuclear atypia from mild to severe

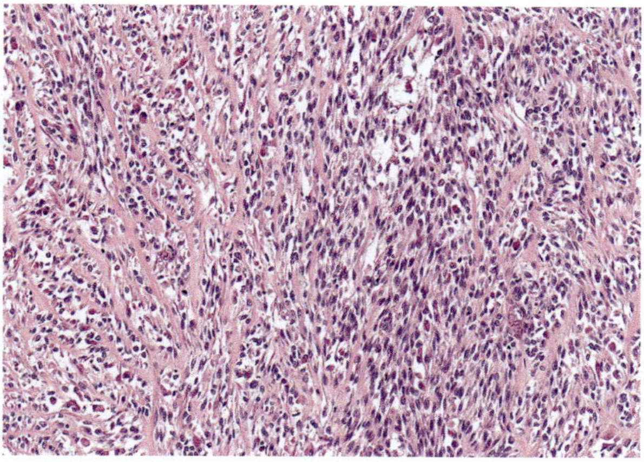

**Fig. 8.79** Spindled rhabdomyoblasts with hyperchromatic nuclei and brightly eosinophilic cytoplasm in spindle cell RMS

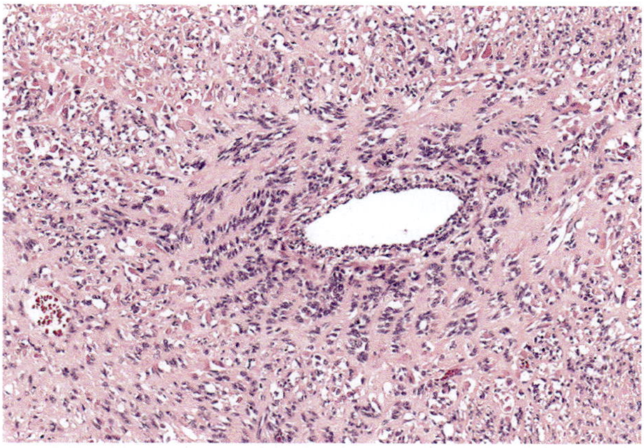

**Fig. 8.80** Sclerosing RMS showing nests, cords, and fascicles of tumor cells embedded in a densely collagenized stroma and imparting a pseudoangiomatous appearance in some areas

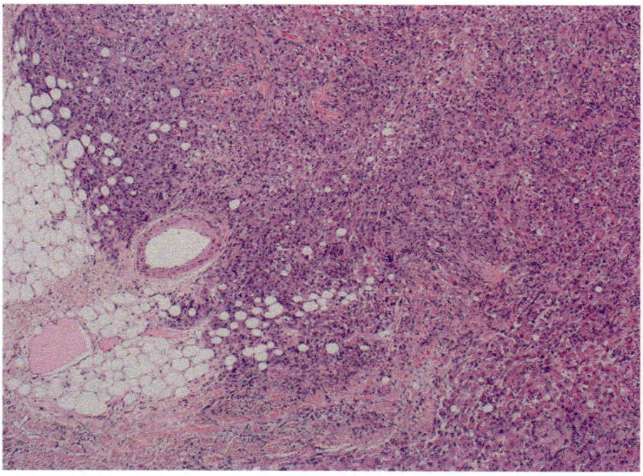

**Fig. 8.81** Pleomorphic (adult) RMS at scanning magnification, showing a high-grade pleomorphic sarcoma with infiltration of the subcutis

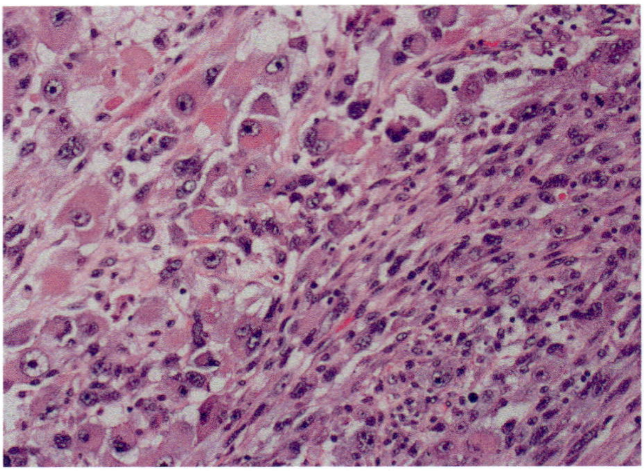

**Fig. 8.82** Pleomorphic RMS with an admixture of undifferentiated pleomorphic spindle cells and brightly eosinophilic pleomorphic rhabdomyoblasts

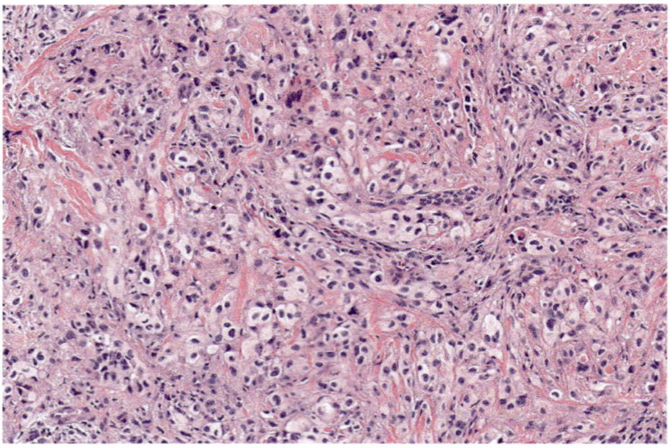

**Fig. 8.83** Epithelioid rhabdomyosarcoma composed of solid sheets of polygonal cells with eccentric nuclei, prominent nucleoli, and eosinophilic cytoplasm resembling carcinoma or melanoma

Epithelioid rhabdomyosarcoma is a variant composed of solid sheets of polygonal cells with eccentric nuclei, prominent nucleoli, and eosinophilic cytoplasm resembling carcinoma or melanoma (Fig. 8.83); recent studies suggest that epithelioid rhabdomyosarcoma represents a distinct molecular subtype of RMS.

## Immunohistochemistry

All forms of rhabdomyosarcoma express desmin and markers of skeletal muscle differentiation in variable proportions, including myogenin and MYOD1. Expression of all of these markers can be quite patchy in ERMS and pleomorphic RMS and is generally strong and diffuse in ARMS. Spindle cell/sclerosing rhabdomyosarcomas tend to express MYOD1 more avidly than myogenin. Undifferentiated pleomorphic sarcomas can be "screened" for myogenic differentiation using desmin and SMA immunostains as part of the initial immunohistochemical workup followed by confirmatory application of myogenin and MYOD1. As an important practical point, rhabdomyosarcomas are often positive for SMA, cytokeratins, neuroendocrine markers, and S100. Epithelioid rhabdomyosarcomas that are associated with *TFCP2* fusions are characterized by a consistent cytokeratin expression and overexpression of ALK protein due to internal deletions of *ALK* gene.

## Genetic and Molecular Findings

Alveolar RMS is characterized by a recurrent t(2;13)(q35;q14) or variant t(1;13)(p36;q14) translocation resulting in a fusion of Forkhead box O1 *(FOXO1)* gene with *PAX3* or *PAX7* genes. Rare variant fusions such as *PAX3-NCOA1*, *PAX3-NCOA2*, and *FOXO1-FGFR1* may occur.

The diagnosis of ARMS requires molecular confirmation by FISH or RT-PCR-based testing, as fusion-defined ARMS are associated with an unfavorable prognosis. Morphologically convincing ARMS that lack the characteristic fusions (formerly referred to as "fusion-negative" ARMS) are now considered to represent embryonal RMS based on the comparable clinical outcomes.

Within the category of spindle cell and sclerosing rhabdomyosarcoma, two prognostically different groups with different genetic alterations have emerged. Spindle cell RMS with *VGLL2* and *NCOA2* gene rearrangements almost exclusively affects newborns, infants, and very young children (<5 y.o.) and is characterized predominantly by cellular spindled cell morphology and a propensity for local recurrence without any significant risk of systemic metastasis. This rhabdomyosarcoma group has superior outcomes even with conservative management and is being constantly expanded by addition of other variant fusions such as recently described RMS with *SRF-FOXO1* and *SRF-NCOA1* fusions. The second group is characterized by spindle cell and/or sclerosing RMS morphology and activating somatic *MYOD1* mutations. These RMS affect both children and adults, often occur in the head and neck region, and are associated with an unfavorable outcome comparable to that of alveolar RMS. Rhabdomyosarcomas with spindle cell morphology that lack the above molecular alterations are classified as spindle cell embryonal RMS.

Embryonal RMS displays a complex array of genetic and molecular abnormalities including copy number alterations, gene amplification, and *KRAS*, *NRAS*, and *HRAS* mutations. It may occur sporadically on in association with other syndromes such as neurofibromatosis type 1, Beckwith-Wiedemann syndrome, Costello syndrome or DICER1 syndrome. The prognosis of embryonal RMS is generally more favorable than that of alveolar RMS or *MYOD1*-mutated spindle cell RMS, providing a significant clinical incentive to correctly classify these different molecular subtypes of RMS based on their molecular signatures.

Pleomorphic rhabdomyosarcoma is associated with a complex array of copy number alterations and point mutations, often involving *TP53*, and may occur in patients with Li-Fraumeni syndrome. No single genetic alteration is pathognomonic for this rhabdomyosarcoma subtype. These tumors have poor prognosis. Epithelioid RMS is an emerging new entity that may be associated with *TFCP2* gene rearrangement and is associated with variable outcomes.

## Differential Diagnosis

From a breast pathology perspective, the principal differential diagnostic consideration for all rhabdomyosarcoma variants, with the exception of alveolar rhabdomyosarcoma, is metaplastic carcinoma and malignant phyllodes tumor with heterologous rhabdomyoblastic differentiation. This distinction can be further complicated by the expression of cytokeratins in rhabdomyosarcoma. The appropriate demographics are very helpful as primary rhabdomyosarcomas tend to occur in much younger patients than any of the above mimics. In difficult cases, extensive sampling might be required to demonstrate an epithelial component or a carcinoma in situ. The more cytologically innocuous examples of spindle cell rhabdomyosarcoma might need to be distinguished from low-grade fibromatosis-like metaplastic carcinoma, nodular fasciitis, inflammatory myofibroblastic tumor, or low-grade myofibroblastic sarcoma (the latter three entities are discussed in the myofibroblastic tumor chapter). This requires a somewhat high index of suspicion due to the overall rarity of spindle cell rhabdomyosarcoma, but the distinction can be easily accomplished by application of skeletal muscle markers that are expected to be negative in the above mimics. Alveolar rhabdomyosarcoma can resemble other small round cell tumors occurring in adults, such as high-grade lymphomas, small cell neuroendocrine carcinoma, Merkel cell carcinoma, and Ewing sarcoma. This distinction can be accomplished using myogenin and MYOD1, which are negative in all of the above mimickers. Alveolar, pleomorphic and epithelioid rhabdomyosarcoma subtypes need to be distinguished from malignant melanoma, which can be accomplished by application of melanocyte-specific markers that are generally negative in rhabdomyosarcoma, with the notable exception of focal S100 expression.

## Treatment and Prognosis

In accordance with the predominantly alveolar subtype, primary breast rhabdomyosarcomas are associated with poor outcomes, with an approximately 30% risk of metastasis and an overall survival of 40%. The treatment for embryonal rhabdomyosarcoma, alveolar rhabdomyosarcoma, and spindle cell rhabdomyosarcoma includes a combination of multiagent chemotherapy, surgery, and radiation therapy, whereas the treatment of adult pleomorphic rhabdomyosarcomas more often conforms to protocols used for soft tissue sarcomas. As outlined above, an accurate classification of rhabdomyosarcoma into these prognostically relevant molecular subsets has practical relevance as it determines the treatment approach and should be attempted in all cases.

## Sarcomas Metastatic to the Breast

In this section, we briefly review select soft tissue sarcomas that are encountered in the breast essentially only in metastatic setting, with an emphasis on their main differential diagnostic considerations and helpful ancillary tests. For a comprehensive review of these tumors, the reader is referred to the respective sections of dedicated soft tissue textbooks.

### Ewing Sarcoma

Classical Ewing sarcoma (ES) is a small round cell tumor occurring predominantly in the bone and soft tissue and characterized by gene fusions between members of the ETS (erythroblast transformation specific) family of genes and members of the FET (*FUS*, *EWSR1*, *TAF15*) family of genes. The most common of these is the *EWSR1-FLI1* fusion, followed by the *EWSR1-ERG* fusion. Tumors harboring identical gene fusions have been described in the head and neck literature as adamantinoma-like ES. These tumors show frequent cytokeratin and p40 expression and their relationship to classical ES remains unclear. Additionally, pathogenetically distinct small round cell tumors of the soft tissue and bone involving other gene fusions have been well characterized in recent years and include *CIC*-rearranged sarcoma, sarcoma with *BCOR* genetic alterations, and round cell sarcoma with *EWSR1*-non-ETS fusions (such as *EWSR1-NFATC2*). For a detailed discussion of these related tumors, the reader is referred to dedicated sources from the soft tissue and head and neck literature.

#### Clinical

Classical ES most frequently presents as a painful bone mass, occasionally with an associated pathological fracture, in children and young adults, in whom it represents the second most common bone sarcoma. Extraskeletal examples of ES also occur in the soft tissue and at visceral sites over a wide anatomical distribution and are more common in adult patients. Metastases are not uncommon in classical ES and rare cases have been reported in the breast.

#### Microscopic

Histologically, classical ES is characterized by sheets of uniform, oval to round tumor cells with a high nuclear-to-cytoplasmic ratio and even, finely stippled chromatin. Nuclear pleomorphism, hyperchromasia, and prominent nucleoli are not common features (Figs. 8.84 and 8.85).

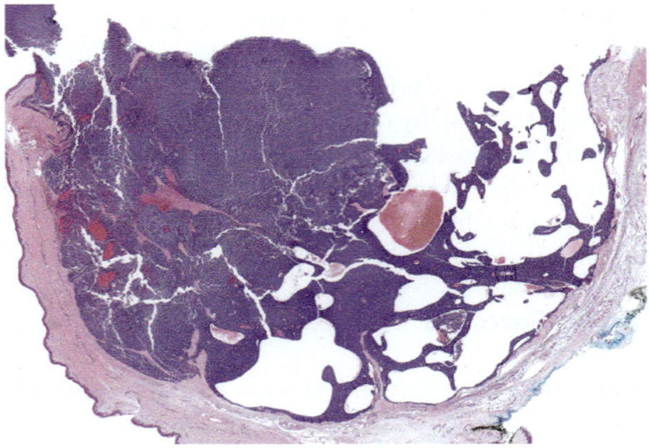

**Fig. 8.84** Extraskeletal Ewing sarcoma is a circumscribed, densely cellular basophilic neoplasm at scanning magnification

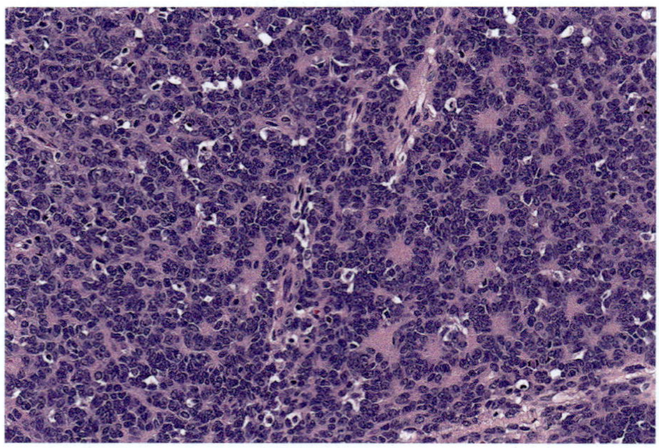

**Fig. 8.85** Extraskeletal Ewing sarcoma composed of uniform, oval to round tumor cells with a high nuclear-to-cytoplasmic ratio and even, finely stippled chromatin. The cells are growing in solid sheets or form rosette-like structures as shown here on the right-hand side

## Immunohistochemistry

Immunophenotypically, the tumor cells show a strong, membranous staining pattern for CD99, but the use of CD99 as a diagnostic marker in classical ES is no longer recommended, due to its very poor specificity. NKX2-2 has greater specificity than CD99, but expression may also be seen in tumors other than classical ES. Cytokeratins, neuroendocrine markers, and S100 may be expressed in classical ES and FLI1 and ERG may be expressed in those tumors harboring fusions involving the respective genes.

## Molecular

As classical ES can aberrantly express many of the immunohistochemical markers used in the diagnosis of these mimickers, molecular ancillary testing for the identification of one of the pathognomonic ETS-FET gene fusions either by FISH, RT-PCR, or a next-generation sarcoma fusion panel is required for a definitive diagnosis.

### Differential Diagnosis

In the adult breast, classical ES can mimic a primary or metastatic small cell neuroendocrine carcinoma, Merkel cell carcinoma,high-grade lymphoma or malignant melanoma. The accurate identification of metastatic ES is important due to disease-specific multimodal therapeutic regimens that can differ from those used in the treatment of its mimickers.

### Treatment and Prognosis

As metastasis is the main factor used for prognosticating patients with ES, its presence in the breast is likely to portend a poor outcome. A case of ES metastatic to the breast reported by Astudillo et al. was associated with aggressive tumor progression despite multimodal therapy.

## Alveolar Soft Part Sarcoma

Alveolar soft part sarcoma (ASPS) is a rare, distinctive mesenchymal neoplasm characterized by an unbalanced translocation, der (17)t(X;17)(p11;q25), which results in a *ASPSCR1-TFE3* gene fusion.

### Clinical

ASPS usually presents as a deep-seated, extremity- or urogenital tract-based mass in teenagers and young adults or as an orbital or tongue tumor in children. Because of its propensity for vascular invasion, ASPS behaves aggressively and tends to metastasize early to the brain, lungs, bone, and a variety of other sites, including the skin and breast.

### Microscopic

Histologically, ASPS is composed of large epithelioid polygonal cells arranged in nests surrounded by delicate capillary vessels (Fig. 8.86). The prototypical pseudoalveolar pattern of this neoplasm is often present due to loss of cellular cohesion

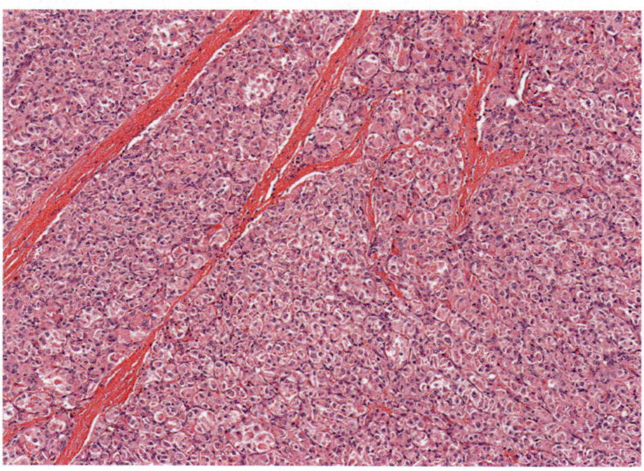

**Fig. 8.86** Alveolar soft part sarcoma composed of large, monotonous polygonal cells arranged in nests surrounded by delicate capillary vessels

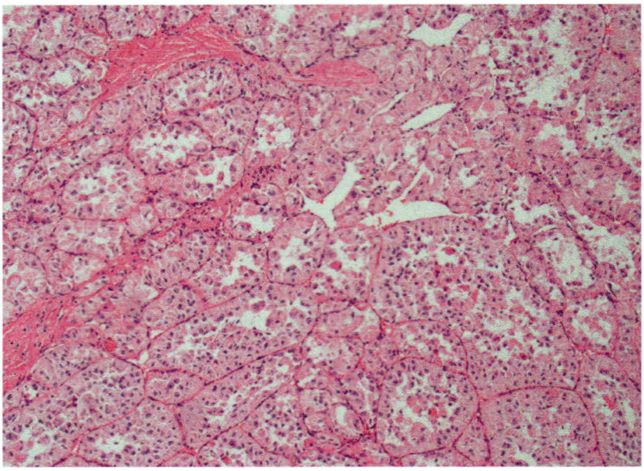

**Fig. 8.87** Alveolar soft part sarcoma showing the prototypical pseudoalveolar pattern due to loss of cellular cohesion in the center of tumor nests

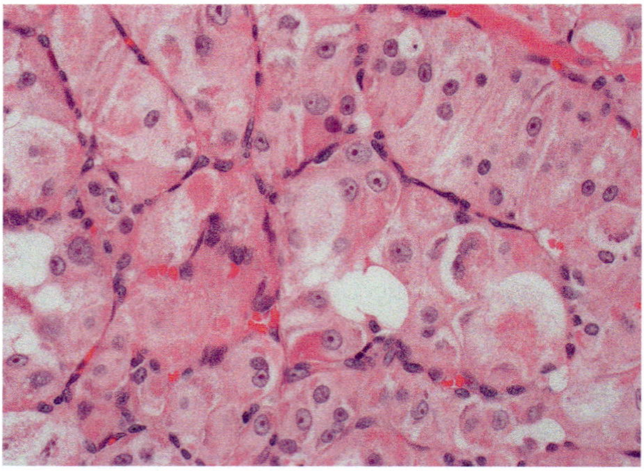

**Fig. 8.88** Alveolar soft part sarcoma composed of epithelioid cells with a large round nucleus, prominent nucleolus, and voluminous eosinophilic or clear cytoplasm containing rod- or rhomboid-shaped crystals

in the center of tumor nests (Fig. 8.87). Cytologically, the epithelioid cells are rather monotonous, with a large round nucleus, prominent nucleolus, and voluminous eosinophilic or sometimes clear cytoplasm, which often contains PAS-positive diastase-resistant rod- or rhomboid-shaped crystals (Figs. 8.88 and 8.89) composed of monocarboxylate transporter 1 (MCT1) protein or rounded precursor granules. Mitotic figures are deceptively rare, but vascular invasion is a consistent finding.

## Immunohistochemistry

Immunohistochemically, the tumor cells are positive for TFE3; the immunoprofile is otherwise completely non-specific and most lineage-based markers in ASPS are negative.

## Molecular

ASPS is characterized by an unbalanced translocation, der (17)t(X;17)(p11;q25), which results in a *ASPSCR1-TFE3* gene fusion.

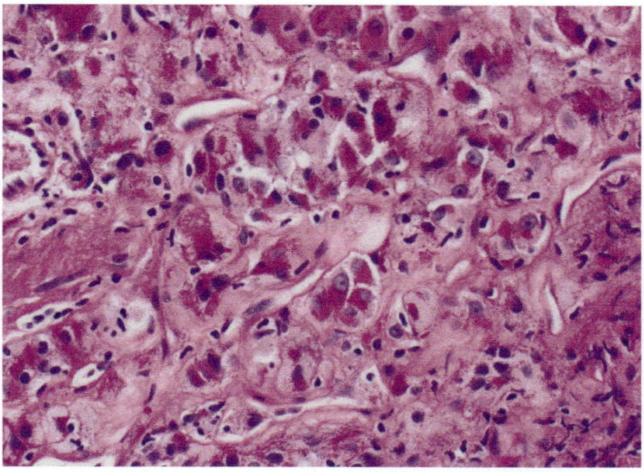

**Fig. 8.89** PAS-positive diastase-resistant rod-shaped and rhomboid crystals and precursor granules in alveolar soft part sarcoma

## Differential Diagnosis

Heightened diagnostic awareness for this entity by breast pathologists is of importance because metastatic ASPS can be mistaken for other tumors with a similar appearance, including glycogen-rich invasive breast carcinoma, PEComa, mammary granular cell tumor, or metastatic renal cell or hepatocellular carcinoma. Glycogen-rich invasive ductal carcinoma can be distinguished from ASPS by diffuse cytokeratin positivity and negative staining for TFE3. Mammary granular cell tumors (GCT) have overlapping morphologic features with ASPS, being composed of large polygonal cells with granular cytoplasm, and like ASPS, are often positive for TFE3 by IHC. GCTs typically lack alveolar architecture and PAS-D-positive crystals (although granular material may be observed) and are usually strongly, diffusely positive for S100 protein, SOX10, and inhibin, unlike ASPS. Metastatic renal cell carcinoma with eosinophilic or granular cytoplasm is another diagnostic consideration. Both tumors can look strikingly similar. This diagnostic dilemma may be resolved by application of cytokeratin Cam5.2, EMA, CAIX, or PAX8 immunostains, which are usually negative in ASPS. TFE3 immunostaining can help confirm ASPS, but caution must be exercised in younger patients since some Xp11-associated pediatric renal cell carcinomas lack expression of various cytokeratins and/or EMA and have the same *ASPSCR1-TFE3* gene fusion and will express TFE3 by immunohistochemistry. In contradistinction to ASPS this translocation is balanced. PEComas (discussed earlier in this chapter) can closely resemble ASPS and may contain PAS-D-positive cytoplasmic material. A subset of PEComas will also express TFE3 as some of them belong to the same family of Xp11 neoplasia as ASPS. But unlike ASPS, PEComas co-express melanocytic and muscle markers, such as desmin and SMA.

## Epithelioid Sarcoma

Epithelioid sarcoma (ES) is a distinctive soft tissue sarcoma with epithelioid cytomorphology and robust expression of cytokeratins. There are two types of ES: the conventional, or distal-type, with pseudogranulomatous growth pattern and a protracted clinical course, and the proximal-type, which has a predilection for proximal or axial locations, rhabdoid morphology, and more aggressive behavior. Both types are characterized by alterations in the *SMARCB1/hSNF5/INI1* gene on chromosome 22q11, which encodes a subunit of the SWI/SNF chromatin remodeling complex. Rarely, other components of the SWI/SNF complex such as *SMARCA4/BRG1* can be involved. Distal-type ES virtually never occurs in the breast and is not discussed here but proximal-type ES, while still exceptionally rare as a primary breast tumor, may be encountered in the metastatic setting or as a primary mass involving chest wall and axilla. From the breast pathology standpoint, the greatest possibility for diagnostic error in this context would be a proximal-type ES in the axilla misclassified as an axillary lymph node metastasis from an occult breast primary carcinoma. Very rare metastases of proximal-type ES to the breast parenchyma have also been reported.

### Clinical Features

Proximal-type ES typically occurs as a deep-seated, rapidly growing mass usually in the fourth decade and above and is slightly more prevalent in men. Common sites of disease include the pelvis and perineum, proximal limbs and limb girdles, axilla, as well as the head and neck region. The tumors can attain a very large size (up to 16–20 cm based on published series).

### Imaging

Proximal-type epithelioid sarcoma has not been specifically characterized by breast imaging modalities. At other sites, it is characterized by rapidly growing, FDG-avid circumscribed or multinodular neoplasm with overtly malignant imaging characteristics; the axillary and groin lesions are often interpreted as metastases of unknown primary.

## Pathologic Features

### Gross Features

Superficial or deep, ill-defined, often multinodular gray-tan fleshy mass with areas of necrosis and hemorrhage.

### Microscopic Features

Proximal-type ES is a large, subcutaneous, or deep-seated mass composed of sheets of large, overtly atypical, and mitotically active epithelioid cells with round nuclei, prominent nucleoli, and dense eosinophilic cytoplasm (Figs. 8.90 and 8.91). A frequent finding is the presence of perinuclear hyaline eosinophilic rhabdoid inclusions (Fig. 8.92). Ultrastructurally, these inclusions are composed of whorls of cytokeratin intermediate filaments.

### Immunohistochemistry

Most cases of proximal-type ES express multiple cytokeratins and EMA, but immunoreactivity for cytokeratin 5/6 is usually absent. Approximately 60% are positive

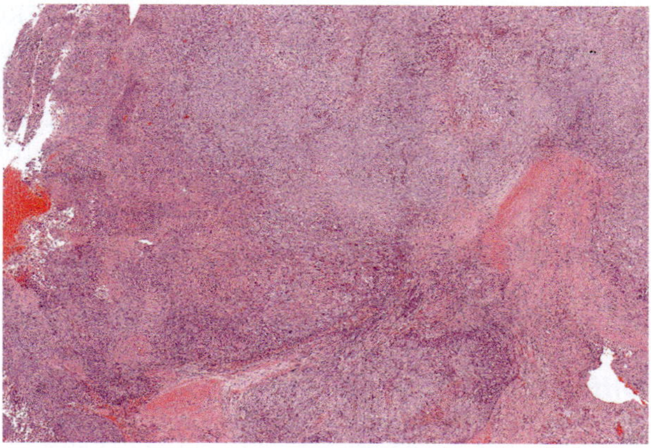

**Fig. 8.90** Proximal-type epithelioid sarcoma showing solid sheets of malignant cells and large areas of necrosis

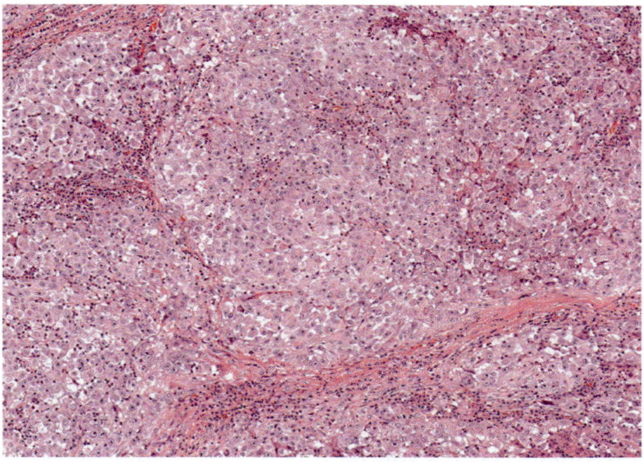

**Fig. 8.91** Proximal-type epithelioid sarcoma composed of large, overtly atypical, and mitotically active epithelioid cells with round nuclei, prominent nucleoli, and abundant eosinophilic cytoplasm

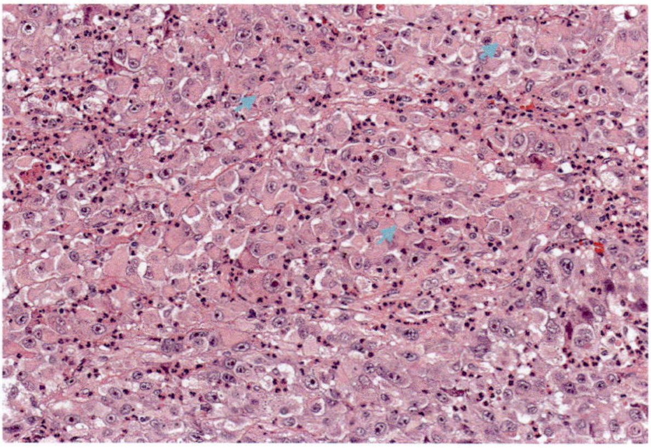

**Fig. 8.92** Eosinophilic perinuclear hyaline eosinophilic rhabdoid inclusions are often present in proximal-type epithelioid sarcoma (arrows). Ultrastructurally, these inclusions are composed of whorls of cytokeratin intermediate filaments

for CD34. Antibody clone-dependent expression of ERG may occur in up to 30% of proximal-type ES. SMA and S100 protein may be focally positive in some cases. SOX10 and estrogen and progesterone receptor expression are not expected. Inactivation of *SMARCB1/hSNF5/INI-1* gene on chromosome 22q11 results in a loss of nuclear expression of SMARCB1 (INI1) by IHC in greater than 90% of all cases. A small subset of proximal ES cases with alterations in other components of the SWI/SNF complex such as *SMARCA4* can be detected by loss of nuclear expression of BRG1. Because INI1 and BRG1 are ubiquitously expressed in normal tissues and in most neoplasms that enter the differential diagnosis in this context, loss of expression of these proteins by IHC is a very useful diagnostic tool.

## Differential Diagnosis

Proximal-type ES can closely mimic breast carcinomas with epithelioid to rhabdoid morphology, including invasive pleomorphic lobular carcinoma, matrix-producing metaplastic breast carcinomas, and high-grade breast carcinoma with apocrine features. The frequent presence of lobular carcinoma in situ in cases of invasive pleomorphic lobular breast carcinoma, together with its consistent nuclear immunoreactivity for GATA3 and retained nuclear expression of INI1 (as well as other components of the SWI/SNF complex), makes this distinction straightforward. Matrix-producing metaplastic carcinoma and high-grade breast carcinomas with apocrine features also retain INI1 and BRG1 expression. All of the above breast carcinomas are typically negative for CD34.

In terms of primary soft tissue sarcomas, epithelioid angiosarcoma of the breast, which may occur both in the primary and – more frequently – in the post-radiation setting, often has a solid growth pattern like proximal-type ES and may express cytokeratins and CD34. These two neoplasms can look astonishingly similar (Figs. 8.93 and 8.94). However, epithelioid angiosarcoma consistently expresses additional vascular markers (particularly ERG and CD31) and retains nuclear INI1 and BRG1 expression. As mentioned above, ERG expression in up to 30% of proximal-type ES can be a diagnostic pitfall in this setting. Epithelioid MPNST

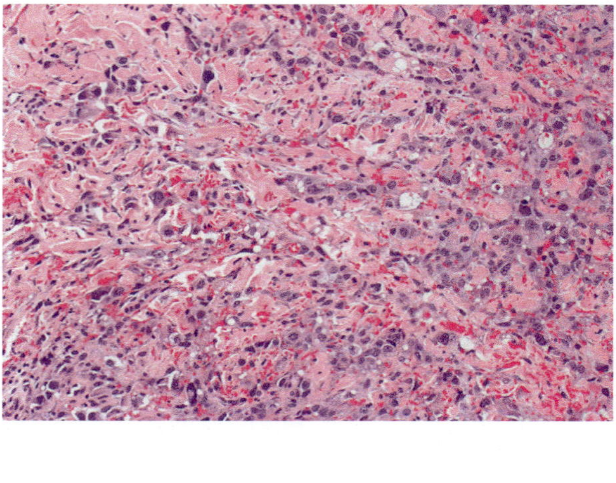

**Fig. 8.93** Proximal-type epithelioid sarcoma with a pseudoangiomatous growth pattern in a hemorrhagic background, closely mimicking epithelioid angiosarcoma

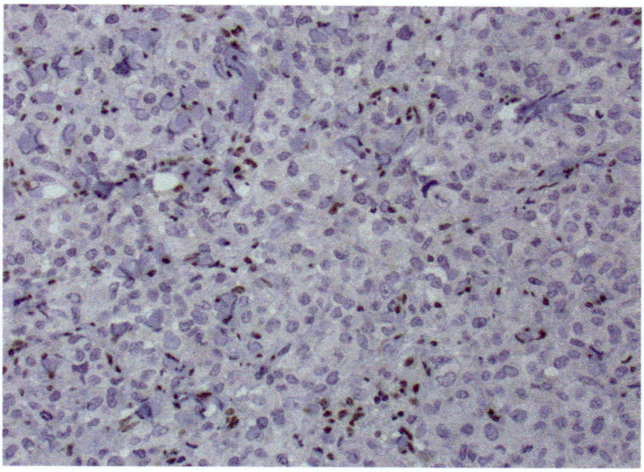

**Fig. 8.94** Most proximal-type epithelioid sarcomas show loss of nuclear expression of INI1, while internal background tissue retains expression (shown here in a case represented in Fig. 8.93)

does have considerable morphologic and immunophenotypic overlap with proximal-type ES, including loss of INI1 expression (70% of cases for epithelioid MPNST); however, epithelioid MPNST is also strongly and diffusely positive for S100 by IHC and is usually negative for cytokeratins. Perhaps the most difficult soft tissue tumor in the differential diagnosis is myoepithelial carcinoma (malignant myoepithelioma), due to its propensity to show proximal-type ES-like morphology, with concurrent cytokeratin expression and INI1 loss (the latter in approximately 50% of cases). Nevertheless, unlike proximal-type ES, myoepithelial carcinomas typically also express markers of myoepithelial differentiation such as p63, SMA, GFAP, S100, and SOX10 and are negative for CD34. A commercial next-generation sequencing assay targeting various sarcoma fusions may be of significant diagnostic value in separating myoepithelial carcinomas from both breast carcinoma and proximal-type ES as most myoepithelial carcinomas are associated with gene rearrangements, the most common being *EWSR1* (approximately 80% of cases). Myoepithelial carcinomas are discussed below.

Malignant melanoma can be distinguished from proximal-type ES by the expression of melanocytic markers, lack of cytokeratin and CD34 expression, retained INI1 and BRG1 expression, and the presence of *BRAF* mutations, which are not typical of proximal-type ES.

## Treatment and Prognosis

Proximal-type ES behaves aggressively with rapid progression, lymph node metastasis, and early systemic metastasis in up to 60% of cases. The reported median overall 5-year and 10-year survival rates are 57% and 37%, respectively. The treatment of choice for proximal-type ES is radical excision; adjuvant radiotherapy and anthracycline and gemcitabine-based chemotherapy regimens have been used with some success. While proximal-type ES can metastasize to lymph nodes, the benefit of lymph node dissection or sentinel lymph node biopsy in epithelioid sarcoma remains uncertain.

## Myoepithelial Tumors of the Breast

### Introduction

Myoepithelial neoplasms represent a morphologically and genetically diverse family of tumors characterized by histologic, immunophenotypic, and ultrastructural features of epithelial and smooth muscle/myoid differentiation. Myoepithelial tumors have a broad anatomic distribution including skin, soft tissue, viscera, salivary glands, bone, and breast. Several types of tumors with myoepithelial differentiation can occur in or around the breast. Primary mixed tumors occurring in the breast parenchyma are histologically analogous to the mixed tumors (pleomorphic adenomas) of the salivary gland and also often show the same *PLAG1* and *HGMA2* gene rearrangements as their salivary gland counterparts. Cutaneous mixed tumors (chondroid syringomas), like primary mixed tumors of the breast, are also morphologically and molecularly analogous to salivary pleomorphic adenomas. Myoepithelial tumors may arise in the soft tissue of the breast region in the form of myoepitheliomas and myoepithelial carcinomas of the soft parts. These tumors typically lack *PLAG1* rearrangements and frequently harbor *EWSR1* rearrangements.

Cutaneous syncytial myoepithelioma is a distinctive subtype with a predilection for intraepidermal growth and *EWSR1-PBX3* fusion that set them apart from other myoepithelial tumors. These tumors have a predilection for the skin of the upper and lower extremities or head and neck, but trunk or chest wall skin can also be involved. Recently, analogous tumors were reported in osseous and deep soft tissue locations. Syncytial myoepitheliomas have not yet been reported in the breast skin, but nonetheless are briefly discussed here to raise awareness of this distinctive appearing and somewhat underrecognized neoplasm.

### Clinical Features

Primary mammary mixed tumors present as a nodule 1–2 cm in size and are most common in adult women, while male cases are rare. Cutaneous mixed tumors (chondroid syringomas) occur in the dermis and subcutis, usually as small (<5 cm), firm, and painless nodules or papules. These tumors usually affect adults, without a gender predilection. Syncytial myoepitheliomas usually present as small (median, 0.8 cm), painless polypoid nodules and are slightly more common in males. Myoepitheliomas and myoepithelial carcinomas usually present as non-tender palpable subcutaneous masses over a broad age range without a sex predilection and are relatively common in pediatric patients in whom they are frequently malignant (nearly half of pediatric cases).

### Imaging

Primary mammary mixed tumors have a radiologic appearance similar to that of fibroadenomas, with a rounded configuration and a well-defined lesional border. If growing within the lumen of a duct, mammary mixed tumors may mimic a cystic lesion. Calcifications can raise suspicion for a malignant tumor. Cutaneous mixed tumors and syncytial myoepitheliomas, being located in the skin, are unlikely to be imaged. Imaging information on myoepithelial tumors of the soft parts is very limited.

## Pathologic Features

### Gross features

Mammary and cutaneous mixed tumors are solid, firm, and well-defined lesions grossly resembling their salivary gland counterparts, with glistening, gelatinous cut surfaces. Mammary mixed tumors typically measure 1–2 cm in size and cutaneous mixed tumors range in size from 0.5–3 cm. Syncytial myoepitheliomas are well-circumscribed but unencapsulated dermal tumors that often abut the overlying epidermis. They are typically less than 3 cm in size (median 0.8 cm). Myoepithelial tumors of the soft tissue may be either circumscribed (in the case of myoepitheliomas) or more infiltrative (in the case of myoepithelial carcinomas) with a cut surface that ranges from a gelatinous pleomorphic adenoma-like appearance to a fleshy sarcoma-like appearance. Tumor sizes vary widely from 1 to 20 cm (mean 4–6 cm) and myoepithelial carcinomas are typically larger than myoepitheliomas.

### Microscopic features

Both mammary and cutaneous mixed tumors, being closely related, have a very similar histologic appearance. Both tumors are well-circumscribed, typically unencapsulated nodules. Like their salivary gland counterparts, however, these mixed tumors may have an infiltrative growth pattern with satellite nodules. The mixed tumors are, by definition, biphasic in that they are composed of both tubuloductal structures and myoepithelial cells, the latter of which are epithelioid, spindled, or plasmacytoid cells arranged in sheets, cords, or nests within a myxoid to hyaline stroma. Heterologous differentiation is often present, usually in the form of hyaline cartilage or bone. Cytologically, the cells have bland oval nuclei, inconspicuous nucleoli, and eosinophilic, amphophilic, or clear cytoplasm (Figs. 8.95, 8.96, and 8.97). Cytologic atypia and pleomorphism are usually not seen in either mammary or cutaneous mixed tumors. In cutaneous examples, squamous metaplasia and folliculosebaceous differentiation may occur (Fig. 8.98).

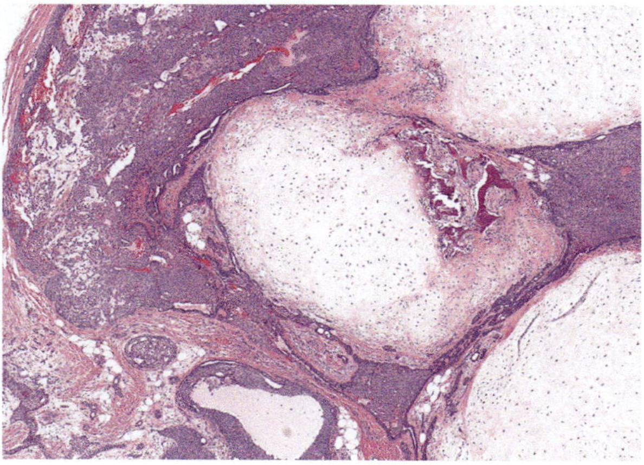

**Fig. 8.95** Mixed tumor showing sheets of myoepithelial cells and ductal structures in a myxohyaline stroma containing heterologous cartilaginous and osseous differentiation

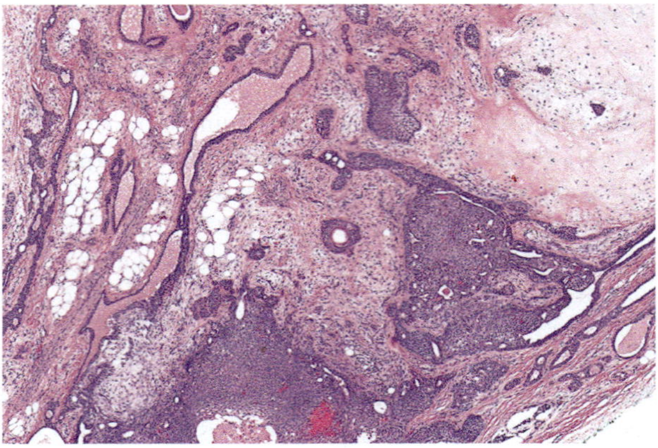

**Fig. 8.96** Architecturally diverse tubuloductal differentiation in mixed tumor

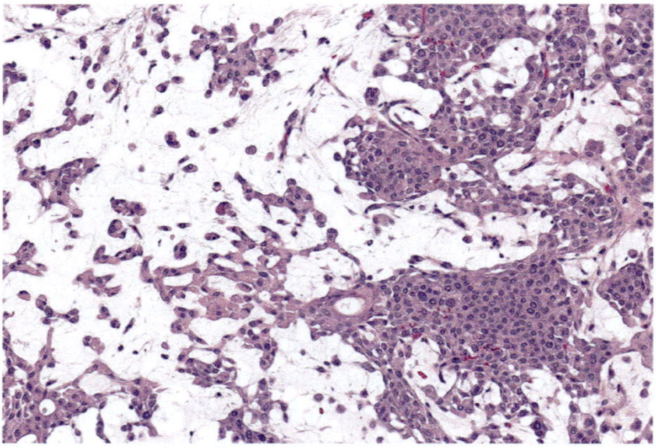

**Fig. 8.97** The ductal and the myoepithelial cells in mixed tumors have bland oval nuclei, inconspicuous nucleoli, and eosinophilic cytoplasm

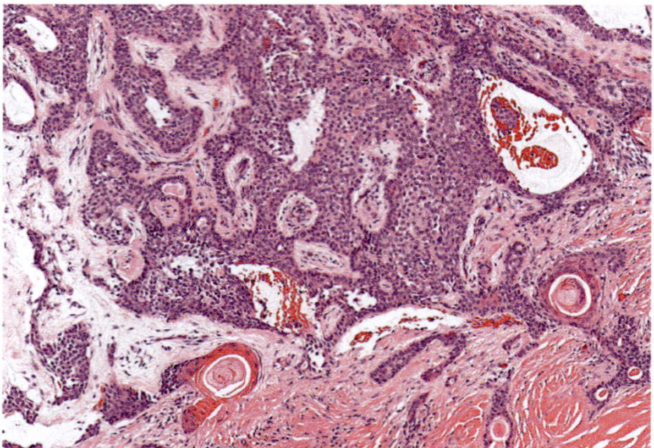

**Fig. 8.98** Cutaneous mixed tumor with tubuloductal differentiation, chondroid areas, and squamous metaplasia

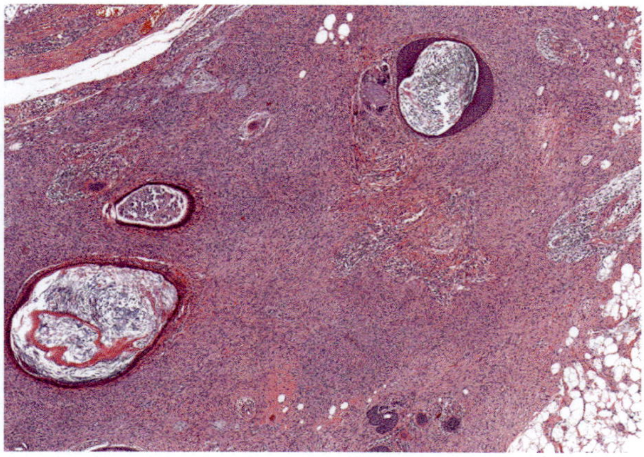

**Fig. 8.99** Syncytial myoepithelioma: a dermal-based neoplasm showing a solid growth at low power, with entrapment of adnexal structures

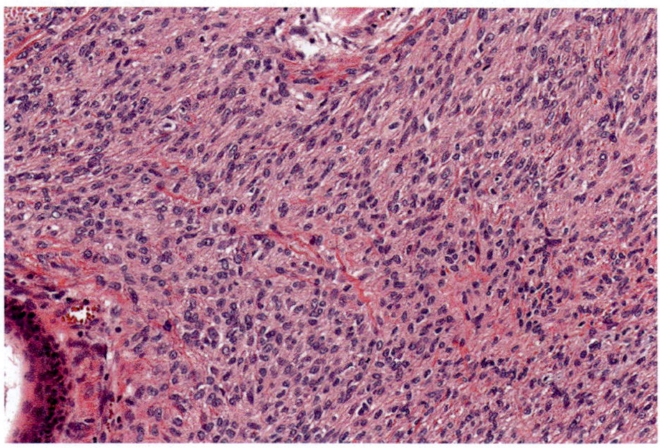

**Fig. 8.100** Syncytial myoepithelioma composed of cytologically banal spindled to histiocytoid cells with oval nuclei and eosinophilic cytoplasm with indistinct cell borders, imparting a syncytial appearance

Syncytial myoepitheliomas are relatively well-circumscribed, unencapsulated nodules usually centered in the dermis and abutting the overlying epidermis, and may show subcutaneous extension. They are composed of solid sheets of spindled, epithelioid, or histiocytoid cells with oval nuclei and eosinophilic cytoplasm without distinct cell borders, imparting a distinctive syncytial appearance at low power. There is no tubuloductal differentiation, though some cases may show entrapped epithelial structures (Fig. 8.99). At high power, the cells have cytologically banal oval nuclei with vesicular chromatin and a slightly granular quality to the cytoplasm, imparting an appearance similar to histiocytes (Fig. 8.100). Multinucleated cells can be noted focally. Mitotic figures are uncommon, and there is no necrosis or vascular invasion. In contrast to other myoepithelial tumors, syncytial myoepitheliomas have very little or no associated myxoid or hyaline stroma. However, wispy collagen fibers and small myxoid islands may be seen, and a third of cases shows chondro-osseous or adipocytic metaplasia (Fig. 8.101). Recognition of adipocytic

**Fig. 8.101** Syncytial myoepithelioma showing adipocytic metaplasia and small myxoid islands

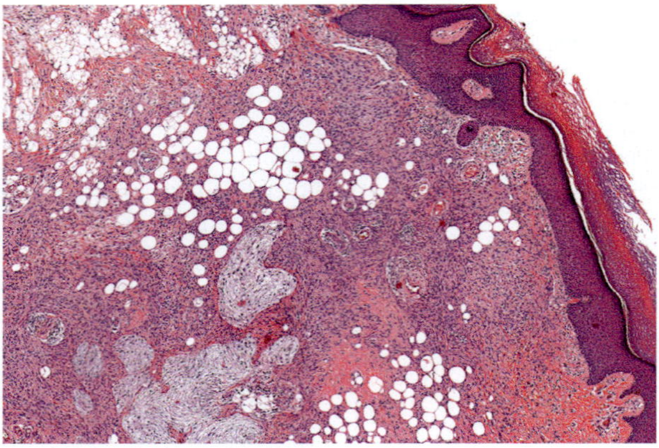

**Fig. 8.102** Syncytial myoepithelioma with lymphoid aggregates at the tumor periphery

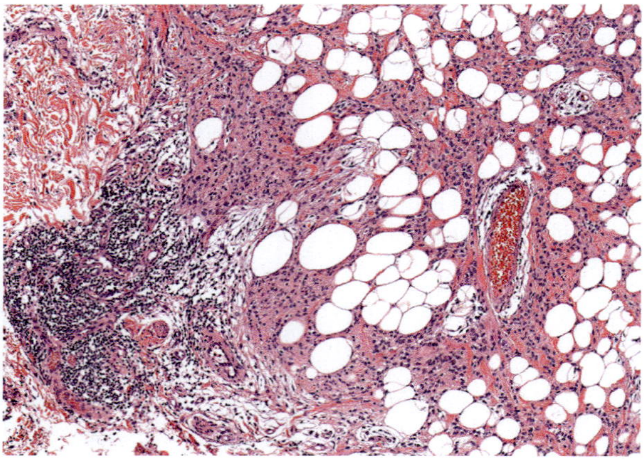

metaplasia and epithelial entrapment in these tumors is important, as these features can be misinterpreted as infiltrative growth, giving the impression of a more aggressive neoplasm. Prominent lymphoid aggregates may be seen, usually at the tumor periphery (Fig. 8.102).

Myoepitheliomas and myoepithelial carcinomas are multilobulated, often infiltrative masses, which are morphologically very heterogeneous. They are typically composed of epithelioid to plasmacytoid to spindled cells arranged in a variety of growth patterns including reticular, trabecular, nested, corded, fascicular, or solid patterns (Figs. 8.103, 8.104, 8.105, and 8.106). The stroma is myxoid, collagenous/hyalinized, or chondroid (Figs. 8.107 and 8.108). Multiple growth patterns are often seen within the same tumor, but in some cases a single pattern predominates. Heterologous differentiation in the form of cartilage, bone, and squamous or adipocytic metaplasia is also often seen in myoepitheliomas, but ductal differentiation is absent. Cytologically, the cells have eosinophilic to amphophilic to clear cytoplasm and round to ovoid, uniform nuclei with inconspicuous or small nucleoli. Cases showing epithelioid cells with voluminous cytoplasm with vacuolization and abundant myxoid stroma used to be referred to as "parachordomas." Myoepitheliomas do not have significant cytologic atypia. Normal mitotic figures may be observed.

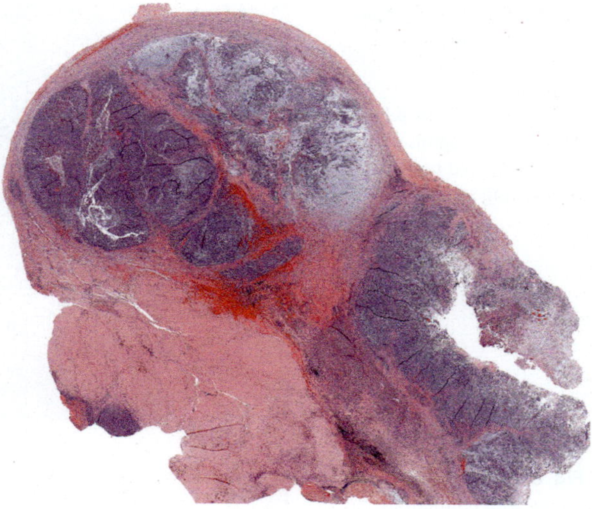

**Fig. 8.103** Myoepithelial carcinoma showing a multilobulated infiltrative growth pattern at low power; myxoid stroma can be readily appreciated

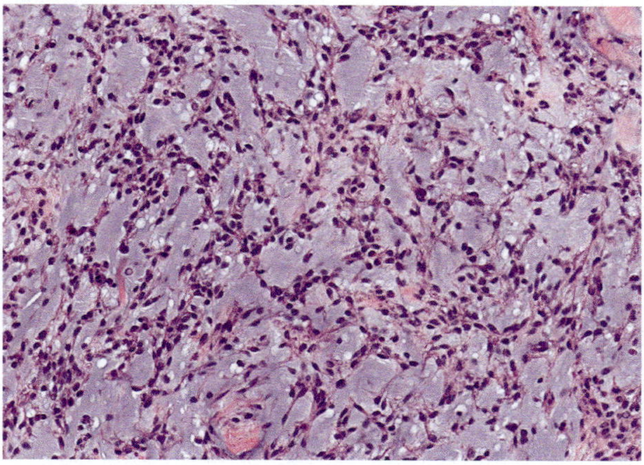

**Fig. 8.104** Myoepithelial tumor with a reticular growth pattern in a myxoid background

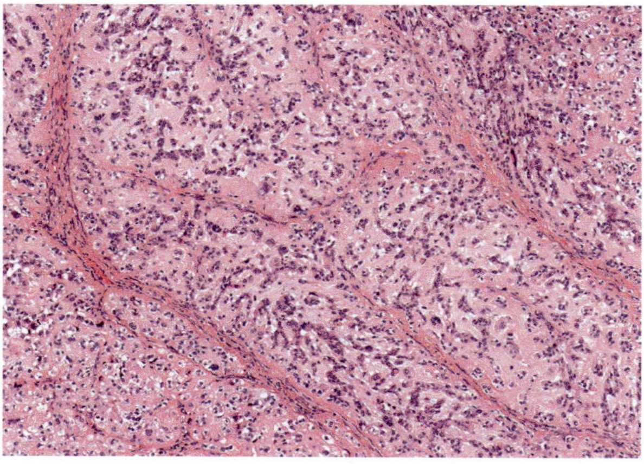

**Fig. 8.105** Myoepithelial tumor with nested and corded growth patterns in a hyalinized stroma

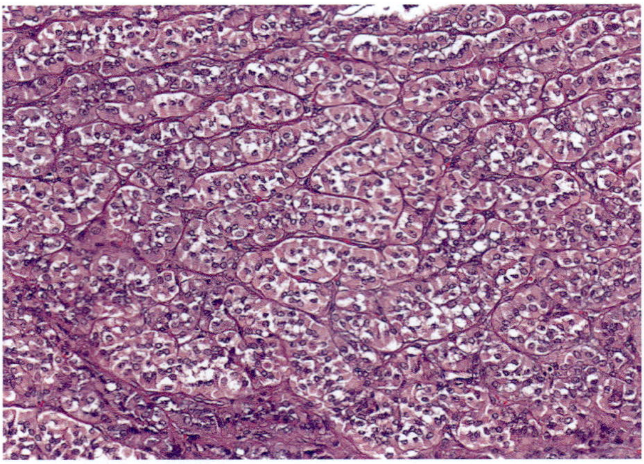

**Fig. 8.106** Myoepithelial tumor composed of uniform nests of plasmacytoid myoepithelial cells with densely eosinophilic cytoplasm, and minimal intervening stroma

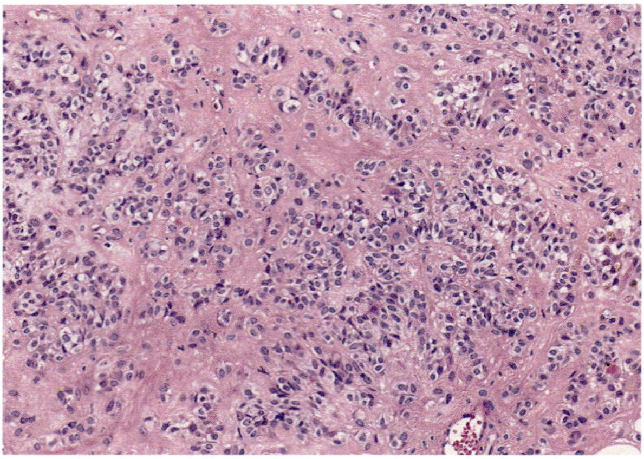

**Fig. 8.107** Myoepithelial tumor with epithelioid myoepithelial cells arranged singly or in small nests in a collagenized stroma. The cells have round to ovoid, uniform nuclei with inconspicuous nucleoli, and no atypia

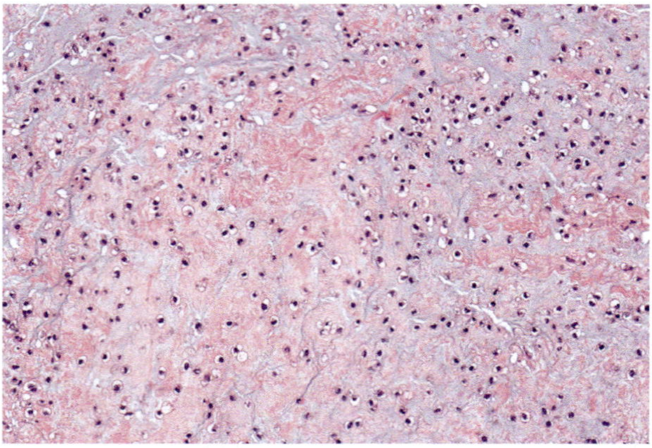

**Fig. 8.108** Myoepithelial tumor composed of myoepithelial cells with clear cytoplasm dispersed within a chondroid background

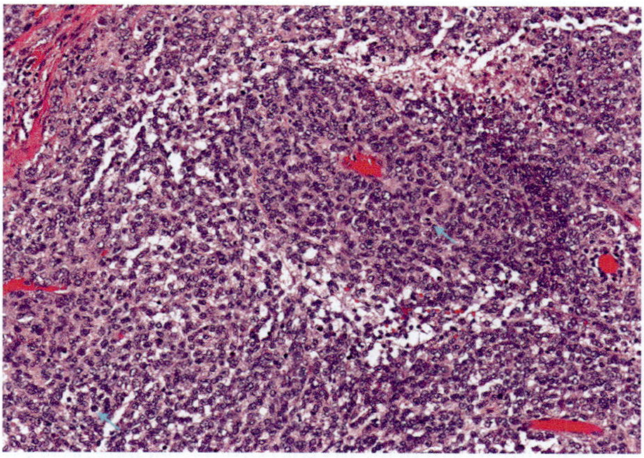

**Fig. 8.109** Malignant myoepithelial tumor (myoepithelial carcinoma) with diffuse nuclear atypia and mitotic figures (arrows)

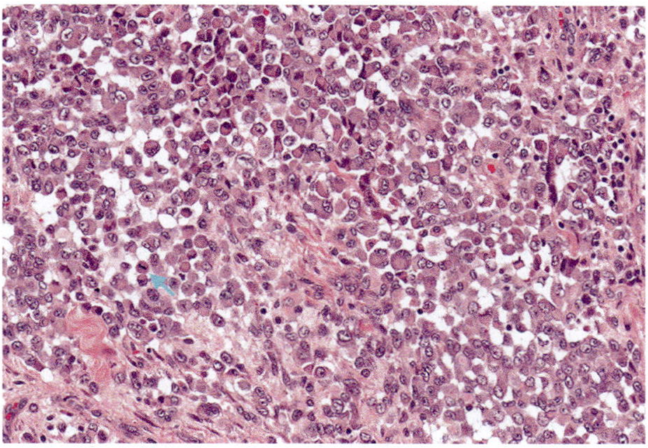

**Fig. 8.110** Another example of myoepithelial carcinoma with rhabdoid features, overt nuclear atypia, and mitotic figures (arrows)

Myoepithelial carcinomas (malignant myoepithelial tumors) have cytoarchitectural features similar to those of myoepitheliomas, but demonstrate morphologic features of malignancy, including nuclear atypia with coarse chromatin, prominent nucleoli or nuclear pleomorphism, increased mitotic activity, atypical mitotic figures, necrosis, and vascular invasion. However, myoepithelial carcinomas are defined largely by their significant nuclear atypia, as this feature most strongly correlates with aggressive behavior (Figs. 8.109 and 8.110). Myoepithelial carcinomas could be further classified as low-, intermediate-, and high-grade based on the degree of nuclear atypia present, but the nuclear grade does not correlate well with behavior. Likewise, necrosis, vascular invasion, frequent mitotic figures, and atypical mitotic figures are more often seen in myoepithelial carcinomas, but these features are not used as criteria for malignancy.

## Immunohistochemistry

By immunohistochemistry, mammary mixed tumors, cutaneous mixed tumors, myoepitheliomas, and myoepithelial carcinomas consistently co-express cytokeratins, EMA, and S100 protein. SOX10, another robust marker of myoepithelial differentiation, can be seen in approximately 80% of mixed tumors and myoepitheliomas, but only in 30% of myoepithelial carcinomas. Expression of other myoepthelial markers such as p63, SMA, GFAP, and calponin is variable. SMARCB1/INI1 loss has been identified by immunohistochemistry in approximately 50% of myoepithelial carcinomas, especially in pediatric myoepithelial carcinomas with rhabdoid morphology.

The cytokeratin and the myoepithelial marker co-expression is an important prerequisite for the diagnosis of myoepithelial tumors as many gene fusion-driven mesenchymal neoplasms, including the OFMT discussed earlier in this chapter, have the "myoepithelial-like" growth pattern with cords and sheets of uniform spindle to epithelioid cells distributed in the myxoid stroma, but they do not represent myoepithelial tumors.

The immunoprofile of syncytial myoepitheliomas is somewhat different. These tumors frequently express EMA, usually diffusely, and S100 protein, which can be either diffuse or focal. Other myoepithelial markers like SOX10, p63, GFAP, and calponin are variably positive. In contrast to other myoepithelial tumors, cytokeratin expression is uncommon (approximately 10%) and is rarely diffuse. The INI1 expression pattern is uncertain.

## Molecular

At the molecular level, both mammary and cutaneous mixed tumors often have *PLAG1* and *HMGA2* gene rearrangements analogous to the mixed tumors of the salivary gland and can show nuclear staining for PLAG1 by immunohistochemistry. Conversely, recurrent *EWSR1-PBX3* gene fusions have been identified in syncytial myoepitheliomas. *EWSR1* and, less often, *FUS* gene rearrangements are also found in approximately 80% of myoepithelial tumors of soft tissue and are more common in myoepithelial carcinomas. *PLAG1* gene rearrangements are usually negative in myoepithelial tumors that lack ductal differentiation, and it appears that *PLAG1*, *EWSR1*, and *FUS* rearrangements are mutually exclusive. A variety of fusion partners have been identified in *EWSR1*-rearranged myoepithelial tumors including *PBX1* and *POU5F1* (most common), *PBX3*, *ZNF444*, *ATF1*, *KLF-15* and *KLF-17*. The latter can also be seen in *FUS*-rearranged cases. Most recent data suggests that these fusions may correlate with different phenotypes. *EWSR1-POU5F1* fusion in deep soft tissue myoepithelial tumors is associated with young patient age, malignant behavior, nested growth pattern and a distinctive clear cell morphology, whereas *PBX1* and *PBX3* translocations are seen in predominantly benign spindle cell examples with sclerotic stroma or bland fascicular growth, including cutaneous syncytial myoepithelioma; *FUS-KLF17* fusions are observed in tumors with trabecular growth of bland epithelioid cells in an abundant myxoid or myxohyaline stroma resembling chordoma (formerly referred to as "parachordoma").

## Differential Diagnosis

The most pertinent differential diagnostic consideration for myoepithelial tumors arising in and around the breast is matrix-producing metaplastic breast carcinoma.

Matrix-producing metaplastic breast carcinomas can have a partial myoepithelial profile, including SOX10 expression, and can show considerable morphologic and immunophenotypic overlap with all of the above-described myoepithelial tumors (Figs. 8.111, 8.112, and 8.113). However, unlike in these tumors,

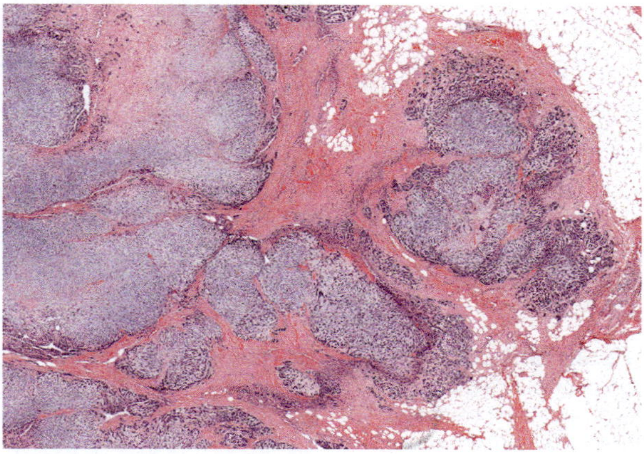

**Fig. 8.111** Matrix-producing metaplastic breast carcinoma showing multinodular configuration and a prominent myxoid stroma, which can be appreciated at scanning magnification

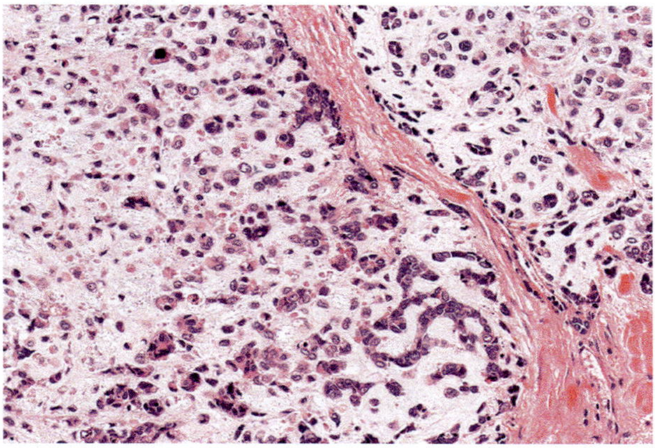

**Fig. 8.112** Matrix-producing metaplastic breast carcinoma composed of atypical epithelioid to plasmacytoid cells arranged in nests, cords, or singly in a myxoid stroma and showing a considerable morphologic overlap with primary myoepithelial carcinoma of soft tissue

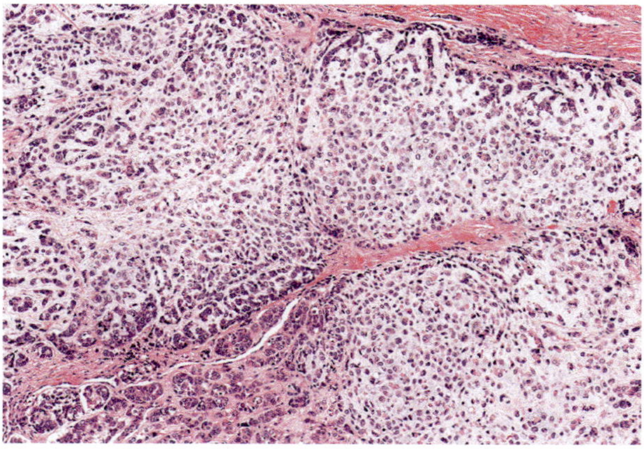

**Fig. 8.113** The presence of the conventional infiltrating breast carcinoma component (bottom left) helps to distinguish matrix-producing metaplastic breast carcinoma from myoepithelial carcinoma

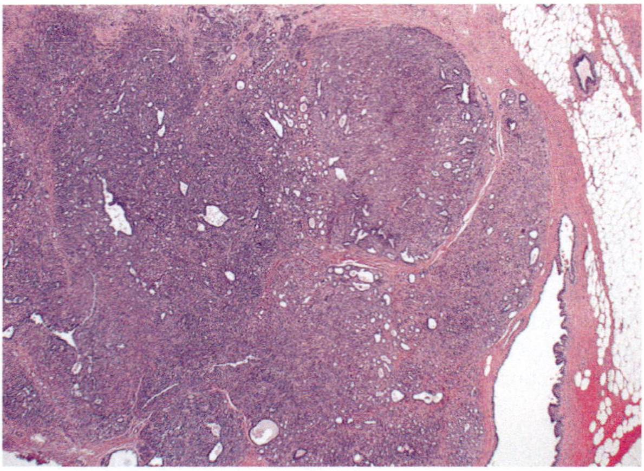

**Fig. 8.114** Breast adenomyoepithelioma: a mildly infiltrative multilobulated neoplasm with a biphasic appearance at scanning magnification

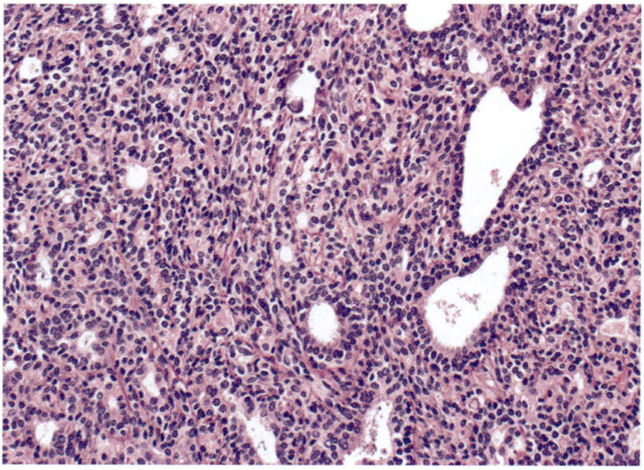

**Fig. 8.115** Breast adenomyoepithelioma: a biphasic lesion composed of glandular structures lined by epithelial cells and surrounded by outer myoepithelial cells

rearrangements in *PLAG1*, *EWSR1*, and *FUS* are not present in matrix-producing metaplastic breast carcinomas. Conversely, the presence of ductal carcinoma in situ (DCIS) would strongly support a diagnosis of matrix-producing metaplastic breast carcinoma.

Adenomyoepitheliomas are another differential diagnostic consideration for primary myoepithelial tumors of the breast. Adenomyoepitheliomas, like both mammary and cutaneous mixed tumors, are biphasic tumors with low recurrent potential composed of both ductal and myoepithelial components (Figs. 8.114, 8.115, and 8.116). In some of these tumors, the myoepithelial component, which may be either epithelioid or spindled in morphology and which has a complete myoepithelial immunoprofile, may predominate. In such cases, the distinction from a primary myoepithelial tumor of soft tissue may be quite challenging. Likewise, malignant adenomyoepithelioma with the malignant myoepithelial component is

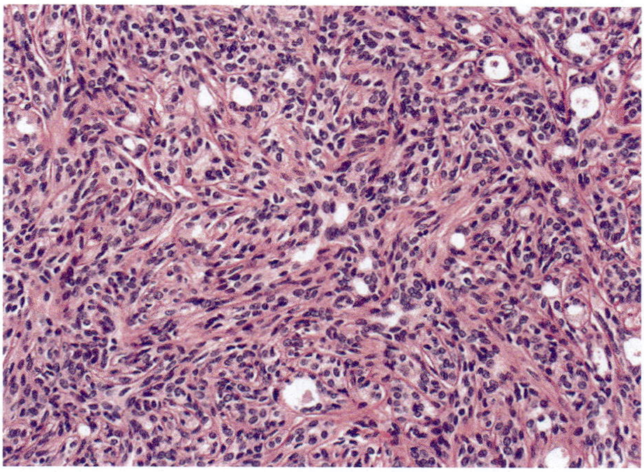

**Fig. 8.116** The myoepithelial cells in adenomyoepithelioma often predominate and can acquire a spindled or an epithelioid configuration

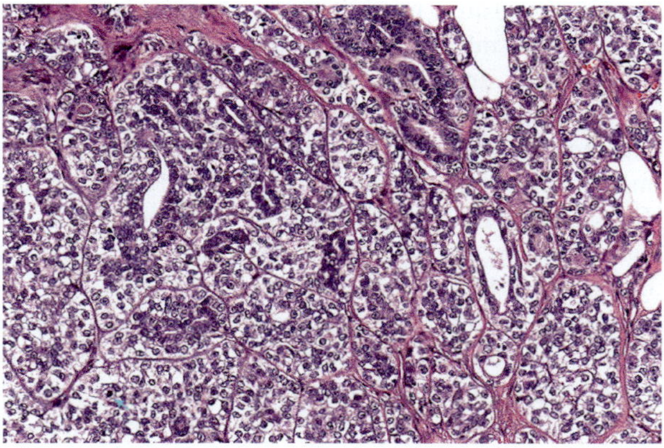

**Fig. 8.117** Malignant adenomyoepithelioma with the malignant component represented by epithelioid myoepithelial cells with diffuse cytologic atypia

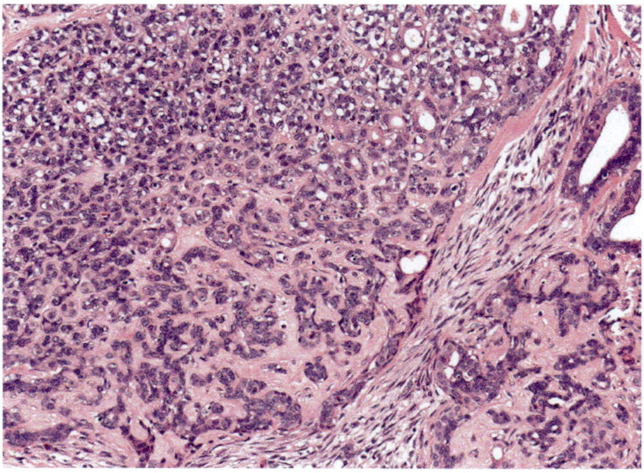

**Fig. 8.118** Malignant adenomyoepithelioma with sclerotic collagenous matrix and nested and corded appearance of the lesional cells resembling primary myoepithelial carcinoma

characterized by diffuse cytologic atypia in the myoepithelial cells; such tumors can closely resemble myoepithelial carcinoma (Figs. 8.117 and 8.118). Of note, *PLAG1*, *HGMA2*, *EWSR1*, and *FUS* rearrangements have not been described in adenomyoepitheliomas, which instead show *PIK3CA*, *AKT1* (in ER-positive cases), and *HRAS* Q61R/K hotspot mutations (in ER-negative cases).

Proximal-type epithelioid sarcoma is a differential diagnostic consideration especially in myoepithelial carcinomas arising in the soft tissue in the vicinity of the axilla. Similar to myoepithelial tumors, proximal-type epithelioid sarcomas are positive for cytokeratins and may show loss of INI1 expression. However, unlike myoepithelial tumors, proximal-type epithelioid sarcomas are typically negative for S100, SOX10, and myogenic markers and lack gene rearrangements in *PLAG1*, *EWSR1*, and *FUS*. Malignant melanomas may also enter the differential diagnosis with myoepithelial carcinomas. The immunoreactivity for SOX10, S100, and p63 in both tumor types can complicate their distinction. However, with the exception of dedifferentiated cases of malignant melanoma, diffuse cytokeratin expression is very rare in melanomas. Additionally, HMB45 and Melan-A, both of which are frequently positive in malignant melanomas, are negative in myoepithelial tumors.

Syncytial myoepitheliomas may pose a diagnostic challenge as they differ morphologically and immunophenotypically from classic myoepithelial tumors and most closely resemble cutaneous lesions. Melanocytic neoplasms, such as nevoid melanomas, can be distinguished based on the expression of melanosome-based melanocytic markers such as HMB45 and Melan-A and, in difficult cases, FISH for *EWSR1* gene rearrangement or RT-PCR for the *EWSR1-PBX3* gene fusion. On the benign end of the spectrum, fibrohistiocytic tumors with epithelioid morphology like epithelioid fibrous histiocytoma (EFH), cellular neurothekeoma, and juvenile xanthogranuloma can resemble syncytial myoepithelioma. EFH usually presents as a well-circumscribed dermal nodule with an epidermal collarette, is composed of cytologically bland epithelioid or plasmacytoid cells with frequent binucleation, and can be positive for EMA. However, EFH lacks a distinctive syncytial growth pattern; rather, the cells are dispersed in a prominent collagenous stroma containing variable vessels. Adipocytic metaplasia is not characteristic of EFH. Immunohistochemistry is helpful as most EFHs show strong diffuse staining with Factor XIIIa and ALK and are consistently negative for S100 protein and other myoepithelial markers. Cellular neurothekeoma has histiocytoid cells that are arranged in a distinctive nodular or plexiform growth pattern separated by fibrous bands rather than forming syncytia; lacks S100 protein, EMA, and other myoepithelial marker expression; and does not have an *EWSR1* gene rearrangement. Juvenile xanthogranulomas might arguably resemble syncytial myoepithelioma if they lack Touton-type giant cells, foamy histiocytes, and inflammatory cells, but these tumors are usually more polymorphous in appearance compared to syncytial myoepithelioma and frequently contain inflammatory cells, such as eosinophils. They are negative for S100 protein, EMA, and myoepithelial markers.

## Treatment and Prognosis

Both mammary and cutaneous mixed tumors behave in an indolent fashion, but may recur locally, particularly when incompletely excised. Accordingly, complete excision is recommended for these tumors. Syncytial myoepitheliomas are benign and only rarely recur if incompletely excised. Simple conservative excision is usually curative in most cases. To date, metastatic examples have not been reported. Myoepitheliomas of soft tissue rarely metastasize, but may recur in 20% of cases; thus, surgical resection is required. Conversely, myoepithelial carcinomas of soft tissue behave more aggressively, with a recurrence rate of approximately 40% and a risk of systemic metastasis ranging from 30% to 50%, and are best treated by a multidisciplinary sarcoma team.

Surgical resection remains the mainstay of therapy of myoepithelial carcinoma, but responses to chemotherapy have been documented. Metastatic sites include lungs, lymph nodes, and soft tissues. As mentioned above, myoepithelial carcinomas of soft parts are defined based on the presence of cytologic atypia but nuclear grade does not appear to correlate well with the biologic behavior of these tumors. Instead, different fusion types in these tumors may correlate with distinct histologic phenotypes and behavior.

## Selected References


1. Adem C, Reynolds C, Ingle JN, Nascimento AG. Primary breast sarcoma: clinicopathologic series from the Mayo Clinic and review of the literature. Br J Cancer. 2004;91(2):237–41. PMID: 15187996.
2. Agaram NP, LaQuaglia MP, Alaggio R, Zhang L, Fujisawa Y, Ladanyi M, Wexler LH, Antonescu CR. MYOD1-mutant spindle cell and sclerosing rhabdomyosarcoma: an aggressive subtype irrespective of age. A reappraisal for molecular classification and risk stratification. Mod Pathol. 2019;32(1):27–36. PMID: 30181563.
3. Agaram NP, Sung YS, Zhang L, Chen CL, Chen HW, Singer S, Dickson MA, Berger MF, Antonescu CR. Dichotomy of genetic abnormalities in PEComas with therapeutic implications. Am J Surg Pathol. 2015;39(6):813–25. PMID: 25651471.
4. Alaggio R, Zhang L, Sung YS, Huang SC, Chen CL, Bisogno G, Zin A, Agaram NP, LaQuaglia MP, Wexler LH, Antonescu CR. A molecular study of pediatric spindle and sclerosing rhabdomyosarcoma: identification of novel and recurrent VGLL2-related fusions in infantile cases. Am J Surg Pathol. 2016;40(2):224–35. PMID: 26501226.
5. Alomari AK, Brown N, Andea AA, Betz BL, Patel RM. Cutaneous syncytial myoepithelioma: a recently described neoplasm which may mimic nevoid melanoma and epithelioid sarcoma. J Cutan Pathol. 2017;44(10):892.
6. Aneiros-Fernandez J, Antonio Retamero J, Husein-Elahmed H, Ovalle F, Aneiros-Cachaza J. Primary cutaneous and subcutaneous leiomyosarcomas: evolution and prognostic factors. Eur J Dermatol. 2016;26(1):9–12.
7. Antonescu CR, Sung YS, Chen CL, et al. Novel ZC3H7B-BCOR, MEAF6-PHF1, and EPC1-PHF1 fusions in ossifying fibromyxoid tumors--molecular characterization shows genetic overlap with endometrial stromal sarcoma. Genes Chromosomes Cancer. 2014;53(2):183.
8. Antonescu CR, Zhang L, Chang NE, et al. EWSR1-POU5F1 fusion in soft tissue myoepithelial tumors. A molecular analysis of sixty-six cases, including soft tissue, bone, and visceral lesions, showing common involvement of the EWSR1 gene. Genes Chromosom Cancer. 2010;49(12):1114.
9. Antonescu CR, Zhang L, Shao SY, et al. Frequent PLAG1 gene rearrangements in skin and soft tissue myoepithelioma with ductal differentiation. Genes Chromosomes Cancer. 2013;52(7):675.

10. Argani P, Zhong M, Reuter VE, Fallon JT, Epstein JI, Netto GJ, Antonescu CR. TFE3-fusion variant analysis defines specific clinicopathologic associations among Xp11 translocation cancers. Am J Surg Pathol. 2016;40(6):723–37. PMID: 26975036.
11. Arias-Stella J Jr, Rosen PP. Hemangiopericytoma of the breast. Mod Pathol. 1988;1(2):98–103.
12. Asirvatham JR, Shah A, Carreon CK, Bhuiya TA, Kahn LB, Kostroff K, Morgenstern NJ. Ossifying fibromyxoid tumor of the breast mimicking fibroadenoma: a case report and differential diagnoses. Arch Pathol Lab Med. 2014;138(8):1098–100.
13. Astudillo L, Lacroix-Triki M, Ferron G, Rolland F, Maisongrosse V, Chevreau C. Bilateral breast metastases from Ewing sarcoma of the femur. Am J Clin Oncol. 2005;28(1):102–3.
14. Atanaskova Mesinkovska N, Buehler D, McClain CM, Rubin BP, Goldblum JR, Billings SD. Ossifying fibromyxoid tumor: a clinicopathologic analysis of 26 subcutaneous tumors with emphasis on differential diagnosis and prognostic factors. J Cutan Pathol. 2015;42(9):622.
15. Audino AN, Setty BA, Yeager ND. Rhabdomyosarcoma of the breast in adolescent and young adult (AYA) women. J Pediatr Hematol Oncol. 2017;39(1):62–6.
16. Bahrami A, Dalton JD, Krane JF, Fletcher CD. A subset of cutaneous and soft tissue mixed tumors are genetically linked to their salivary gland counterpart. Genes Chromosomes Cancer. 2012;51(2):140.
17. Baranov E, McBride MJ, Bellizzi AM, Ligon AH, Fletcher CDM, Kadoch C, Hornick JL. A novel SS18-SSX fusion-specific antibody for the diagnosis of synovial sarcoma. Am J Surg Pathol. 2020;44(7):922–33. PMID: 32141887.
18. Barco I, González C, Vallejo E, Pessarrodona A, Giménez N, García-Fernández A. Malignant solitary fibrous tumour of the breast mimicking a benign tumor. Clin Pathol. 2019;8:12. PMID: 31448370.
19. Boland JM, Folpe AL. Hemosiderotic fibrolipomatous tumor, pleomorphic hyalinizing angiectatic tumor, and myxoinflammatory fibroblastic sarcoma: related or not? Adv Anat Pathol. 2017;24(5):268.
20. Buza N, Zekry N, Charpin C, Tavassoli FA. Myoepithelial carcinoma of the breast: a clinicopathological and immunohistochemical study of 15 diagnostically challenging cases. Virchows Arch. 2010;457(3):337–45. Epub 2010 Jul 24.
21. Carter CS, Patel RM. Ossifying fibromyxoid tumor: a review with emphasis on recent molecular advances and differential diagnosis. Arch Pathol Lab Med. 2019;143(12):1504–12.
22. Carter JM, Sukov WR, Montgomery E, et al. TGFBR3 and MGEA5 rearrangements in pleomorphic hyalinizing angiectatic tumors and the spectrum of related neoplasms. Am J Surg Pathol. 2014;38(9):1182.
23. Charli-Joseph Y, Saggini A, Vemula S, Weier J, Mirza S, LeBoit PE. Primary cutaneous perivascular epithelioid cell tumor: a clinicopathological and molecular reappraisal. J Am Acad Dermatol. 2014;71(6):1127.
24. Chaudhary KS, Shousha S. Leiomyoma of the nipple, and normal subareolar muscle fibres, are oestrogen and progesterone receptor positive. Histopathology. 2004;44(6):626–8. PMID: 15186281.
25. Cheah AL, Billings SD, Goldblum JR, Carver P, Tanas MZ, Rubin BP. STAT6 rabbit monoclonal antibody is a robust diagnostic tool for the distinction of solitary fibrous tumour from its mimics. Pathology. 2014;46(5):389.
26. Chen L, Wang L, Zhang X, Yao M, Fu P. Ipsilateral breast metastasis after axillary dissection caused by epithelioid sarcoma: a case report and pathological investigation. Diagn Pathol. 2019;14(1):111.
27. D'Alfonso TM, Subramaniyam S, Ginter PS, Mosquera JM, MacDonald TY, Noorzad Z, Orta LY, Liu YF, Rubin MA, Shin SJ. Characterization of the leiomyomatous variant of myofibroblastoma: a rare subset distinct from other smooth muscle tumors of the breast. Hum Pathol. 2016;58:54–61.
28. D'Angelo P, Carli M, Ferrari A, Manzitti C, Mura R, Miglionico L, Di Cataldo A, Grigoli A, Cecchetto G. Bisogno G; AIEOP soft tissue sarcoma committee. Breast metastases in children and adolescents with rhabdomyosarcoma: experience of the Italian soft tissue sarcoma committee. Pediatr Blood Cancer. 2010;55(7):1306–9.

29. Davis JL, Horvai AE. Special AT-rich sequence-binding protein 2 (SATB2) expression is sensitive but may not be specific for osteosarcoma as compared with other high-grade primary bone sarcomas. Histopathology. 2016;69(1):84–90.
30. Demicco EG, Harms PW, Patel RM, et al. Extensive survey of STAT6 expression in a large series of mesenchymal tumors. Am J Clin Pathol. 2015;143(5):672.
31. Demicco EG, Wagner MJ, Maki RG, et al. Risk assessment in solitary fibrous tumors: validation and refinement of a risk stratification model. Mod Pathol. 2017;30(10):1433.
32. Doyle VJ, Bateman AC, Theaker JM. An unusual breast mass: primary synovial sarcoma. BMJ Case Rep 2013 19;
33. Dubois C, Nika E, Hoffmann P, Delouche A, Michy T, Philippe AC. Solitary fibrous tumor of the breast: a rare entity. Breast J. 2020;26(2):289–90.
34. El Beaino M, Araujo DM, Lazar AJ, Lin PP. Synovial sarcoma: advances in diagnosis and treatment identification of new biologic targets to improve multimodal therapy. Ann Surg Oncol. 2017;24(8):2145.
35. Filho OG, Gordan AN, Mello Rde A, Neto CS, Heinke T. Myoid hamartomas of the breast: report of 3 cases and review of the literature. Int J Surg Pathol. 2004;12(2):151–3.
36. Flucke U, Palmedo G, Blankenhorn N, Slootweg PJ, Kutzner H, Mentzel T. EWSR1 gene rearrangement occurs in a subset of cutaneous myoepithelial tumors: a study of 18 cases. Mod Pathol. 2011;24(11):1444.
37. Folpe AL, Kwiatkowski DJ. Perivascular epithelioid cell neoplasms: pathology and pathogenesis. Hum Pathol. 2010;41(1):1.
38. Folpe AL, Mentzel T, Lehr HA, Fisher C, Balzer BL, Weiss SW. Perivascular epithelioid cell neoplasms of soft tissue and gynecologic origin: a clinicopathologic study of 26 cases and review of the literature. Am J Surg Pathol. 2005;29(12):1558.
39. Folpe AL, Weiss SW. Ossifying fibromyxoid tumor of soft parts: a clinicopathologic study of 70 cases with emphasis on atypical and malignant variants. Am J Surg Pathol. 2003;27(4):421.
40. Folpe AL, Weiss SW. Pleomorphic hyalinizing angiectatic tumor: analysis of 41 cases supporting evolution from a distinctive precursor lesion. Am J Surg Pathol. 2004;28(11):1417.
41. Frezza AM, et al. Anthracycline, gemcitabine, and Pazopanib in epithelioid sarcoma: a multi-institutional case series. JAMA Oncol. 2018;4(9):e180219.
42. Frezza AM, Sbaraglia M, Lo Vullo S, Baldi GG, Simeone N, Frenos F, Campanacci D, Stacchiotti S, Pasquali S, Callegaro D, Gambarotti M, Barisella M, Palomba A, Mariani L, Casali PG, Dei Tos AP, Gronchi A. The natural history of epithelioid sarcoma. A retrospective multicentre case-series within the Italian Sarcoma Group. Eur J Surg Oncol. 2020;46(7):1320–6.
43. Fritchie KJ, Carver P, Sun Y, Batiouchko G, Billings SD, Rubin BP, Tubbs RR, Goldblum JR. Solitary fibrous tumor: is there a molecular relationship with cellular angiofibroma, spindle cell lipoma, and mammary-type myofibroblastoma? Am J Clin Pathol. 2012;137(6):963–70.
44. Fukunaga M. Giant cell tumor of the breast. Virchows Arch. 2002;441(1):93–5.
45. Gajdzis P, Laé M, Choussy O, Lavigne M, Klijanienko J. Fine-needle aspiration features of ossifying fibromyxoid tumor in the breast: a case report and literature review. Diagn Cytopathol. 2019;47(7):711–5.
46. Gebre-Medhin S, Nord KH, Moller E, et al. Recurrent rearrangement of the PHF1 gene in ossifying fibromyxoid tumors. Am J Pathol. 2012;181(3):1069.
47. Geyer FC, et al. Recurrent hotspot mutations in HRAS Q61 and PI3K-AKT pathway genes as drivers of breast adenomyoepitheliomas. Nat Commun. 2018;9(1):1816. PMID: 29739933.
48. Goldstein-Jackson SY, Gosheger G, Delling G, Berdel WE, Exner GU, Jundt G, Machatschek JN, Zoubek A, Jürgens H, Bielack SS, Cooperative Osteosarcoma Study Group COSS. Extraskeletal osteosarcoma has a favourable prognosis when treated like conventional osteosarcoma. J Cancer Res Clin Oncol. 2005;131(8):520–6.
49. Graham RP, Weiss SW, Sukov WR, et al. PHF1 rearrangements in ossifying fibromyxoid tumors of soft parts: a fluorescence in situ hybridization study of 41 cases with emphasis on the malignant variant. Am J Surg Pathol. 2013;37(11):1751.

50. Guillou L, Gebhard S, Coindre JM. Lipomatous hemangiopericytoma: a fat-containing variant of solitary fibrous tumor? Clinicopathologic, immunohistochemical, and ultrastructural analysis of a series in favor of a unifying concept. Hum Pathol. 2000;31(9):1108.
51. Guillou L, Wadden C, Coindre JM, Krausz T, Fletcher CD. "Proximal-type" epithelioid sarcoma, a distinctive aggressive neoplasm showing rhabdoid features. Clinicopathologic, immunohistochemical, and ultrastructural study of a series. Am J Surg Pathol. 1997;21(2):130.
52. Haiges D, Kurz P, Laaff H, Meiss F, Kutzner H, Technau-Hafsi K. Malignant PEComa. J Cutan Pathol. 2018;45(1):84–9.
53. Hammer P, White K, Mengden S, Korcheva V, Raess PW. Nipple leiomyoma: a rare neoplasm with a broad spectrum of histologic appearances. J Cutan Pathol. 2019;46(5):343–6.
54. Hasegawa T, Matsuno Y, Shimoda T, Umeda T, Yokoyama R, Hirohashi S. Proximal-type epithelioid sarcoma: a clinicopathologic study of 20 cases. Mod Pathol. 2001;14(7):655–63.
55. Hayes-Jordan A, Stoner JA, Anderson JR, Rodeberg D, Weiner G, Meyer WH, Hawkins DS, Arndt CA, Paidas C, Children's Oncology Group. The impact of surgical excision in chest wall rhabdomyosarcoma: a report from the Children's Oncology Group. J Pediatr Surg. 2008;43(5):831–6. PMID: 18485948.
56. Hays DM, Donaldson SS, Shimada H, Crist WM, Newton WA Jr, Andrassy RJ, Wiener E, Green J, Triche T, Maurer HM. Primary and metastatic rhabdomyosarcoma in the breast: neoplasms of adolescent females, a report from the Intergroup Rhabdomyosarcoma Study. Med Pediatr Oncol. 1997;29(3):181–9.
57. Hornick JL, Dal Cin P, Fletcher CD. Loss of INI1 expression is characteristic of both conventional and proximal-type epithelioid sarcoma. Am J Surg Pathol. 2009;33(4):542.
58. Hornick JL, Fletcher CD. Myoepithelial tumors of soft tissue: a clinicopathologic and immunohistochemical study of 101 cases with evaluation of prognostic parameters. Am J Surg Pathol. 2003;27(9):1183.
59. Huang SC, Chen HW, Zhang L, et al. Novel FUS-KLF17 and EWSR1-KLF17 fusions in myoepithelial tumors. Genes Chromosomes Cancer. 2015;54(5):267.
60. Hussien M, Sivananthan S, Anderson N, Shiels A, Tracey N, Odling-Smee GW. Primary leiomyosarcoma of the breast: diagnosis, management and outcome. A report of a new case and review of literature. Breast. 2001;10(6):530–4.
61. Iwata J, Fletcher CD. Immunohistochemical detection of cytokeratin and epithelial membrane antigen in leiomyosarcoma: a systematic study of 100 cases. Pathol Int. 2000;50(1):7–14.
62. Jo VY, Antonescu CR, Zhang L, Dal Cin P, Hornick JL, Fletcher CD. Cutaneous syncytial myoepithelioma: clinicopathologic characterization in a series of 38 cases. Am J Surg Pathol. 2013;37(5):710.
63. Jo VY, Mariño-Enríquez A, Fletcher CD. Epithelioid rhabdomyosarcoma: clinicopathologic analysis of 16 cases of a morphologically distinct variant of rhabdomyosarcoma. Am J Surg Pathol. 2011;35(10):1523–30.
64. Jour G, Wang L, Middha S, Zehir A, Chen W, Sadowska J, Healey J, Agaram NP, Choi L, Nafa K, Hameed M. The molecular landscape of extraskeletal osteosarcoma: a clinicopathological and molecular biomarker study. J Pathol Clin Res. 2015;2(1):9–20. PMID: 27499911.
65. Jung MJ, Alrahwan D, Dubrovsky E, Baek D, Ayala AG, Ro JY. Solitary fibrous tumor of breast with anaplastic areas (malignant solitary fibrous tumor): a case report with review of literature. J Breast Cancer. 2019;22(2):326–35. PMID: 31281733.
66. Kallen ME, Sanders ME, Gonzalez AL, Black JO, Keedy VL, Hande KR, Homlar KC, Halpern JL, Holt GE, Schwartz HS, Coffin CM, Cates JM. Nuclear p63 expression in osteoblastic tumors. Tumour Biol. 2012;33(5):1639–44.
67. Kao YC, Sung YS, Zhang L, Chen CL, Huang SC, Antonescu CR. Expanding the molecular signature of ossifying fibromyxoid tumors with two novel gene fusions: CREBBP-BCORL1 and KDM2A-WWTR1. Genes Chromosomes Cancer. 2017;56(1):42.
68. Karanian M, Pissaloux D, Gomez-Brouchet A, Chevenet C, Le Loarer F, Fernandez C, Minard V, Corradini N, Castex MP, Duc-Gallet A, Blay JY, Tirode F. SRF-FOXO1 and SRF-NCOA1 fusion genes delineate a distinctive subset of well-differentiated rhabdomyosarcoma. Am J Surg Pathol. 2020;44(5):607–16.

69. Kebudi R, Koc BS, Gorgun O, Celik A, Kebudi A, Darendeliler E. Breast metastases in children and adolescents with rhabdomyosarcoma: a large single-institution experience and literature review. J Pediatr Hematol Oncol. 2017;39(1):67–71.
70. Kenerson H, Folpe AL, Takayama TK, Yeung RS. Activation of the mTOR pathway in sporadic angiomyolipomas and other perivascular epithelioid cell neoplasms. Hum Pathol. 2007;38(9):1361–71. PMID: 17521703.
71. Kilpatrick SE, Hitchcock MG, Kraus MD, Calonje E, Fletcher CD. Mixed tumors and myoepitheliomas of soft tissue: a clinicopathologic study of 19 cases with a unifying concept. Am J Surg Pathol. 1997;21(1):13.
72. Kohashi K, Yamada Y, Hotokebuchi Y, Yamamoto H, Taguchi T, Iwamoto Y, Oda Y. ERG and SALL4 expressions in SMARCB1/INI1-deficient tumors: a useful tool for distinguishing epithelioid sarcoma from malignant rhabdoid tumor. Hum Pathol. 2015;46(2):225–30.
73. Kohashi K, Yamamoto H, Yamada Y, Kinoshita I, Taguchi T, Iwamoto Y, Oda Y. SWI/SNF chromatin-remodeling complex status in SMARCB1/INI1-preserved epithelioid sarcoma. Am J Surg Pathol. 2018;42(3):312–8.
74. Kosemehmetoglu K, Vrana JA, Folpe AL. TLE1 expression is not specific for synovial sarcoma: a whole section study of 163 soft tissue and bone neoplasms. Mod Pathol. 2009;22(7):872.
75. Kraft S, Fletcher CD. Atypical intradermal smooth muscle neoplasms: clinicopathologic analysis of 84 cases and a reappraisal of cutaneous "leiomyosarcoma". Am J Surg Pathol. 2011;35(4):599–607. https://doi.org/10.1097/PAS.0b013e31820e6093.
76. Le Loarer F, et al. A subset of epithelioid and spindle cell rhabdomyosarcomas is associated with TFCP2 fusions and common ALK upregulation. Mod Pathol. 2020;33(3):404–19.
77. Lee JC, Liang CW, Fletcher CD. Giant cell tumor of soft tissue is genetically distinct from its bone counterpart. Mod Pathol. 2017;30(5):728–33.
78. Lee JS, Fetsch JF, Wasdhal DA, Lee BP, Pritchard DJ, Nascimento AG. A review of 40 patients with extraskeletal osteosarcoma. Cancer. 1995;76(11):2253–9.
79. Leiner J, Le Loarer F. The current landscape of rhabdomyosarcomas: an update. Virchows Arch. 2020;476(1):97–108.
80. Lidang Jensen M, Schumacher B, Myhre Jensen O, Steen Nielsen O, Keller J. Extraskeletal osteosarcomas: a clinicopathologic study of 25 cases. Am J Surg Pathol. 1998;22(5):588–94.
81. Liegl B, Hornick JL, Fletcher CD. Primary cutaneous PEComa: distinctive clear cell lesions of skin. Am J Surg Pathol. 2008;32(4):608.
82. Lin L, Skacel M, Sigel JE, et al. Epithelioid sarcoma: an immunohistochemical analysis evaluating the utility of cytokeratin 5/6 in distinguishing superficial epithelioid sarcoma from spindled squamous cell carcinoma. J Cutan Pathol. 2003;30(2):114.
83. Llamas-Velasco M, Mentzel T, Requena L, Palmedo G, Kasten R, Kutzner H. Cutaneous PEComa does not harbour TFE3 gene fusions: immunohistochemical and molecular study of 17 cases. Histopathology. 2013;63(1):122.
84. Luangxay T, Osako T, Yonekura R, Sugiura Y, Kikuchi M, Gomi N, Ueno T, Ohno S, Machinami R, Takeuchi K, Akiyama F. Giant cell tumor of soft tissue of the breast: case report with H3F3A mutation analysis and review of the literature. Pathol Res Pract. 2020;216(2):152750. PMID: 31784095.
85. Magro G, Angelico G, Righi A, Benini S, Salvatorelli L, Palazzo J. Utility of STAT6 and 13q14 deletion in the classification of the benign spindle cell stromal tumors of the breast. Hum Pathol. 2018;81:55–64. PMID: 29940288.
86. Mancini I, Righi A, Gambarotti M, Picci P, Dei Tos AP, Billings SD, Simi L, Franchi A. Phenotypic and molecular differences between giant-cell tumour of soft tissue and its bone counterpart. Histopathology. 2017;71(3):453–60.
87. Massi D, Franchi A, Alos L, Cook M, Di Palma S, Enguita AB, Ferrara G, Kazakov DV, Mentzel T, Michal M, Panelos J, Rodriguez-Peralto JL, Santucci M, Tragni G, Zioga A, Dei Tos AP. Primary cutaneous leiomyosarcoma: clinicopathological analysis of 36 cases. Histopathology. 2010;56(2):251–62.

88. May SA, Deavers MT, Resetkova E, Johnson D, Albarracin CT. Giant cell tumor of soft tissue arising in breast. Ann Diagn Pathol. 2007;11(5):345–9.
89. McCart Reed AE, et al. Phenotypic and molecular dissection of metaplastic breast cancer and the prognostic implications. J Pathol. 2019;247(2):214–27.
90. Mentzel T, Reisshauer S, Rutten A, Hantschke M, Soares de Almeida LM, Kutzner H. Cutaneous clear cell myomelanocytic tumour: a new member of the growing family of perivascular epithelioid cell tumours (PEComas). Clinicopathological and immunohistochemical analysis of seven cases. Histopathology. 2005; 46(5): 498.
91. Miettinen M, McCue PA, Sarlomo-Rikala M, et al. Sox10--a marker for not only schwannian and melanocytic neoplasms but also myoepithelial cell tumors of soft tissue: a systematic analysis of 5134 tumors. Am J Surg Pathol. 2015;39(6):826.
92. Miettinen M, Wang Z, Sarlomo-Rikala M, Abdullaev Z, Pack SD, Fetsch JF. ERG expression in epithelioid sarcoma: a diagnostic pitfall. Am J Surg Pathol 2013;37(10):1580–1585. PMID: 23774169.
93. Minami S, Matsuo S, Azuma T, Uga T, Hayashi T, Eguchi S, Kanematsu T. Parenchymal leiomyoma of the breast: a case report with special reference to magnetic resonance imaging findings and an update review of literature. Breast Cancer. 2011;18(3):231–6.
94. Mosquera JM, Fletcher CD. Expanding the spectrum of malignant progression in solitary fibrous tumors: a study of 8 cases with a discrete anaplastic component--is this dedifferentiated SFT? Am J Surg Pathol. 2009;33(9):1314.
95. Mujtaba B, Nassar SM, Aslam R, Garg N, Madewell JE, Taher A, Hanafy AK, Whitman G. Primary osteosarcoma of the breast: pathophysiology and imaging review. Curr Probl Diagn Radiol. 2020;49(2):116–23.
96. Naujokas A, Charli-Joseph Y, Ruben BS, et al. SOX-10 expression in cutaneous myoepitheliomas and mixed tumors. J Cutan Pathol. 2014;41(4):353.
97. Nogi H, Kobayashi T, Kawase K, Tabei I, Toriumi Y, Suzuki M, Kawakami M, Morikawa T, Uchida K. Primary rhabdomyosarcoma of the breast in a 13-year-old girl: report of a case. Surg Today. 2007;37(1):38–42.
98. Oliveira AM, Dei Tos AP, Fletcher CD, Nascimento AG. Primary giant cell tumor of soft tissues: a study of 22 cases. Am J Surg Pathol. 2000;24(2):248–56.
99. Pan CC, Chung MY, Ng KF, Liu CY, Wang JS, Chai CY, Huang SH, Chen PC, Ho DM. Constant allelic alteration on chromosome 16p (TSC2 gene) in perivascular epithelioid cell tumour (PEComa): genetic evidence for the relationship of PEComa with angiomyolipoma. J Pathol. 2008;214(3):387–93.
100. Panagopoulos I, Gorunova L, Andersen HK, Pedersen TD, Lømo J, Lund-Iversen M, Micci F, Heim S. Genetic characterization of Myoid hamartoma of the breast. Cancer Genomics Proteomics 2019;16(6):563–568. PMID: 31659109.
101. Pareja F, Weigelt B, Reis-Filho JS. Problematic breast tumors reassessed in light of novel molecular data. Mod Pathol. 2021;34(Suppl 1):38–47.
102. Robinson DR, Wu YM, Kalyana-Sundaram S, et al. Identification of recurrent NAB2-STAT6 gene fusions in solitary fibrous tumor by integrative sequencing. Nat Genet. 2013;45(2):180.
103. Salemis NS. Solitary fibrous tumor of the breast: a case report and the review of the literature. Breast J. 2018;24(1):78–81.
104. Schmitz KJ, Losch M, Agaimy A. Myositis ossificans mimicking metaplastic breast cancer on core needle biopsy. Hum Pathol. 2019;93:97–102.
105. Shin J, Kim HJ, Kim DY, Gong G, Cho KJ. Primary Rhabdomyosarcoma of the Breast: Study of Three Cases at One Institution with a Review of Primary Breast Sarcomas. J Pathol Transl Med. 2019 Sep;53(5):308–316. PMID: 31370385; PMCID: PMC6755652.
106. Sidoni A, Lüthy L, Bellezza G, Consiglio MA, Bucciarelli E. Leiomyoma of the breast: case report and review of the literature. Breast. 1999;8(5):289–90.
107. Silver SA, Tavassoli FA. Primary osteogenic sarcoma of the breast: a clinicopathologic analysis of 50 cases. Am J Surg Pathol. 1998;22(8):925–33.
108. Stafyla V, Kotsifopoulos N, Grigoriadis K, Bakoyiannis CN, Peros G, Sakorafas GH. Myoid hamartoma of the breast: a case report and review of the literature. Breast J. 2007;13(1):85–7.

109. Suurmeijer AJH, Dickson BC, Swanson D, Zhang L, Sung Y-S, Fletcher CD, Antonescu CR. A morphologic and molecular reappraisal of myoepithelial tumors of soft tissue, bone, and viscera with EWSR1 and FUS gene rearrangements. Genes, Chromosomes and Cancer. 2020;59(6):348–56.
110. Suurmeijer AJH, Song W, Sung YS, Zhang L, Swanson D, Fletcher CDM, Dickson BC, Antonescu CR. Novel recurrent PHF1-TFE3 fusions in ossifying fibromyxoid tumors. Genes Chromosomes Cancer. 2019;58(9):643–9.
111. Tallarigo F, Squillaci S, Putrino I, Zizzi N, Bisceglia M. Pleomorphic hyalinizing angiectatic tumor of the male breast: a heretofore unreported occurrence. Pathol Res Pract. 2009;205(1):69–73.
112. Tavassoli FA, Weiss S. Hemangiopericytoma of the breast. Am J Surg Pathol. 1981;5(8):745–52.
113. Tavassoli FA. Myoepithelial lesions of the breast. Myoepitheliosis, adenomyoepithelioma, and myoepithelial carcinoma. Am J Surg Pathol. 1991;15(6):554–68.
114. Terada M, Gondo N, Sawaki M, Hattori M, Yoshimura A, Kotani H, Adachi Y, Iwase M, Kataoka A, Sugino K, Mori M, Horisawa N, Ozaki Y, Iwata H. A case of giant cell tumor of the breast, clinically suspected as malignant breast tumor. Surg Case Rep. 2019;5(1):77. PMID: 31076887
115. Thampi S, Matthay KK, Boscardin WJ, Goldsby R, DuBois SG. Clinical features and outcomes differ between skeletal and Extraskeletal osteosarcoma. Sarcoma. 2014;2014:902620. PMID: 25294959.
116. Thway K, Fisher C. Synovial sarcoma: defining features and diagnostic evolution. Ann Diagn Pathol. 2014;18(6):369.
117. Tormo V, Andreu FJ. Primary breast synovial sarcoma: a rare primary breast neoplasm. Clin Transl Oncol. 2009;11(12):854–5.
118. Varela-Duran J, Enzinger FM. Calcifying synovial sarcoma. Cancer. 1982;50(2):345.
119. WHO Classification of Tumours Editorial Board. Breast tumours. Lyon (France): international agency for research on cancer: 2019. 5th ed; vol 2.
120. WHO Classification of Tumours Editorial Board. Soft tissue and bone tumours. Lyon (France): international agency for research on cancer. 2020. 5th ed; vol 3.
121. Zaborowski M, Vargas AC, Pulvers J, Clarkson A, de Guzman D, Sioson L, Maclean F, Chou A, Gill AJ. When used together SS18-SSX fusion-specific and SSX C-terminus immunohistochemistry are highly specific and sensitive for the diagnosis of synovial sarcoma and can replace FISH or molecular testing in most cases. Histopathology. 2020;77(4):588–600.
122. Zhong E, Swistel A, Viswanathan K, Hoda SA. Leiomyoma of the nipple: a common neoplasm in an uncommon location. Breast J. 2020;26(3):529–30. https://doi.org/10.1111/tbj.13572. Epub 2019 Sep 4.

# Index





J. J. Rowe, E. Downs-Kelly (eds.), *Mesenchymal Tumors of the Breast and Their Mimics*, https://doi.org/10.1007/978-3-030-74474-8

Printed by Printforce, the Netherlands